An analysis of primary medical care:
an international study

AN ANALYSIS OF

Primary Medical Care

AN INTERNATIONAL STUDY

W.J.STEPHEN

General Practitioner

CAMBRIDGE UNIVERSITY PRESS

CAMBRIDGE

LONDON · NEW YORK · MELBOURNE

CAMBRIDGE UNIVERSITY PRESS
Cambridge, New York, Melbourne, Madrid, Cape Town, Singapore, São Paulo, Delhi

Cambridge University Press
The Edinburgh Building, Cambridge CB2 8RU, UK

Published in the United States of America by Cambridge University Press, New York

www.cambridge.org
Information on this title: www.cambridge.org/9780521218603

First published 1979
This digitally printed version 2008

A catalogue record for this publication is available from the British Library

Library of Congress Cataloguing in Publication data
Stephen, William John, 1932–
An analysis of primary medical care.

Includes bibliographical references.
1. Family medicine. 2. Ambulatory medical care.
I. Title. [DNLM: 1. Family practice. 2. Delivery
of health care.   W89 S831a]
R729.5.G4S73   362.8′2   77–83999

ISBN 978-0-521-21860-3 hardback
ISBN 978-0-521-10230-8 paperback

CONTENTS

To my long-suffering wife and children

FOREWORD

The British National Health Service is in difficulties now, partly for lack of money, partly for factors in the administrative structure, partly because of defects in the structure of the professions, especially of medicine, but most of all because these things together have greatly undermined morale. Nevertheless the public generally believes in the Service and receives from it a high standard of care with fewer gaps than could be found in most other countries. The Service is not at the point of dissolution, as occasional disgruntled doctors have been announcing for the last twenty-five years, and its very real defects can be remedied. The real reason why it was viable in 1948 and has been only moderately damaged by the dissensions of recent years is the stability and effectiveness of the primary care system which is its main support. General medical practice has evolved a long way since 1948 and primary care in Britain has become mainly group medical practice of doctors with nurses and other professionals. As at the time of the Collings Report, it is uneven in quality and still requires continuing effort to raise its standards. Other countries organise primary care in other ways and some of them provide examples which could assist development here. Dr Stephen's study covers more countries than any other now available and his book will, at the least, suggest opportunities for closer examination of such differences.

Dr Stephen has not only read widely about his subject but has devoted much time and energy, with only limited outside help, to visits which have given him uniquely wide personal acquaintance with primary care in other countries. He has some personal convictions which influence his assessments of other countries, as his chapter on the United Kingdom reveals. There is much in that chapter with which, in common with many others, I would disagree. That does not invalidate the large amount of factual information he has brought together from other countries, though it may influence his assessment. Because the area covered is so wide it is inevitable that there should be evidence of some misinterpretation of local situations – for example, full investigation by Danish general practitioners is said to have produced a low rate of hospital use. In fact the admission rate in Denmark is well above that in Britain where availability of diagnostic services has been wider and earlier than the text implies. There is a problem, too, with the reconciliation of statistics from widely differing sources and with their interpretation. It is nonetheless remarkable to find so much collected together in one volume.

One reservation about the views expressed must be made. The author himself writes 'Primary care cannot be considered in isolation from the rest of the health service and without good secondary care in hospitals it will founder'. This is the underlying truth of the British NHS; but he goes on to say later that primary care must do better than hospital, when its real object is to do best with whatever contribution is best made by 'hospital'. It is quite artificial to judge what has been done for one side or the other by comparing the proportions of total expenditure and changes in them over the years. The fact is that the lesser needs of general practice for capital in absolute terms have been preferred to the far greater needs of secondary care ever since British doctors have come round to acceptance of health centres. In general his emphasis on the greater need of primary care, especially in developing countries, is justified but the even greater urgency of providing safe water supplies and safe disposal of human wastes could have been given even stronger emphasis. Any reader will surely regard this as a small matter only to be expected in so large a single-handed achievement.

This book is an important contribution to the review of primary care and its relation to secondary or specialist care in any country. Relationships within medicine and between medicine and the other professions have changed much in the last thirty years and must change much more under the pressure of both scientific and social advance. Shared responsibility, rather than autocratic medical control, must be the pattern of the future and the general practitioner of medicine with his other professional colleagues in primary care is at the focal point.

The most important relationship of all is the continuing family doctor relationship with patients in health as in illness, whether minor or major. The answers we have now in Britain are far from perfect and there is much in Dr Stephen's book from which we can all learn. It is a special feature of this study that it has been made by one who throughout has been engaged in primary care himself. To have encompassed the review of the relevant literature alone is a considerable achievement; to have undertaken the travelling, with a valuable contribution from Eric Gambrill, and surmounted the language problems as well makes it monumental.

At the end of my reading of this book, despite the inevitable reservations on points of emphasis, I was left feeling that my own knowledge of health care in other countries – even those well known to me – had been enlarged. There is nothing quite like it in print now. If it is written from an essentially general practitioner point of view, that is in its favour for it brings with it a deeper appreciation of the health care needs of people than a writer with an administrative or hospital background might have. Yet the historical perspective, so often ignored in descriptions of health service organisation, and the statistical background are there. This is an achievement in a class of its own.

Sir George Godber
Formerly Chief Medical Officer,
Department of Health and Social Security

PREFACE

The health of any given population depends more on the availability of good primary health care than on the advanced technical resources of modern hospitals; and it is generally accepted that a properly organised system of primary care can deal with a very large proportion of all demands for health care: a figure of 80 per cent is commonly quoted, and many would put it a good deal higher. It has been claimed also that the treatment of illness through a primary care system leads to economy of money and resources, though in a situation of potentially unlimited demand for health care services, this represents a better use of resources, rather than an actual saving of money. A contrast is, however, sometimes drawn between the high cost of providing hospital and specialist services for a relatively small number of people, and the relatively much lower expenditure on the provision of primary care required by the great bulk of the population. In consequence, there has, not unnaturally, been a tendency to question the disproportionate amount of resources made available for the institutional forms of care, particularly hospital care, compared with the much smaller amount devoted to primary care.

No independent, fair-minded observer could disagree with this extract from a report of the World Health Organisation, following a meeting in Moscow in July 1973 on 'Trends in the development of primary care'.

During the last twelve years, I have been studying the difficulties and problems of primary care in a world-wide context. This has not been easy, as I have found little interest in universities, medical schools or the Department of Health and Social Security, and certainly no financial support has been available from these organisations for this type of research.

Between 1966 and 1968, I spent five weeks in Eastern Europe, visiting Bulgaria, Czechoslovakia, Hungary, Poland and Romania, followed by two weeks in Canada in 1969, and a further five weeks in the USSR during 1971/2. This was organised under the auspices of the Anglo/Soviet Cultural and Scientific Agreement, with the help of the British Council. In 1972, I spent two months in Japan, which was made possible by a Nuffield Foundation Travelling Fellowship. Three-week visits to Cuba and Chile in 1974, followed by Norway, Sweden and Finland in 1976 and the USA in 1977 completed my studies, except for brief visits to Belgium, France, the Netherlands, Italy and the World Health Organisation in Geneva. I have also collected material through the European office of the World Health Organisation in Copenhagen, and its headquarters in Geneva, and from official sources in many countries. Since 1960, I have been in active general practice, working in the National Health Service which, while it has made me acutely aware of our own domestic problems and difficulties, has also made me aware of our strengths.

Throughout the last twelve years, I have felt the need for a book which would give an account of the different methods of organisation in operation throughout the world. None is available. This book is, therefore, an attempt to fill the gap; it includes many of the major industrialised countries and one chapter considering in general principles the problems of the developing world. It is obviously an incomplete and personal account, and has dealt almost entirely with the structure and organisation of primary care, rather than with its clinical and technical aspect. I hope I have not fallen into the trap of drawing too many facile conclusions from such a comparative study, as the organisation of any country's health service depends on so many variable factors – political, social, historical, educational and financial – each specific to the country under consideration, that it makes direct comparisons almost meaningless. Rather, my aim has been to collect the facts, in the hope that, in spite of all its defects and limitations, or perhaps because of them, it may stimulate a much more detailed and comprehensive study in the future. It is intended for anyone who is interested in improving health care – politicians, patients, doctors, health service administrators, journalists, university departments of community medicine and general practice, students and other health workers – so that, by illuminating and focusing on each other's problems and dilemmas, a rational discussion can take place and progress can be made.

John Stephen

Wells, Somerset 1978

ACKNOWLEDGEMENTS

Space does not allow me to mention by name all those people who, during the last twelve years, have helped to plan my visits and arrange programmes of study, or those who have given so generously of their time, knowledge and hospitality, or those who have willingly given advice and letters of introduction. A list is, therefore, included in an appendix: inevitably this has omitted many people whose views and opinions have helped to formulate this book. I would ask them to accept my apologies and I hope that they will realise how much their assistance has been valued.

The suggestion that I should write this book came from Dr František Ošanec, Department of Foreign Health Services, Prague, who encouraged an idea which I had been pondering for several years. His encyclopaedic knowledge of the organisation of health services is known in many parts of the world, and to him I readily express my thanks and admiration, and acknowledge his influence.

To Dr Eric Gambrill, who has not only written Chapter 9, but has also read the manuscript, I am extremely grateful. His sound and helpful comments on the initial draft have proved invaluable. Also I wish to thank Mr Alan Quilter, Headmaster, Wells Cathedral School, for his advice and suggestions regarding style and grammar. The guidance I have received from the Cambridge University Press has been greatly appreciated. The considerable knowledge and pertinent criticisms of Dr John Fry have been of particular value. Finally I owe a special debt to Mrs Susan Record and Mrs Lisbeth Bull, assisted by Mrs Pauline Penney, who have miraculously converted my illegible scrawl into an orderly typescript.

1

INTRODUCTION

The need to provide medical care has stirred the imagination of man throughout the world from the earliest records of history, but the organisation of medical care is an activity which has only interested governments, patients and doctors since the end of the nineteenth century, and only seriously since the end of the Second World War.

What are the reasons for this? European culture and tradition have been based on the Christian ethic, even if, at the present time, most countries in Europe and throughout the rest of the world are largely secular. Basic to this belief is the absolute importance of man as an individual, and this idea was reinforced by the concept of 'post-Renaissance man', which was also fired by the same philosophy. For nearly two thousand years, at least, in Western Europe, and subsequently in those parts of the world which came under the influence of European civilisation, the best in medicine was always closely associated with the Christian tradition. Consequently, the highest standards in medicine and nursing have been synonymous in most people's minds with devoted attention to individual patients. Paradoxically, this compassionate caring for the individual has tended to obscure the needs of the community, at least from the eyes of many doctors and nurses, even if not from patients. There has been a delay in understanding, or even appreciating, the issues involved in providing health care for large numbers of people, and this failure to recognise the problems has been a major obstacle to progress.

Of course, no-one would pretend that this is the whole story, and to many it is merely a reflection on the nature of society. The USSR has succeeded in providing a comprehensive service for its entire popula-

1

tion, virtually starting from nothing, following the revolution of 1917, while the USA is still debating about a health service. The different philosophies of health care in Cuba and Chile, or India and China, also highlight the political nature of the problem. But equally, in Scandinavia, New Zealand or the UK, the organisation of medicine has altered to a considerable extent, without any fundamental change in the structure of government or society. But what would seem certain is that in countries which fail to provide appropriate care there is a danger that medicine may become a political issue and nothing else.

A great responsibility thus lies with the medical profession, at least to try to meet the needs of the people, and thus prevent a polarisation of opinions and a general atmosphere of distrust, which imposes an impossible strain on patients, government and doctors. Patients have the right to be treated with the highest ethical and clinical standards; governments have the right to expect the cooperation of doctors in providing a fair distribution of care and resources to the benefit of all, and doctors have the right not to be used as a political tool. It will require the highest standards of integrity and motivation between government and profession, also considerable understanding and cooperation from patients, if a satisfactory solution is to be found.

A new force has recently entered into the arena of health care, whose advocates claim that medicine in fact does more harm than good! (Illich, 1975) Many people would agree that much modern, sophisticated therapy is of doubtful value, and may sometimes be harmful; that much aggressive, heroic surgery produces very little benefit for the unfortunate patient; that medicine has fostered and encouraged an overdependence on the part of many patients; that the value of early diagnosis, and therefore the hope of better treatment, is often illusory, and that many investigations and treatments are an expensive luxury, even a total charade. But to claim, as some do, that poor people who cannot afford any health care are probably better off than those who are rich enough to run the risk of seeing a doctor, is surely a perverted view of medicine. It is not without interest that such views are often paraded by those people who, in reality, live in the secure knowledge that medical care is at hand for them should they need it. And so it is accepted that there is a demand and need for people to have some form of health care, and to argue otherwise is to ignore reality and to misinterpret their expectations. But where should the emphasis be placed and the resources allocated? There is no health service in the world today which can meet all the demands made on it, and it is in this context that resources must be allocated. How necessary, therefore, is primary care and how should it be organised? This surely will be the essence of much deliberation on the future planning of health services. If, of course, universal care for the entire population is not accepted, then medicine can remain a commercial enterprise, governed by the rules of the market place. In such a situation, only the rich or privileged can afford the luxury of medical care and others will have to rely on chance or patronage.

It is a fact that in all developed countries hospital services take a very much larger proportion of money than primary care; this is inevitable. It is also true that the number of physicians employed in the hospital service has increased greatly compared with the number of general practitioners; this is inevitable with the present-day emphasis on technological medicine. Even in the UK, where it is claimed there is a strong primary care sector, the figures show only too clearly the magnetic effect of the hospital service and its dominant role (Table 1).

TABLE 1 *Increase in number of hospital doctors and general practitioners in the National Health Service*

Category	Number of doctors		
	1959	1973	Increase (%)
Consultants	5 322	8 988	+69
Senior registrars	931	1 821	+96
Registrars	2 787	4 408	+58
Senior house officers	2 315	6 292	+172
House officers	2 436	2 351	− 3
Total hospital doctors	13 791	23 860	+73
General practitioners	22 091	21 358	− 3

Based on DHSS statistics

Governments and health service administrators, encouraged and advised by the medical profession, still expand the hospital service at the expense of primary care, even though it is realised that there is a definite need for an effective system of first-contact care. It is difficult to believe that this situation can continue for much longer, and in the near future personal long-term continuing care, as far as possible within the context of the family, will be seen as one of the major priorities of medicine today. Minor ailments, self-limiting diseases, the problem of incurable disease and the inevitability of the ageing process all require help and advice from a physician (or medical auxiliary) working in the community. But the advocates of primary care or general practice must be able to demonstrate that their claims are attainable, desirable and necessary. The next chapter will attempt to describe the aims, requirements and essential ingredients of good primary care and the differing methods of organisation.

What is a good health service and how can it be measured? Can good health care be provided without a sound organisation of primary care? What is a sound pattern of organisation and who should provide the service: a family doctor or specialist, working individually or in a team? Are doctors prepared to carry out general practice which is *accessible*, *available* and provides *continuity*, and are they capable of carrying it out? Is there a satisfactory method of paying doctors? Does the method of payment influence the quality of service received by the patient? How appropriate is the medical education of most primary care physicians?

Subsequent chapters will focus on individual countries in an endeavour to answer these questions and to show how successful or unsuccessful they have been in organising their own system of first-contact care within the context of their differing political, economic and social backgrounds.

2

PRIMARY MEDICAL CARE

Function, requirements and special features of primary care

The role of the general practitioner, both now and in the future, has been the subject of endless conferences, working parties and reports, both nationally and internationally, over the last twenty years. Speculation and controversy have raged, regarding not only the differing approach of various countries – the specialist or 'specialoid'* in the USA and USSR (Fry, 1969) as compared to the firmly rooted family doctor philosophy of the Netherlands, Denmark, New Zealand, the Republic of Ireland and the UK – but also whether primary care might disappear from the medical scene altogether; this seemed a distinct possibility during the 1950s. Since then there has been a renaissance of general practice throughout most of the world and to quote Professor James Knox (1970), Department of General Practice, University of Dundee, 'For too long general practice has been considered to be an ailing patient whose demise is expected hourly. The patient has refused to die. The severity of the illness is no longer at issue, but the crisis is passed and the patient is on the long road to recovery, even if the understanding of the complex aetiology is still important.'

An all embracing definition of general practice or primary care and of general practitioners/family physicians/primary physicians is difficult, particularly when considered in relation to the differing political, economic and social structures of the countries involved. There have been many attempts of which the following are examples.

* See footnote on p. 246.

(*a*) World Health Organisation:

> Primary health care consists of the advice given to a person or a group
> of persons for preventative or therapeutic purposes by one or more
> members of the health or related professions, acting alone or as a
> team. (WHO, 1970)

(*b*) The Report of the Committee on Medical Schools and the American
Association of Medical Colleges in relation to training for Family Practice (Pellegrino Committee) defines the functions of the primary care
physician as follows:

> He must be capable of establishing a profile of the total needs of the
> patient and his family. This evaluation should include social, econ-
> omic and psychological details as well as the more strictly 'medical'
> aspects. He should then define a plan of care, deciding which parts
> are to be carried out by himself and which by others. The plan should
> have a long-range dimension. It should be understandable to the
> patient and his family and it should include a follow-up on whether
> they have been effective. (Jonas, 1973)

(*c*) British Medical Association:

> primary care deals with the work of the doctor whom the patient first
> approaches when he wants advice or medical treatment. The disci-
> pline of primary medicine is based on a particular synthesis of know-
> ledge drawn from clinical and social (including preventive) medicine,
> psychology and sociology. The clinical skills of the primary physician
> should enable him, not so much to attach a diagnostic label as to
> unravel the undifferentiated, clinical problem, which is often a com-
> plex of physical, emotional and social factors, and to take immediate
> and appropriate action. (BMA, 1970)

(*d*) The following job definition from a book on current general practice:

> The general practitioner provides personal, primary and continuing
> medical care to individuals, families and a practice population, irres-
> pective of age, sex and illness. He will attend his patients in his
> consulting room and in their homes, and sometimes in a clinic or
> hospital. His aim is to make early diagnoses. He will include and
> integrate physical, psychological and social factors in his considera-
> tions about health and illness. He will make an initial decision about
> every problem which is presented to him. He will undertake the
> continuing management of his patients with chronic, recurrent or
> terminal illnesses. He will practice in cooperation with other col-
> leagues, medical and non-medical. He will know how and when to

intervene through treatment, prevention and education to promote the health of his patients and their families. He will recognise that he also has a professional responsibility to the community. (Fry, 1977)

These definitions would seem to cover every eventuality and to be all embracing, even Utopian, and yet most general practitioners know that in some ways they say nothing, and the indefinable quality of good practice has been omitted. 'You have to be half dead before he'll come.' 'I can't get an appointment to see him for weeks!' 'He doesn't care; all he's interested in is doing all the tests so he can get the money.' 'He's always in a hurry and doesn't want to listen.' 'He said bring the child down to the office or emergency room even though she had been delirious all night.' Such comments or accusations are commonplace, so perhaps the best definition, at least the one most readily understood by patients, was by Dr Roger Cohen, Department of Community Medicine at Stony Brook, New York State, who said 'Primary care is what everybody needs and can't get'. (Jonas, 1973) or, put in another way by the Planning unit report of the British Medical Association (1970), 'Patients find it helpful to have a doctor who, come what may, will accept immediate responsibility; a doctor who may say "We need someone else to help here", but will never say "I am afraid your problem is not in my department".'

What are, then, the minimum requirements considered necessary for the adequate organisation of primary care which may help to prevent such criticism? Probably no system, even with medical audit, can legislate against the idle or greedy or professionally incompetent physician but, nevertheless, a basic framework can render such occurrences less likely. There is no universal 'best buy' service, but there are a number of fundamental principles without which primary care would be hopelessly inefficient and unlikely to serve the needs of the majority of people.

1. *Basic triad*: to provide *continuous* comprehensive care which is *accessible* and easily *available* at the time of need. Without these three qualities, primary care is nothing. With the change in the spectrum of disease from acute infectious illnesses to the chronic degenerative and malignant diseases of middle and old age, and with the increase in emotional and psychiatric illness, in part produced by the 'false gods' of the consumer-orientated society and the repetitive, pointless monotony of so many jobs in industrialised countries, it is no surprise that

there should be a change in emphasis from 'curing' to 'caring', and a desire by patients to seek some continuity in their medical care.

There is mounting anxiety and doubt expressed about the hospital service, with its ever-increasing use of sophisticated technology and the impersonal attitudes which so often accompany 'modern medicine', and in some ways seem an inevitable consequence of it. When as many as ten, and often more, doctors may be concerned with the clinical care of one patient, it is perhaps to be expected. 'You're only an interesting case or a number in there, nobody knows who you are'; 'Are these tests necessary?'; 'Is this treatment safe? Are there any side-effects?'; 'I think they're just experimenting'; 'Nobody told me anything and when they did I couldn't understand': such remarks are heard frequently by practising general practitioners. Patients feel a need to be protected from over-zealous investigation and treatment, so throughout the world people are looking for a point of stability, an anchor-man in medicine; there can be very few who at some time in their lives have not felt such a need.

This can only be provided by a physician who knows not only the patient's physical problem, but also his family and social background, and is thus in a position to interpret the technical advice of the specialist or hospital service. In some countries where the specialist himself also provides the primary care, the patient is less likely to get independent advice, particularly if there is a financial incentive for unnecessary investigation, treatment or operation.

A major social problem in most industrialised societies, though found much less frequently in the USSR or Eastern Europe, is the dispersed 'nuclear' family, always on the move, with no roots, giving rise to the inevitable anxieties, tensions and insecurity that such a life brings. For the elderly, bereft of the family, a feeling of loneliness and despair is common and it is often accompanied by a belief that they are not wanted, either by society or the family. Such psycho/social *malaise* is now a major drain on health services, and underlines the need for some continuity at the primary care level. Socialist countries maintain that they do not have these problems to such an extent because of the nature of their society; undoubtedly families move around much less frequently, which leads to the presence of the 'extended family' in the community, and all the benefits this can bring.

Accessibility is of great importance to the young and the very old. Each country's solution will depend to a large extent on such factors as the relationship between public and private transport, the density and distribution of the population, and whether the primary care physicians work in solo or group practice (including health centres and polyclinics). Rural areas present more clearly delineated problems and often involve expensive and dramatic remedies, for example the Australian Flying Doctor Service, with similar organisations in Siberia, the Soviet Far East and Northern Canada.

Availability is a deceptively vague and innocuous word, but in the context of primary care it pinpoints one of the unsolved problems of many health services: how to provide 24-hour cover for 365 days of the year. General practitioners are following the rest of society in their desire to make the working day shorter and not to work at weekends. This trend would appear to be increasing so that, at the end of the century, it is conceivable that the majority of the working population will spend more time at leisure than at work! Here then is one of the major dilemmas of primary care: how to maintain availability without sacrificing the principle of continuity. Doctors and patients must decide together a workable and satisfactory compromise within the context of their own society.

2. With the increasing strains being placed on all health services, it is mandatory for each country to define various levels of health care (Table 1). As a principle, the more specialised the care a patient may require, the further it should be from the patient's point of entry into the service. The reasons for this are obvious. To have a neuro-surgeon or radiotherapist in a position where he is required to provide primary care is manifestly absurd, both from the patient's and doctor's point of view. This, of course, is an extreme example, but the same principle also applies to less highly specialised physicians as in Belgium, Canada, France, the Federal Republic of Germany, Italy, Japan and the USA. Unless there is some basic organisation, there will inevitably be overlapping and gaps in medical care, with a wasteful and inappropriate use of medical manpower.

The initial visit which a patient makes to a doctor or other health worker should be restricted, wherever possible, to the primary level only, should rarely occur at the secondary level and never at the tertiary. Although the population covered at the primary level may be as many as 100 000 people, the individual doctors working in such a catchment area, whether they are single-handed or in groups working from a polyclinic, will be looking after a relatively small number of patients varying between 1000 and 4000. Until relatively recent times, populations were fairly static, particularly in rural areas, and this helped to provide a good doctor/patient relationship. Unfortunately, this is no longer the case, with a consequent fragmentation of this relationship which has led to problems, both for patient and doctor alike.

TABLE 1 *Level and flow of care*

Population	Level of care	Premises or personnel providing care
Up to 50 000	Primary	Single-handed general practitioner Group practice Health centre practice Polyclinic
50 000–500 000	Secondary	General hospital, including general medicine and surgery, orthopaedics, paediatrics, obstetrics and gynaecology as a minimum
500 000–5 000 000 or more	Tertiary	Super-specialist hospital, or super-specialist department in a general hospital

As a consequence of dealing with a small population, the spectrum of clinical conditions encountered will be limited and will, of course, be entirely different from that encountered in hospital practice. 'Common diseases occur commonly, rare diseases happen rarely, and patients with chronic diseases are always present. This represents the picture of disease in the community, mirrored so well in general practice.' (JRCGP, 1973) Furthermore, it is important to understand the basic content of general practice, in relation to both the actual severity of illness and the broad spectrum of disease, if rational planning in the organisation of primary care is to be carried out. Health is extremely difficult to define and does not lend itself to any objective measurements: almost all measurements of health are actually measurements of disease and general ill health. The severity of conditions seen in general practice in the UK are shown in Table 2. Comparable data for other countries are not available, but there is no evidence to suggest

that they would differ to any great extent: in fact a report on the content
of family practice from Virginia USA (Marsland, Wood & Mayo, 1976)
although not directly comparable, does show great similarities in the
content of conditions seen and diagnoses made.

Of the conditions recorded, 64 per cent are classified as 'minor',
which means there is no risk to life or permanent disability, but they
are not necessarily self-limiting. From this it should not be inferred that

TABLE 2   *Severity of conditions seen in different general practices
(percentages)*

Condition	(1954)	(1959)	(1960)	(1962)	(1966)	(1968)	(1970)	(1972)
Minor	54	51	75	53	68	56	54	61
Major	16	16	17	14	6	13	17	18
Chronic	30	33	8	33	26	21	19	21

Source: *JRCGP* (1973)

TABLE 3   *Persons consulting for minor illnesses per year in a hypothetical
average practice (2500)*

Minor illness	Consultations per 2500 patients
Conditions	
General	
Upper respiratory infections	500
Emotional disorders	300
Gastrointestinal disorders	250
Skin disorders	225
Specific	
Acute tonsillitis	100
Acute otitis media	75
Cerumen	50
Acute urinary infections	50
'Acute back' syndrome	50
Migraine	30
Hay fever	25

Source: *JRCGP* (1973)

they are trivial or unimportant. What it does mean is that they are conditions which should be dealt with by a primary care physician and do not require the attention of a specialist colleague. Chronic conditions account for 21 per cent, and require long-term medical supervision, again by the primary care physician, while the acute cases representing 15 per cent will often need either immediate hospital admission, or certainly specialist advice.

In a hypothetical 'average' practice of 2500, the consultations for minor, acute, chronic and congenital disorders are given in Tables 3, 4 and 5. Again, there are no equivalent statistics for other countries, but

TABLE 4 *Persons consulting for acute major illnesses per year in a hypothetical average practice (2500)*

Acute major (life-threatening) illness	Consultations per 2500 patients
Conditions	
Acute bronchitis and pneumonia	50
Severe depression	12
Acute myocardial infarction	7
Acute appendicitis	5
Acute strokes	5
All new cancers	5
Cancer of lung	1–2 per year
Cancer of breast	1 per year
Cancer of large bowel	2 every 3 years
Cancer of stomach	1 every 2 years
Cancer of bladder	1 every 3 years
Cancer of cervix	1 every 4 years
Cancer of ovary	1 every 5 years
Cancer of oesophagus	1 every 7 years
Cancer of brain	1 every 10 years
Cancer of uterine body	1 every 12 years
Lymphadenoma	1 every 15 years
Cancer of thyroid	1 every 20 years
Suicidal attempts	3
Deaths in road traffic accidents	1 every 3 years
Suicide	1 every 4 years

Source: *JRCGP* (1973)

it is certain they would only differ in emphasis rather than principle.

3. As previously stated, efficient and well-organised primary care needs adequate diagnostic and therapeutic facilities, so that as many patients as possible can be investigated, treated and looked after in the community. The reasons for this policy are varied. First, specialist colleagues and hospitals can be protected from unnecessary referrals, and anything which reduces hospital admissions saves money. Second, it is more convenient for the patient to be investigated, and if possible treated, within his own community. Finally, primary care physicians can use the skills they have been taught, which leads to a greater degree of 'job satisfaction'. This is a rational and economic approach which few people will dispute, and indeed most developed countries are organised in this way, the main exceptions being the Republic of Ireland and the UK.

TABLE 5 *Congenital disorders expected in a population of 2500*

Congenital disorders	Expected occurrence in a population of 2500	
Conditions		
Congenital heart lesion	1 new patient every	5 years
Pyloric stenosis	1 new patient every	7 years
Talipes	1 new patient every	7 years
Spina bifida	1 new patient every	7 years
Mongolism	1 new patient every	10 years
Anencephaly	1 new patient every	10 years
Cleft palate	1 new patient every	20 years
Dislocation of hip	1 new patient every	20 years
Phenylketonuria	1 new patient every	200 years

Source: *JRCGP* (1973)

4. Lastly, if primary care is to encompass not only curative medicine but also health education, preventive medicine and the coordination of all social welfare and public health services for the patient and for his family as well, such an enormous undertaking can be fulfilled only by a team of health workers rather than doctors working in isolation. A number of countries (Australia, Belgium, France, Italy and the USA)

certainly do not accept such a total commitment, and there is only enthusiasm for the team concept from a minority of doctors in these countries.

Who else provides primary care besides the doctor?
The use of other health personnel in the work of primary care is not a new idea. Certainly the practice of obstetrics has remained in the hands of midwives for the last two hundred years and they have continued to dominate this branch of primary care. In Russia, until the middle of the nineteenth century, there was no organised medical profession and it was Peter the Great in about 1700, who introduced the *feldscher* (from the German 'field-barber') into the army; gradually they became an accepted part of the medical scene throughout Russia, particularly in rural areas.

Linnaeus, in 1751, advocated that rural clergy in the State Church of Sweden should be given training in medicine to enable them to bring treatment to the virtually undoctored country population. There is evidence of similar discussions in other European capitals, but the most comprehensive of the proposals was put forward at Halle in Germany, in 1804, by the Professor of Medicine, Johann Christian Reil (1759–1813). He advanced a plan providing for medical auxiliaries to be trained to serve in the rural areas and underprivileged quarters of the large cities. The doctors would still follow the long curriculum in the universities and university hospitals, but the auxiliaries would have a three-year training in separate institutions developed for the purpose, but whereas the doctor would continue to be trained in the basic 'scientific philosophy' of medicine, the auxiliaries would be taught differently and with the emphasis on practical needs. He even antici-pated one of the biggest difficulties of achieving the desired results in the Third World, not to speak of many of the developed countries. He wrestled with the difficulty of inducing the auxiliaries to remain in the outlying rural areas without resorting to compulsion (Heller, 1976).

What is new, therefore, in the present-day attitudes towards medi-cal auxiliaries? In the developing world, and also more recently in the advanced industrialised countries, two serious shortages have plagued health care – money and manpower – and a realistic solution has to be found for these two parallel problems. The training of medical auxiliaries who can act as a substitute or alternative for a doctor is a logical answer. It must be stressed that an auxiliary is not a poorly trained or second-rate doctor, but someone who has a special training to meet the needs of the particular country in which he or she works. In other words, each country must decide its own priorities and devise its own educational programme. According to the World Health Organisation (WHO), such an auxiliary is defined as 'a technical worker in a certain field with less than the full professional qualifications'. Doctors are the most expensive personnel to train in any health service and, particularly in poorer countries, there is a much better return for money by training a greater number of auxiliaries rather than very few doctors. This means that a small number of doctors working in co-operation with auxiliaries, are able to care for a much larger population than would have been possible if training had been restricted to doctors alone (Gish, 1971). In this way the expensively trained doctors can be used more rationally with work that actually requires their high degree of skill and knowledge. Delegation of responsibility to appropriately trained personnel is an absolute prerequisite for the success of any health service.

Developed countries

Partly as a result of the shortage of doctors prepared to work in general practice, partly because of the expense of training doctors and partly because of the obvious benefits produced by the use of auxiliaries in developing countries (p. 337), a number of advanced industrialised nations have been reconsidering the ways in which primary care can be provided.

Countries can be divided into two groups – those which use medical auxiliaries within the definition of the WHO, and those which use paramedical staff – district nurses, health visitors, midwives – as a form of intermediate technology in primary health care.

Group 1

USSR. The *feldscher* is probably the best known of all medical auxiliaries as she (or he) has been in existence for nearly three hundred years and her future is assured as an essential and integral part of health care, even though the USSR has the greatest number of doctors per population of any country in the world (USSR, p. 168).

USA. The first training programme of physicians' assistants started in 1966 at Duke University, North Carolina. It was in response to the growing alarm about the state of primary care in the USA. In 1967, a scheme was started in Denver at the University of Colorado Medical Centre for the training of special paediatric nurses for the provision of primary care in those areas without a doctor, or as a substitute for a paediatrician. It is estimated that each nurse allows a physician to increase his potential by one third (Elliott, 1971). Yet another sub-specialty of nurses involved in primary care has recently entered the medical scene: the neonatal nurse practitioner in Arizona. She is trained to examine newborn babies and to understand medical technology (X-rays and blood tests) and, in fact, acts as a neonatal paediatrician.

Group 2

Canada. The practice nurse who is attached to, or rather works under the direction of, a general practitioner, is beginning to extend her role away from general reception duties, book-keeping, answering the telephone and dealing with repeat prescriptions to supervising preventive medicine and screening clinics, for example hypertension, diabetes, cervical smear as well as baby clinics. This is intended to liberate the physician from routine work and thus enable him to concentrate on problems requiring his special diagnostic and therapeutic skills.

A further development has been the remarkably successful scheme in Ontario, where the practice nurse has been used in carrying out initial home visits – in other words, in a diagnostic role previously felt to be the province of the doctors and no-one else (Spitzer *et al.*, 1974).

Sweden. Largely because primary care has been neglected for a long period of time, there has been a need to provide first-contact care in many parts of the country by nurses, who carry out diagnostic as well as preventive work under the overall supervision of the district medical officer. Although they are trained as nurses, in many ways their function is similar to the *feldscher* in the USSR.

Recently, in urban areas, specialist nurses have been trained to care specifically for various chronic, long-term diseases – diabetes, hypertension and chronic urinary-tract infections (Haglund, 1974).

UK. With the blessing of the Royal College of Nursing and the Royal College of General Practitioners, following recommendations made in 1963 about attachment of district nurses, midwives and health visitors to general practitioners, in the last decade there has been a steady growth in this type of team work. It is interesting to note that initially the Royal College of Nursing was against the use of district nurses in anything but accepted nursing procedures, but this has changed gradually and at the present time in many practices much routine measurement and investigation (BP recording, urine testing, venepuncture, cervical smears, electrocardiology, audiometry), also assessment and diagnosis, both in the surgery and in the home (infectious diseases, tonsillitis, influenza,) are carried out by the nurse or health visitor. In 1968, it was estimated that at least 15 per cent of the doctor's working time could be freed by sensible and appropriate delegation of his work to attached nurses. A number of important and extremely valuable papers have been produced on the use of nurses in general practice and the attitude of patients to home visits by nurses and health visitors (Weston-Smith & Mottram, 1967; Marsh, 1969; Weston-Smith & O'Donovan, 1970; Marsh *et al.*, 1972).

Variations in organisation of primary care

1. The single-handed physician
This is still the commonest type of doctor involved in primary care throughout the world, particularly in Western Europe and those countries which have been influenced by the European tradition, both culturally and socially as well as medically, for example Australia, New Zealand, the USA, many South American countries and, of course, densely populated cities of Africa and parts of southeast Asia.

Today he may be either a generalist or a 'specialoid' physician.* If he is a generalist, very often he will look after the whole family. As a 'specialoid' he is much less likely to do this; rather he will attend patients according to his own specialty, for example paediatrician, internist or gynaecologist (Fry, 1969).

Place of work. Normally general practitioners work from their private houses, although this is gradually changing in cities where they have separate offices or clinics containing the minimum of consulting rooms, office and secretarial space. In the UK some single-handed general practitioners work from health centres, alongside groups of doctors who are working in partnership.

* See footnote, p. 246.

Ancillary staff. Here there is tremendous variation, from the direct personal involvement of the doctor's own family, his wife and/or daughter acting as his nurse-receptionist at one end of the scale, to the employment of nurses, midwives, social workers, receptionists and secretaries at the other.

Diagnostic and therapeutic facilities. These also vary from one extreme to another. If practising from his own house, a general practitioner's facilities can be described as basic, with equipment limited to stethoscope, auriscope, ophthalmoscope, and arrangements for simple urine testing. In many countries such as Australia, Canada, France, the Federal Republic of Germany and the USA, the doctor will have a more extensive examination room where he can perform minor gynaecological operations and some minor surgery; often he will have a small laboratory and X-ray facilities. The extreme is reached in Japan where over 70 per cent of all primary care physicians have contrast X-ray equipment on their own premises.

In most countries in the developed world there is a growing tendency to centralise pathology facilities in private or jointly owned laboratories thus providing a more comprehensive and better service; alternatively specimens are sent direct to the local hospital.

Advantages and disadvantages of generalist and 'specialoid'. In this context, the term generalist means a family doctor or general practitioner. There are sound practical reasons for the view that the general practitioner is better able to provide comprehensive care than his specialist colleague; they have been expressed as follows (McWhinney, 1964).

(a) Many infections and children's illnesses have a strong family tradition.

(b) The care of chronic disease often requires a close knowledge of other members of the family. A patient may frequently be best helped by a relative with whom the doctor has already established a close *rapport.*

(c) Nearly all emotional disorders have their origin in the family. In addition, any organic illness often has a most profound effect on the health of the other members of the family.

The general practitioner is more likely to be able to deal with the open-ended, unsystematic, non-categorised pattern of illness with which the first-contact doctor is confronted. If the family situation is well known, he is much more aware of the interplay of emotional, social, financial, sexual and work factors on the presentation of illness. He is less likely to take symptoms on their face value and to embark on a whole series of unnecessary tests and investigations which are often expensive in time, money and resources.

The generalist is more likely to have a wider outlook on medicine, and is better able to protect the patient from the dangers of over-specialisation. He is able to distil for the patient the advice received from specialists, and to recommend the wisest course of action for that particular patient and his family.

The advantages of the 'specialoid' and specialist are that they are likely to have a greater knowledge of their own particular specialty, and have immediate access to a wider variety of investigatory and diagnostic equipment. They may be more up to date with the latest advances in their subject and, because of all these factors, their treatment should be quicker and of better quality. Of course this argument presupposes that the patient is capable of deciding which symptoms require which specialist. This basic assumption is just not true and although there may be no danger to the patient if he chooses wrongly, it is an inappropriate use of highly trained and scarce resources.

Advantages and disadvantages of single-handed practice. The obvious disadvantage is that the practitioner is isolated from his professional colleagues and, with the rapid advances in medicine, he will find it increasingly difficult to keep up to date. He may also become unaware of his own limitations and delay referral to the appropriate specialist. This is a theoretical rather than a practical danger, and is not necessarily confined to the single-handed doctor. In addition, the cost of diagnostic equipment (e.g. ECG machine, microscope) and the employment of ancillary staff (nurses, receptionists and secretaries) is more expensive for the single-handed doctor.

Perhaps the main disadvantage from the doctor's point of view is the fact that, by definition, primary care is a continuing and continuous responsibility which means a 24-hour service throughout the year – at nights, at weekends and during holiday periods. This imposes almost impossible demands on the doctor and his family, and leads to tiredness, loss of interest and increasing staleness. But from the patient's point of view, knowing that the doctor is on duty all the time creates great confidence and reassurance in times of emergency. Equally, the doctor, if he knows his patients really well, has a great advantage and is able to assess, advise and treat his patients more effectively and realistically.

Finally, the feelings of the patients are ambivalent – on the one hand there is the security that most patients experience in knowing that 'their' doctor is always available, on the other is the doubt that it is possible for him to keep thoroughly up to date.

2. *Group and health centre practice*

These will be considered together because basically they involve the same principles, the only difference being in the ownership of the premises, and sometimes in the variety and scope of ancillary help and diagnostic facilities.

The number of doctors involved varies enormously: from two (which is still the commonest type of partnership) up to six in a group practice, and even twelve to twenty in some health centres in Australia, Canada, Sweden and the UK, while in the USA there may be as many as fifty. The physicians involved may be general practitioners, general practitioners with special interests (psychiatry, paediatrics, family planning, obstetrics), 'specialoids', and even specialists, all of whom provide some primary care. In some health centres in Finland and the UK, specialists from the nearest hospitals may provide regular referral consultation sessions (i.e. secondary care only).

Place of work. This comprises an office including consultation and examination rooms, with space available for the use of nurses, health visitors, midwives, receptionists and secretaries, and for the storage of records. There is often a special treatment or minor-operation room, where casualties can be dealt with and surgery carried out.

Ancillary staff. It is customary to have a staff of nurses, midwives, health visitors, secretaries and receptionists, the ratio being better than in most single-handed practices. This has given rise to the idea of the *practice team* with which social workers have in some instances become involved. It is being felt increasingly that, under present-day conditions, comprehensive care can be provided only on this basis, rather than by each worker operating separately and in isolation. It prevents duplication of work, and enables manpower to be used efficiently and effectively. It is beginning to make all primary health care workers redefine their roles, so that everyone is performing the job for which he has trained, and no-one is doing something which could be better done by someone else. There are two types of team in operation throughout the world: the *interdisciplinary* team, composed of a variety of health workers (Finland, Sweden and the UK), and the *intradisciplinary* team, composed of members of the same discipline, i.e. a team of doctors, usually a variety of specialists working together as a team (Australia, p. 281; France, p. 80; the USA, p. 247).

The basic members or nucleus of a health or practice team are the doctor, nurse, social worker and secretary. The requirements and expectations of countries differ, and a wide variety of additions can be made, forming a multiple team: for example dentist and dental auxiliary, physiotherapist, chiropodist, occupational therapist, radiographer, pharmacist and dietician (Finland, p. 133; Sweden, p. 160). The most important aspect of the team should be flexibility, and the ability to change as the needs of the community change. If the team is particularly large, an administrator, who will probably be non-medical, is necessary.

Diagnostic and therapeutic facilities. Most large group practices or health centres will possess an ECG machine, microscope, equipment for undertaking minor surgery, haemoglobinometer, laryngoscope, proctoscope and, perhaps, sigmoidoscope, steriliser, cautery apparatus and audiometer. Physiotherapy departments are usually present in Finland and Sweden, while in Australia, Canada and the USA, all large groups, and even small ones, will have X-ray equipment and a pathology laboratory.

Advantages and disadvantages of group or health centre practice. The ability to provide both better premises with more staff and a wider range of diagnostic equipment is an advantage both to the patient and the doctor. In theory it should be easier to provide comprehensive 24-hour cover at weekends, holidays and during sickness, which again helps both patient and doctor.

For the doctor, it is easier to organise his life both professionally and domestically. He can attend postgraduate courses and professional meetings, and lead a normal family life with adequate leisure and recreation. He can be ill without the worry of finding a deputy. His expenses are shared and his worries are alleviated. There is more likely to be an interchange of ideas, both with the doctors in the team and with the other professional workers, thus helping his continuing education. New horizons should appear as the functions and roles of the team are continually examined.

The greatest potential and real disadvantage is concerned with the doctor/patient relationship. A health centre is more likely to have the cold, clinical, out-patient atmosphere of the hospital, which is not conducive to easy relationships; many patients feel that this is too high a price to pay for the sake of efficiency and a comprehensive service. There are often criticisms about the impersonal approach of doctors and staff, leading to a breakdown of confidence. If an appointment system is run it is often difficult to see the doctor quickly and this gives rise to complaints. The danger of this situation is that patients are forced to turn away from primary care and go straight to the hospital out-patient or emergency department.

3. Polyclinic

In some socialist countries the polyclinic provides the facilities for both primary and secondary medical care. In the USSR and Cuba and under certain circumstances in Eastern Europe (pp. 192, 199, 204) it is the focus of primary medical care, as well as providing specialist and 'specialoid' services. The paediatric, adult and industrial services each have separate polyclinics with different catchment areas for each specialty. In rural areas, there are general polyclinics covering the adult and paediatric population, usually attached to a small rural hospital.

Staff. All doctors of first contact restrict their working to a particular age group or sex of patient. Dentists are always included at this primary care level. In addition, all polyclinics, except in rural areas, contain physicians in all the major specialities.

Ancillary staff. Each *uchastok* doctor has a nurse attached to his clinic. She acts partly as a nurse, helping in the clinic and with home visits, and partly as a secretary. There is the usual receptionist staff involved in the storage and distribution of patient's notes. *Feldschers/* midwives are often found in rural areas (USSR, p. 179).

Diagnostic and therapeutic facilities. There are always X-ray, laboratory and physiotherapy departments with all the necessary and appropriate staff.

4. District or community medical/health centre

These provide the setting of the basic services for giving medical care in eastern Europe (Bulgaria, p. 192; Czechoslovakia, p. 198; Hungary, p. 204). As in the USSR, the doctors concerned in first-contact care restrict their work to a particular age group or sex of patient. The basic staff consists of a community or district paediatrician, internist and gynaecologist (usually working part-time and serving several centres) with the appropriate nurses. A dentist is also included as a statutory member of staff, although this is not always possible due to shortages.

Such units are simply housed and equipped with the minimum of clinical and diagnostic aids. On some occasions, they are geographically attached to a polyclinic. In rural areas, a small number of maternity beds are usually provided.

Diagnostic and therapeutic facilities. These are provided at the local polyclinics which, in Eastern Europe, usually provide only secondary care, i.e. all specialised ambulatory services, X-ray, laboratory and physiotherapy departments.

Relationship between primary care and hospital service

In almost every developed country in the world where there is poor primary care in inner-city areas, the emergency departments of hospitals provide this service, particularly at night, at weekends and during public holidays. They are not only used by the poor and underprivileged, but also often by ordinary patients who are unable to find a doctor.

In parts of rural France, the UK, Finland, Norway, throughout the USA, Canada, Australia and in rural areas of the USSR, primary care physicians have the opportunity to admit patients to hospital under their own care, exercising full clinical responsibility. Such hospitals have a wide variety of names – rural, general practitioner, cottage or community, while in urban areas, particularly of the USA and Canada, there are general hospitals to which primary care physicians have the right to admit patients. The function and purpose of all these hospitals is the same: to service the needs of the local community by providing hospital care for patients who are too ill to be looked after at home, and yet do not require the sophisticated facilities found in major centres, or because the general practitioner cannot or will not make home visits. In some places, these hospitals may be so remote from the nearest specialist centre that the type of treatment and facilities required will be much more extensive, including acute surgery and obstetrics. Obviously, the functions and objectives will vary from country to country, even from one area to another. They are all staffed by primary care physicians, sometimes with the help of visiting specialists (Finland, p. 134; UK, p.

44). It can be seen that their main feature is variety, and it is hoped that in the future flexibility will be the watchword in planning.

In some countries (the Republic of Ireland, New Zealand, Norway and the UK) X-ray facilities and also physiotherapy departments are provided at the local hospital rather than in the doctor's private office, in the health centre, or in private diagnostic centres. There are two great disadvantages: first, patients may live at a great distance from the hospital, and second, if there is a pressure on the X-ray or laboratory departments, then the first curtailment of service is usually to the referrals from general practitioners. As a principle, it should be accepted that such facilities must be the right of all general practitioners, and not a privilege. Only in this way can rational clinical decisions be made about diagnosis, effective treatment and the need for specialist referral.

The relationships between general practitioners/family physicians and specialists is far from satisfactory. This is to the detriment of both, but more particularly it affects the general care of patients. The blame must be shared by both. The specialists have tended to denigrate and belittle the value of the general practitioner; to underestimate the importance of the family and social background of the patient which can so readily be provided by the general practitioner; and to fail to supply the doctor in the community with information about patients' investigations and treatment after discharge from hospital. The general practitioners have very often failed lamentably in adequately communicating information to the specialists, and have suffered from a feeling of inferiority because of their poor training, apprehensive that they will be unwelcome and feel 'out of their depth' in the hospital environment, often giving the impression that they are thankful to see patients admitted and thus removed from their care and their responsibility. Where these problems exist, poor communication is felt to be the basic problem. If this could be improved, then better cooperation would follow. Cooperation between hospital doctor and primary care physician is best in rural areas and small towns, and worst in the large urban sprawl. The reasons for this are obvious: doctors know each other personally and this tends to remove unnecessary suspicion. It follows that patient care is also likely to improve in such situations.

Continuing postgraduate education is generally considered to be the responsibility of the large hospital. There is a wide variety of response, from almost no involvement in France and Italy, to total responsibility in Eastern Europe and the USSR, where primary care physicians are recalled to hospital training for varying periods of time during the year. In Australia, Canada, Denmark, the Netherlands, Norway, New Zealand, the UK and the USA, there is now tremendous encouragement for general practitioners to attend postgraduate courses, often centred in the local hospital or postgraduate centre.

Education and training usually take the form of formal lectures, short courses on particular subjects and clinical meetings, but inevitably they are of only limited value because they are organised primarily by specialists who perpetuate the disease-orientated interests of hospital medicine. Often the subjects under discussion are largely irrelevant to primary care, although undoubtedly they will be of academic interest. In order that postgraduate education for primary care physicians should be more worthwhile, they themselves should be involved to a far greater degree – as lecturers, as organisers of courses and by active participation in hospital rounds, clinical meetings and case conferences.

3

UNITED KINGDOM

The United Kingdom of England, Wales, Scotland and Northern Ireland is a constitutional monarchy with power in the hands of Parliament. It has a population of 55 million, of whom 46 million live in England, 2.5 million in Wales, 5 million in Scotland and 1.5 million in Northern Ireland. The population is homogenous, and although during the last fifteen years there has been an increased immigration from India, Pakistan, Bangladesh and the West Indies, immigrants account for only about 5 per cent of the population. The UK has many problems which are similar to Japan: it is overpopulated, with England having the highest population density figure in Europe, and 80 per cent of the population living in 20 per cent of the land mass; it is highly industrialised and is dependent on trade for survival. Parliament at Westminster has sovereignty over the whole of the UK, although there has been devolution to Scotland and Northern Ireland, and more recently to Wales, in such matters as education, health, housing and social policy. In practice, the general organisation of the health service and the facilities provided are fairly uniform and therefore in the following account it is assumed that each country is similar unless specifically stated otherwise.

Although the UK became a member of the European Economic Community in 1975, its National Health Service is to be considered in rather more detail than the health services of the other eight countries. This is because the introduction of the National Health Service marked a significant milestone in the evolution of medical care in the non-Communist world. Whether it has been successful, or whether it can continue in its present form, is a matter which is argued in many parts of the world. Few countries are more concerned with tradition and custom, or appear to be more conservative in their general attitudes than the UK, so to the outside observer the introduction of such a service probably seemed unexpected and completely 'out of character'. But a superficial knowledge of English history shows that although there may be initial resistance to new ideas, gradually they are introduced by evolution and compromise. Now tradition in medicine is very strong, and in order to understand the changes which have overtaken the medical profession and produced the present situation, it is necessary to delve briefly into the past.

Historical background

In medieval times, as in the rest of Western and Central Europe, the care of people was basically in the hands of the Church and monastic orders. Many hospitals were started in the Middle Ages, and St Thomas's and St Bartholomew's hospitals in London are descended directly from religious foundations. As early as the fourteenth century, barber–surgeons had organised themselves into guilds and, in 1540, it was decided by Royal Assent that surgeons should no longer be barbers and that barbers should restrict their surgery to dentistry. Thus was born the Royal College of Surgeons in London. At the same time, apothecaries realised that clerics and all manner of imposters were becoming involved in the practice of medicine and Henry viii was persuaded to give his Royal Assent to the foundation of an independent organisation to control the practice of medicine; thus, in 1551, the Royal College of Physicians in London was founded. From that moment right up until the present time the Royal Colleges, later to be supported by the College of Physicians (1681) and the College of Surgeons (1778) in Edinburgh, have been concerned with maintaining standards; they have also wielded great 'political' power, forming an 'establishment' through their original royal patronage. Apothecaries, who were not members of the College of Physicians, formed their own society in 1617 and evolved to become the general practitioners of the present day.

With the dissolution of the monasteries in 1536, many hospitals were destroyed, and over two hundred years elapsed before the next period of hospital growth in the eighteenth and nineteenth centuries. During this time, the voluntary hospital appeared – founded and financed locally by public contributions for the good of local people. Obviously, such hospitals only arose where there was sufficient money and interest, and so the distribution was haphazard and uneven. An important tradition grew up at this time which was maintained until 1948. All medical staff were unpaid for the services they gave to the hospital, and made their living from private practice in the local community. Thus hospitals in the UK have always been non-profit-making institutions, and specialists have never been paid on an 'item-of-service' basis. Gradually, with the spread of scientific medicine, apothecaries began referring difficult cases to the specialists, and another unwritten law arose over the years whereby patients could only be seen by a specialist if they had first been referred by a general practitioner. This is now a completely accepted code of behaviour and to transgress it is very much frowned on by specialists and family doctors alike. It has placed the family doctor in the UK in a strong position compared with almost all other primary care physicians in the world, giving them a virtual monopoly of first-contact care. Such a situation also occurs in Denmark, the Republic of Ireland and the Netherlands.

Before the National Health Service

For all practical purposes there were no organised medical services until the end of the nineteenth century. Up to this time, personal doctoring was paid for over the counter by the patient. Some enlightened doctors started 'clubs' in which the working man paid a small amount each week, which entitled him to some medical treatment in time of need. Simultaneously, a number of other organisations grew up which contracted with a doctor to look after its members. This was a start, but obviously not nearly enough, and it was not until the government became involved that the beginnings of an effective primary care service grew up. In 1912, Lloyd George introduced the National Health Insurance Scheme, which aimed to provide a general practitioner service for all workers earning less than £160 per annum. This gave no entitlement to hospital services, nor was there any provision for families or old people. Less than half the population were covered under this scheme, and the rest were committed to direct payment or subscription to a number of already existing 'sick clubs' and 'approved societies' run by the trade unions or private insurance companies. The outcome of this was that the sickness benefits varied considerably and serious anomalies arose in the medical services provided. General practitioners participating in the National Health Insurance Scheme were paid on a capitation fee system: in other words, a patient registered with a doctor who was then responsible for providing medical care and was paid an annual fee for doing so. The amount which was paid did not vary, irrespective of whether the patient was seen frequently or not at all.

In 1918, the Maternity and Child Welfare Act was passed, which gave local authorities the right and duty to set up clinics for expectant mothers and young children. This was an attempt to fill in the obvious gap in a deficient primary care service, and clinics continued in this manner until 1948 or shortly afterwards when, by law, everyone in the country had the right to register with a general practitioner.

During the Second World War the Emergency Medical Service (EMS) was set up and all hospitals were taken over by the state; in some ways, therefore, the hospital service was prepared for the final state take-over in 1948. The Coalition Government welcomed and fostered a proposal about a welfare state, and the Beveridge Report on Social Services setting out these views was published in November 1942. In this report the need for a comprehensive health service was proposed, and in 1943 discussion between the government and the profession started. It would be quite wrong to believe that the National Health Service was the brain child of the Socialist Medical Association, or the Fabians, or Sir William Beveridge, although they were perhaps its most enthusiastic and persistent advocates. Even the British Medical Association had seen the need and set up a Medical Planning Commission in 1940 which had concluded that some form of organised health care was needed. Rather, there was an awareness on the part of many people, and the idea certainly had the unanimous support of the three political parties. On the other hand, it is fair to say that the National Health Service would never have been introduced so quickly and so comprehensively if it had not been for the determination and political competance of one man, Aneurin Bevan.

Main features of the National Health Service

The National Health Service was started on 5 July 1948, after a considerable amount of initial opposition, both on the part of the hierarchy of the Royal Colleges of Surgeons and Physicians, the great majority of general practitioners and the leaders of the British Medical Association. The intentions of the new service were:

(*a*) To ensure that everybody in the country – irrespective of means, age, sex or occupation – should have equal opportunity to benefit from the best and most up-to-date medical and allied services available.

(*b*) To provide for all who needed it a comprehensive service covering every branch of medical or allied activity, from care of minor ailments to major medicine and surgery, including mental as well as physical health, all specialist services, all general services (family doctor, dentist, optician, midwife, nurse and health visitor) and all necessary drugs and medicines, and a wide range of appliances.

(*c*) To divorce the care of health from questions of personal means or other factors relevant to it, and thus encourage the obtaining of early advice and the promotion of good health rather than the treatment only of ill health.

Furthermore, a number of principles were to be observed and safeguarded (DHSS, 1970):

(*a*) There was to be no compulsion into the new service, either for patients or the profession. People were to be free to use or not to use, as they wished, the facilities placed at their disposal. The right was maintained to make private arrangements at private cost for those who wished to do so.

(*b*) People were to be free to choose their own family doctors and family doctors free to decide whom they accepted on their list.

(*c*) Doctors were to be free to treat their patients in their own individual ways, without being subject to any interference in clinical matters.

(*d*) The traditional doctor/patient relationship was to be safeguarded, and the family doctor was to be the link between his patient and the hospital and the local authority services which he might need to use.

(*e*) These principles were to be combined with the degree and kind of public organisation needed to ensure that the service was properly provided, that resources were properly distributed and that scope was given to new methods and developments.

The cost of the service was to be met from a variety of sources as shown in Table 1. Central taxation is the main provider of funds, while compulsory social insurance payments are very small compared with our European neighbours; whether this is right or wrong, desirable or undesirable is a matter for endless argument amongst economists. Direct payment by the patient has always been an emotive and doctrinaire issue and has rarely exceeded more than 4 per cent.

Private practice plays a small part in total health expenditure. This may well change if standards in the health service continue to fall with ever-increasing waiting lists for specialist out-patient appointments and non-urgent surgery

TABLE 1   *Source of health-service financing (as a percentage)*

	Finance (%)		
Source	1958/59	1967/68	1972/73
Central government tax	70.7	74.4	70.7
Local government tax	12.0	14.0	18.8
National Health Insurance	12.7	9.4	7.3
Direct payment by patient	4.4	2.0	2.9
Miscellaneous	0.2	0.2	0.3

Source: Ministry of Health and Social Services, *Annual Statistics, 1974*

In 1974, the total spending on private practice was barely over 1 per cent of the total health budget. Basically, private practice involves the specialists and hospital services, as 'only 5 per cent of family doctors have a hundred or more private patients, about a third have none at all and the rest rarely more than twenty' (Cartwright, 1967). There is nothing to suggest that the situation in general practice has altered since that investigation and almost certainly it is steadily getting less. But one thing is certain and beyond doubt: the total cost of the service has risen beyond anyone's wildest fears, and the fallacy of the idea that if the health of the nation were improved, so eventually the cost of the service would decrease has been brutally exposed (Table 2).

It was the intention that the service should be uniform throughout the UK. In fact, there are differences in the standards and provision of care within the different regions, for example industrialised Northern England or Scotland compared with the South-east England or South Wales with the South-west England. 'The widest disparity – that between expenditure on the hospital service in Scotland compared with England and Wales – has increased materially in the last decade so that *per capita* expenditure is now 25 per cent greater in Scotland. Even Wales spends £1 *per capita* more than England on Health and Social Services.' (Godber, 1975) It is perhaps worth noticing that, in spite of this increased expenditure, Scotland stands lower in the international table of health statistics (infant and maternal mortality, etc.) than England.

TABLE 2   *The total cost of the NHS and percentage of GNP*

Year	Cost of NHS (£ million)	Cost of NHS as percentage of GNP
1951	503	3.87
1953	546	3.61
1957	720	3.67
1961	981	4.01
1963	1092	4.00
1967	1592	4.52
1971	2371	4.87
1973	3092	4.89

Source: Office of Health Economics, *Compendium of Health Service Statistics*, 1975

After the National Health Service
The service was basically divided into three quite separate parts:
(a) family doctor service,
(b) specialist and hospital service,
(c) local authority public health service.

Each of these services was totally independent until 1974. This independence was carried to the point of absurdity and it made rational planning on a regional basis almost impossible. For most people working at 'ground level' in the service, it became increasingly obvious that 'the right hand didn't know what the left hand was doing'. There was little communication between the administrator of the hospital, the family doctor or the public health service, and such planning as there was appeared to be initiated in a piecemeal fashion. The allocation of resources tended to go to the institution, hospital or doctor who shouted loudest, and the decision about priorities remained firmly in the lap of the medical establishment, with the inevitable emphasis on the specialist and hospital service. In spite of the fact that successive Ministers of Health and numerous politicians and health administrators have repeated with monotonous regularity that the family doctor is the corner-stone of the service, he has been allocated a steadily decreasing percentage of money (Table 3 shows that between 1951 and 1973 the proportion of money spent on the hospital service increased by 10.5 per cent, while that spent on general practice decreased by just over 2 per cent). At the same time, the number of physicians working in the hospital service has dramatically increased, while general practice has remained virtually static (Table 4 shows that between 1949 and 1973, the total hospital medical staff more than doubled, while the total number of general practitioners increased by one-third).

TABLE 3   *NHS expenditure: proportion (as a percentage) spent on each service*

Service	Percentage of NHS expenditure					
	1951	1957	1961	1967	1971	1973
Hospital	55.7	56.8	57.0	59.9	65.3	66.2
GP	9.5	9.7	9.6	7.9	8.1	7.4
Dental	7.8	5.5	6.2	5.0	4.9	4.4
Pharmaceutical	9.7	9.7	9.8	10.6	9.8	9.4
Ophthalmic	2.8	2.2	1.8	1.5	1.3	1.1
Local health	8.5	8.8	9.3	10.4	7.0	6.9
Others	6.0	6.4	6.3	4.7	3.6	4.6

Source: Office of Health Economics, *Compendium of Health Service Statistics*, 1975

TABLE 4   *Hospital and general medical practitioners employed in the NHS (England and Wales)*

	1949	1959	1969	1973
All hospital staff	11 735	16 033	22 001	26 152
Consultants	3 488	5 322	7 763	9 496
Senior registrars	1 430	931	1 431	1 910
Junior registrars	1 523	2 787	4 467	4 667
Senior house officers	797	2 315	4 761	6 606
House officers	2 613	2 436	2 405	2 430
General practitioners	approx.17 000	22 091	21 505	22 686

Source: Ministry of Health Statistics, 1974

The reorganisation of the health service in 1972 coincided with plans to redraw local government boundaries. It was decided that health service areas should coincide with the new county boundaries, although in practice this has led to much confusion, inefficiency and considerable overmanning. After endless discussion and much fore-boding on the part of the majority of doctors, the reorganised health service became law in April 1974. The basic intention was to eliminate the tripartite structure which had existed since 1948 and replace it with a unified hospital, family doctor and public health service at regional, area and district levels. In England there are 14 regions and 90 areas, while in Scotland, Wales and Northern Ireland the regional level has been omitted, leaving 14 (Scotland), 7 (Wales) and 4 (Northern Ireland) Area Health Boards. The day-to-day running of the service, which is the responsibility of the Area Health Board, is based on health districts with populations varying between 150 000 and 300 000. The Depart-ment of Health and Social Security (DHSS) is concerned with overall planning and policy, while the Regional (England) or Area (Scotland, Wales and Northern Ireland) Boards are responsible for deciding priorities and allocating money and manpower. (For a more detailed description of the reorganisation (DHSS, 1973, 1974a).) Thus it is hoped that already scarce funds will be distributed more rationally rather than according to previously held traditional values. One new departure is the setting up of Community Health Councils intended to represent the views of the patients. They are established at district level and at least one-half of their members are appointed by the local authorities, another third by voluntary bodies concerned locally with the health service and the remainder by the regional health authority. They are seen by some as a threat to the medical profession, by others as a welcome and necessary development in any health service, while there are those who fear that the councils will have no influence at all. It is too early to know whether 1974 will be remembered as a great step forward or merely as a sideways move: probably neither view will prove accurate, and things will just muddle through in a typically British compromise fashion; but the omens are not good. There has been an enormous increase in the number of administrators (non-medical, medical and nursing):

(a) Between 1949 and 1971 the hospital administrative and clerical staff in England and Wales increased from 23 797 to 47 690 – an increase of 100.4 per cent.

(*b*) Between 1971 and 1973 the hospital administrative and clerical staff in England alone increased from 45 091 to 51 632 – an increase of 14.5 per cent.

(*c*) Figures for the Executive Council Staff (in charge of administration of general practice) are not available prior to 1964. However, between 1964 and 1973 the Executive Council Staff in the UK increased from 4326 to 5634 – an increase of 30.2 per cent.

(*d*) Between 1949 and 1973 the administrative and clerical staff of Regional Hospital Boards increased from 1320 to 8359 – an increase of 533 per cent!

(*e*) Figures for 1974–7 are not available, but few people believe that the hospital administrative and clerical staff, plus the medical and nursing administrations have increased by less than 25 per cent in this three-year period.

(*f*) Between 1971 and 1975 the full-time equivalent number of administrative and clerical staff, including community health staff previously employed by the local health authorities, increased in England from 70 396 to 91 865 according to a written answer on 24 March 1977 by Mr Eric Deakins, Under-secretary of State, DHSS.

(*g*) Executive Council Staff figures for 1974–7 are also not available, but the increase is less than in the hospital service.

The doctor or nurse working in either the hospital or community feels totally impotent about dealing with this growth which is spreading like an uncontrolled cancer. The bureaucracy is stunning, with two or three people doing one man's job; overmanning is accepted as an inevitable consequence of the present organisational structure. In the three years following reorganisation there has been an ominous drop in morale amongst doctors and nurses, more particularly amongst those working in the hospital service. There is a feeling that the service is now being increasingly organised and run by those who are, in fact, remote from the day-to-day needs of patients. The majority of doctors feel that reorganisation is perpetuating the very things it was claimed would be eliminated, and it is no wonder that disenchantment is rife. It will take more than administrative reorganisation to alter the traditional attitudes of both doctors and the general public towards technological, scientific medicine.

> If hospital doctors are to be involved in future in the determining of clinical policy, then not only will a collective view be required of where priorities lie, but this view should also be based on an appraisal

of existing and proposed procedures. Cochrane, drawing attention to the finding that some costly technical innovations may be no more effective than established cheaper regimes, goes so far as to suggest that no new procedures should be introduced unless their effectiveness has been established. This is an extreme view, but it is a challenging approach to the change in attitude which will be required among clinicians. (Forsyth, 1973).

General practitioners, who for the first time in their lives are to have more say in policy-making decisions, must show that they are capable of discerning problems in their widest context, and that they are also able to withstand misplaced patient pressures at the district level.

Primary medical care

The UK is totally committed to the concept of the general practitioner, or family doctor as he is now more commonly known. He provides continuing and comprehensive care for the whole family and attempts to restrict his work to one particular age group or sex of patient have been resisted (McKeown, 1965). Even the idea of family doctors within a group practice developing their own particular special interest has not been followed up with much enthusiasm. The National Health Service did not change the tradition of British medicine, where the family doctor has the monopoly of primary care. What did change was the extent of this monopoly so that the general practitioner service covered not only the working population but also their families and all who previously paid by insurance or private fees. Within a year, 95 per cent of the population had registered with a family doctor and this has risen to just over 97 per cent.

A patient is entitled by law to register with a family doctor. In theory, there is a free choice of doctor by the patient, but this is obviously not possible in some rural areas and is becoming less common in towns, where doctors are attempting to restrict and localise their practice areas. Doctors can refuse to accept patients, and at the present time patients and doctors can part company without giving a reason. Once a patient is registered, a doctor accepts 24-hour responsibility for providing all necessary and appropriate care, both in the consulting room and the patient's home, including emergency 'out of hours' services. This is an enormous commitment and something which is not readily understood by anyone who has not had first-hand knowledge of what it means. Obviously few doctors are continuously 'on call', but it is the doctor's responsibility and not the government's to find a deputy. The reason for this burden is that family doctors have always insisted on having an independent contractor status within the health service as opposed to the rest of the profession who are paid by salary.

What does the independent contractor status mean, and what benefits does it give the doctor? He is free to appoint the colleague with whom he works without any interference from the state; he can resign from the health service and still continue to practise from his own premises; he is able to practise medicine and organise his day as he wishes without interference from the state; he can undertake salaried hospital and industrial work, private and insurance work in addition to his routine tasks. On the other hand, he is responsible for finding and paying a deputy at all times when he is away from his practice, even during illness, postgraduate training and holidays. Some family doctors feel that the so-called independence is an illusion, and is rather more of a 'millstone' than anything else, with all the disadvantages of independence and none of the advantages of a salaried service. Nevertheless, the majority cling passionately to this form of contract, as it at least leaves the loophole of resignation available: salaried doctors in the hospital service do not have this safeguard.

Payment agreed by the government and the profession in 1965 was known as the Charter for the Family Doctor Service. This was one of the turning points in the history of the health service. Mass resignation was threatened, and prevented by the acceptance of the charter, which has done much to improve the organisation of general practice by encouraging the employment of secretarial staff. The payments are as follows:

(*a*) Basic practice allowance to recognise commitments and obligations which do not vary proportionately to the size of the list.

(*b*) Special allowances to recognise seniority, group practice, practice in unpopular areas and special training for general practice.

(*c*) Capitation fee for each patient on a doctor's list with special additional payments for those over 65 years. This is a continuation of the principle started by the National Health Insurance Scheme in 1912.

(*d*) Fee for item-of-service payment for vaccination, immunisation and cervical cytology.

(*e*) Payment in respect of (i) employment of ancillary help, whereby 70 per cent of the salary is reimbursed to the doctor. This has been recognised as one of the most enlightened moves by any government, as the payment involves a direct improvement in the standards of practice; (ii) rent and rates of premises.

Administration

The responsibility for the general administration of primary care is in the hands of the Family Practitioner Committee, of which there are 90 in England; one for each area health authority. They have no direct influence on planning or research, nor have they any power to influence the clinical work of doctors within their area. One of their most important tasks is to keep a record of the patients on each individual doctor's list and to arrange for the transfer of all clinical notes and documents when a patient moves to another area, therefore changing his doctor. This facility is of great value to both patient and doctor in helping to maintain some degree of continuity, and is another unique feature of the British primary care system. The Family Practitioner Committees are responsible for maintaining as even a distribution of family doctors as possible throughout the UK, but this policy has had only limited success, even allowing for additional payments being made to doctors working in unpopular areas (Tables 5 and 6), but compared with France (p. 76) or the Federal Republic of Germany (p. 88) maldistribution of personnel is not a major problem. The country is divided into a number of differently classified practice types: 'restricted', where no further doctors are considered necessary and no further appointments will be allowed; 'intermediate', where doctors are required; 'designated', where doctors are required and extra payments will be given to them for coming to such a practice.

TABLE 5   *Size of lists (England)*

	1963	1967	1973
Number of principals	19 065	18 617	19 997
Average list size	2 343	2 490	2 398

Source: Ministry of Health Statistics, 1974

The actual appointment of a doctor to a single-handed practice, because of death or resignation, is the responsibility of the Family Practitioner Committee. In the case of partnership, it is a private matter between the applicant and the doctors concerned.

The location of general practice is very varied, from isolated rural practice in the Highlands of Scotland to the densely populated, industrialised areas of England. Between these extremes, there are old residential areas, vast new housing estates often built on the edge of industry, and small country towns. Each has its own particular problems and patterns of work, while the expectations of patients are equally variable, usually determined by what has gone before, whether it was good or bad.

TABLE 6 *Classification of areas (England and Wales)*

	1963		1970		1971	
	Number of principals	Average list size	Number of principals	Average list size	Number of principals	Average list size
Designated	3305	2742	6482	2791	6207	2781
Open	12 888	2382	7554	2480	7543	2458
Intermediate	2375	1942	3991	2223	4501	2248
Restricted	1767	1659	2330	1884	2382	1896

Source: Ministry of Health Statistics, 1974

Organisation

Single-handed practice dominated the scene in 1948, with the doctor usually practising from his private house and his wife and family often acting as secretary or receptionist and, in country areas, as his dispenser as well. Gradually, the spread of partnership or group practice has gathered momentum (Table 7). The reasons for this are well documented (Chapter 2), but are primarily concerned with the 24-hour responsibility and the need for relief over night work, off-duty and holiday times, and the general desire to improve the social and family life of the doctor.

One of the chief characteristics of general practice in the UK over the last 25 years has been the formation of partnerships, followed by group practice and, finally, health centres and the concept of the team approach to primary care. This has been fostered and encouraged by the government with special allowances for group practice, in the belief that this is the correct direction for general practice to develop.

What is the difference between partnership and group practice? In partnership, two, three or four (but rarely more) doctors work from their individual practice premises, often a private house, and keep their own list of patients, arranging to cover each other for off-duty, night work and holidays. In group practice, two or more doctors work from a central location and in this way are more likely to provide better premises with more secretarial and receptionist help and usually attachment with district nurses and health visitors. They are able to benefit from mutual discussion and by the joint examination of individual cases. Group practice premises are privately owned by the doctors themselves.

TABLE 7   *Analysis by practice structure of principals providing unrestricted general medical services. Changes in proportions of doctors practising single-handed and in partnership*

	Percentages of principals practising single-handed and in partnership					
	No. in partnership					
Year	1	2	3	4	5	6 or more
1952	43.6	33.0	15.0	5.7	1.6	1.1
1959	31.2	35.7	19.5	9.3	3.3	2.0
1966	24.0	31.1	24.0	12.9	4.5	3.5
1968	22.7	27.3	25.4	14.4	6.0	4.2
1970	20.7	24.7	25.9	16.0	7.4	5.3
1971	20.0	23.5	25.4	17.0	7.7	6.4

Source: Ministry of Health Statistics, 1974

The next development was health centres, which in effect are group practice premises, owned by the area health authority and rented to the family doctors. In the UK, group or health centre practice only involves general practitioners and their ancillary staff, so the question of multispecialty or single-specialty groups does not arise.

A catchphrase in an easy substitute for thought. Group practice and health centres are often spoken of as universal cures for the ills of general practice. It is clear that general practice can reach the highest level without anything in the nature of a group, and that grouping, *per se*, even when combined with a common working place, does not necessarily produce the best. It is often said that the greatest single advantage of group practice is that it raises the standard of medical work done. This is easy to say but hard to prove. Of the disadvantages of group practice, the possibility of the group pulling down standards rather than raising them must not be forgotten. Two great enemies of good medical work are failure to keep notes and to examine properly, usually brought about by laziness or fatigue. The temptation to succumb to either is greater for the individual working alone, since he often lacks any ancillary help and always lacks the critical stimulation of colleagues. But inside a group, slovenly medical practice may be infectious, just as good practice is infectious. In fact, much more experiment will be needed before the value of health centres (or group practice) can be finally assessed. (Taylor, 1954)

It is more than twenty years since these words were written and although the benefits of group and health centre practice, both to doctor and patient, are beyond doubt, there are certain matters which are giving cause for concern and will be considered later in the chapter.

Health centres

One of the most visionary documents on the organisation of health care was produced over fifty years ago (Dawson, 1920). That so many of its far-sighted recommendations were largely ignored for so long has been one of the major follies of this century for which both doctors and the Department of Health are responsible. To quote from the report:

The changes which we advise are rendered necessary because the organisation of medicine has been insufficient, and because it fails to bring the advantages of medical knowledge adequately within the reach of the people. This insufficiency of organisation has become more apparent with the growth of knowledge.

Preventive and curative medicine cannot be separated on any sound principle, and in any scheme of medical services must be brought together in close cooperation. They must likewise both be brought within the sphere of the general practitioner, whose duties should embrace the work of communal as well as individual medicine.

We begin with the home, and the services, preventive and curative, which revolve round it, viz. those of the doctor, dentist, pharmacist, nurse, midwife and health visitor. A health centre is an institution wherein are brought together these various personnel.

The domiciliary services of a given district would be based on a primary health centre which would be equipped for services of a curative and preventive nature to be conducted by the local general practitioners in conjunction with an efficient nursing service and with the aid of visiting consultants and specialists.

A group of primary health centres should in turn be based on a secondary health centre. Here cases of difficulty or cases requiring special treatment would be referred from primary centres. The equipment of the secondary centres would be more extensive and the medical personnel more specialised. The distinguishing feature of the primary centre would be that it would be staffed by general practitioners in contradiction to the secondary centres staffed by specialists.

Secondary health centres should in turn be brought into relation with a teaching hospital. This is desirable, first in the interest of the individual patient, that in difficult cases he may have the advantage of the highest skill available, and secondly in the interest of the medical men attached to the primary or secondary centres.

Nothing new or original has been written about health centres since 1920, and yet still the basic structure and facilities of the majority remain inadequate with no specialist clinics, X-ray or physiotherapy facilities (compare Scandinavia, pp. 135, 160; USSR, p. 172).

In 1948, the National Health Service Act gave power to the local authority to build health centres: in fact, it was an essential part of government policy. But there was to be no cohesion and, predictably, the vast majority of general practitioners were sceptical about the value of this new venture in health care. More important than this, they were afraid of the motives of the government. Once they were practising from health centres, which were owned by the local authority, most doctors felt that should they wish to resign from the health service they would find it extremely difficult to find or build new accommodation. To many, the health centre concept led directly to a state-controlled, salaried service, and very few wanted this. Of course, the government and local authorities were secretly delighted by the profession's attitude, as it saved them a great deal of money.

Over the last fifteen years, there has been a steadily increasing demand for health centres (Table 8), so that at the present time the government is unable to keep pace with applications. What has brought about this change in heart on the part of family doctors? First, younger doctors feel that there are quite definite medical benefits from practising in a health centre; second, rapidly rising costs with high interest rates make it almost impossible for doctors to borrow enough capital to build adequate group practice premises. Third, many doctors in the cities were and are in danger of losing their premises because of redevelopment and are unable to find other practical sites.

TABLE 8   *Number of health centres built in the UK*

Year	UK	Number of health centres			
		England	Wales	Scotland	N. Ireland
1948–63	28	21	4	3	0
1964–7	32	23	4	3	2
1968	50	36	4	4	6
1969	60	46	5	3	6
1970	81	62	7	6	6
1971	119	86	9	16	8
1972	144	116	12	10	6
1973	–	104	11	14	–
1974	–	102	–	–	–

Source: *British Health Centre Directory*, 1973, King Edward's Hospital Fund, London

The number of family doctors working in health centres at the end of 1973 expressed as a percentage of all family doctors was England 13.9 per cent, Wales 18.3 per cent, Scotland 17.7 per cent and Northern Ireland 31.6 per cent. By the end of 1975, 3500 family doctors (17 per cent) in England and Wales were practising in health centres compared with about 3000 (15 per cent) at the end of 1974 (DHSS, 1976).

The average numbers of family doctors per health centre in the UK are as follows:

1964–7	1968	1969	1970	1971	1972	1973	1974	1975
5.0	4.3	4.8	5.9	5.0	5.2	5.7	5.5	5.9

There are very wide variations throughout the country as no less than 6 of the Scottish centres are for twenty or more family doctors, while there are only 2 centres in the rest of the UK with provision for this number. At the other end of the scale is Wales with an average of four doctors per centre.

The basic services are fairly standard, with consulting room suites for the doctor and his team (nurse, midwife, health visitors) plus receptionists and secretaries. In addition, the local authority often provides chiropody, speech therapy, dental, health-education and family-planning facilities (the family-planning facilities were transferred in 1975 to the family doctor service). The main criticism of health centre planning lies in the inadequacy of readily available X-ray facilities and the almost total lack of specialist out-patient sessions. There has always been the anxiety which has grown into a belief that if family doctors were given direct access to X-ray (and pathology) examination their demand would be limitless and even irresponsible. In fact, this does not occur as various studies have shown (Barber *et al.*, 1974; Howie, 1974). Likewise, the lack of specialist involvement in providing an out-patient service is inexplicable. A recent study showed that 85 per cent of patients seen in a general medical out-patient department could have had the consultation at a health centre (Wade & Elmes, 1969). In Scotland, however, the Health Department has been much more forward-looking in the actual concept of health centres and the obvious advantages of out-patient facilities and, where possible, X-ray services have been appreciated. It is accepted that when the catchment area of a health centre rises above a certain number, then various additional services are required over and above the purely family doctor team. At the level of 20 000 population physiotherapy is needed; at 30 000 population specialist out-patient sessions are of great benefit to both doctors and patients, and at 40 000 every effort should be made to provide a good X-ray department (although at the moment with no thought of providing contrast media examinations). In the rest of the UK, the only places in which these additional and absolutely essential facilities are provided are where the health centre has been built next to a general practitioner hospital. The high standard of comprehensive care which can be attained by family doctors either working from fully equipped health centres or a general practitioner hospital/centre complex has been well documented (Stranraer Health Centre, 1968; Burns, 1971). It would behove all health planners to remember that good primary care cannot be carried out without the tools to do the job or adequate support from specialist services.

What do patients feel about health centres? Usually they have had no say whatsoever on the introduction of a health centre to their area, and in most cases it has been foisted upon them. It is interesting that in recent surveys of patients' attitudes to health centres and their assessment of their benefits a fairly constant figure of 70–75 per cent stated that they preferred and approved of health centres and found their facilities satisfactory (McDonald, Morgan & Tucker, 1974; Woods *et al.*, 1974; Patterson, 1975). Whether this proves that health centres provide a good service or confirms the view that patients are notoriously uncritical and accept whatever is put before them, it is difficult to say. There were some doubts expressed and these related mainly to the problems of appointment systems.

Facilities

In the early 1960s, one of the main weaknesses of primary care in the UK was the lack of diagnostic tools with which the family doctor was asked to carry out his work. The situation was worst in those areas surrounding the large district or teaching hospital where the local family doctors were not given access to the pathology, radiology or electrocardiograph departments. Thus it was impossible to provide an adequate service, and, not surprisingly, the morale of general practice reached a very low ebb and the hospital out-patient departments became overloaded with unnecessary referrals. Unfortunately, the idea of anything better or different was not understood by the average patient who had been indoctrinated into accepting second best. Gradually it was realised that no family doctor could provide first-class care without easy access to such facilities, and it was also appreciated that it would save some specialists from carrying out work that should have been done at the primary care level. In all health services, it is important to define levels of care and to make sure that everyone in the service is able to work to his fullest potential, thus avoiding the unsatisfactory situation which was commonplace in general practice in the UK until fairly recently. There was no other developed country in the world (except the Republic of Ireland) where the primary care physician lacked such facilities, and very few would have tolerated such an absurdity. Uneven progress has been made, although, of course, not nearly enough (Table 9).

Pathology services are usually provided at the local hospital, the specimens either being sent direct to the laboratory or collected from group practice premises or health centres. Very few family doctors carry out anything but the very simplest tests.

TABLE 9 *Availability (in percentages of general practitioners questioned) of diagnostic facilities*

Investigation	1963	1968	1969
Haematology and biochemistry	94	96	88
Bacteriology	88	94	83
Radiology:			
Chest	92	95	88
Skeletal	61	72	58
Contrast media	40	72	58
ECG	8	39	40

Source: Report from general practice No. 16. *Journal of Royal College of General Practitioners* (1973)

Radiology departments are either in the local hospital or, exceptionally, in some of the newer, large health centres. Many investigations have now been carried out which prove conclusively that family doctors do not overload X-ray departments with excessive or thoughtless examinations, and that in fact a higher percentage of abnormalities are found in patients referred by family doctors than by out-patient departments (Lennon, 1971; Wallace *et al.*, 1973; Mair *et al.*, 1974).

Electrocardiograph facilities have improved, but they are far from satisfactory. A recent survey (Bradford, 1975) has suggested that 34 per cent of partnerships or health centres own their own electrocardiographs, while 52 per cent of family doctors have open access to a referral service which, although not as satisfactory as practice ownership, undoubtedly allows the doctor to give a quicker and better service to his patients.

Finally, brief mention must be made of the almost complete lack of physiotherapy facilities for the family doctor. There are no definite figures available, but it is estimated that less than 5 per cent have open access. Such a situation is quite appalling as it means that the majority of patients in the community requiring active treatment receive nothing at all. It has been shown that such facilities are not abused or squandered (Freedman *et al.*, 1975; Norman *et al.*, 1975; Waters *et al.*, 1975).

If a general practitioner feels a patient requires physiotherapy treatment, the only way in which this can be arranged is for the patient to be seen first by an orthopaedic surgeon or by a private physiotherapist. As the average waiting time to see an orthopaedic surgeon is in fact at least six to eight weeks, the situation is even more ludicrous than it would first appear.

The team
The evolution of the team approach to general practice has been developing steadily over the last fifteen years. It is one of the major contributions of the UK to solving the problem of providing adequate primary care. The value of a nurse working in cooperation with a family doctor is well known (Crombie, 1957; Cartwright & Scott, 1961; Weston-Smith & Mottram, 1967; Marsh, 1969), and gradually it was appreciated that an extension of this idea to involve health visitors (Connolly, 1966) and, more recently, social workers (Lord, 1965; Evans, 1969) should increase the comprehensiveness and effectiveness of family care in the community. It was an entirely logical and necessary step as 'the physician can no longer work alone to provide the care required and expected at first-contact level, for if he is to devote his time to conditions, problems and situations requiring the medical skills for which he has been trained, he must be able to delegate some of his present tasks to paramedical colleagues' (Fry, 1969).

The paramedical staff can be employed directly by the family doctor (since 1966, the government has reimbursed 70 per cent of the salaries) or on attachment from the local authority. The single most important factor in any successful team is for everyone to be *en rapport* and for there to be no conflict of personality. Next, everyone must have clearly defined roles, otherwise it is difficult to delegate effectively. Finally, nurses, midwives, health visitors and social workers should be treated as colleagues by the doctor, so that patients can be referred to them in the same way as to the specialist services. There are dangers in the team approach: the patient may feel that no-one is ultimately responsible, that confidentiality has been impaired, that there has been a loss of the personal doctor/patient relationship, that the doctor does not care particularly if the nurse or health visitor does first visits and is involved in diagnosis. If it is to be a success, patients must be educated about what, for them, is a new idea in health care, and these innovations should be brought in gradually.

Finally, in group or health centre practice, the receptionist/secretary plays a vital role in the management of patients, particularly in relation to the vexed problem of appointment systems which have become increasingly popular on the part of doctors – 64 per cent of family doctors in 1972 had such systems (DHSS, 1974b). There is some controversy, usually in relation to the lack of flexibility which sometimes prevents a patient from obtaining an urgent appointment which he believes to be necessary. In the view of many, the receptionist has the most difficult task of all: to please both the patient and the doctor at the same time.

Hospital service and primary care

The relationship between the family doctor and the hospital service is far from satisfactory. Although between the two World Wars a number of general practitioners, usually those living in small country towns, did work as part-time specialists in hospitals, in 1948, when the National Health Service Act became law, they ceased to do so. Hospital beds were given to the specialists, the family doctors were excluded from the hospital and the separation of the hospital from the community was almost complete, to the detriment of patients, family doctors and often, unknowingly, to the specialists as well. It has been known for many years by the few family doctors who have the advantage of looking after their patients in hospital how much this improves the scope and quality of patient care (Weston-Smith & O'Donovan, 1970; Kyle, 1971). Equally, there is no doubt that the lack of hospital facilities, including beds, has a direct effect on recruitment into general practice (Horder, 1969), while in a survey of medical students 67 per cent felt that both beds and diagnostic facilities were absolutely necessary for effective general practice (Stephen, 1969). This of course, will be no surprise to readers from as far afield as Australia, Canada or the USA.

Family doctors at the present time have access to hospitals in the following ways:

1. They may help as clinical assistants, where they work under the surveillance of a specialist in out-patient clinics – paediatrics, general

medicine, obstetrics, psychiatry and casualty being the commonest. There is no question of their looking after their own patients, and although it does help to develop their own special interests, cynics would say the scheme is more concerned with helping to overcome the manpower shortage in hospitals than assisting with the needs of primary care. Some clinical assistants, for instance in anaesthetics, work in smaller hospitals away from the supervision of specialists.

2. About 5000 family doctors work in 400 cottage hospitals or general practitioner hospitals where they have direct access to beds and are able to look after their patients in hospital. The practices which are attached to these hospitals are eagerly sought after and have many applications for partnership vacancies. In 1962, the Hospital Plan for England and Wales decided that all hospital care should be provided in district general hospitals, and this culminated in the report of the DHSS which outlined the plan in more detail (DHSS, 1969). As a result of this 'steam roller' policy which manifestly ignored the wishes of the patients and the reality of the situation, it was decided to close as many general practitioner hospitals as possible, not to mention general hospitals with under 300 beds. A number of family doctors who were outraged at this unbelievable folly set up an Association of General Practitioner Hospitals (Roberts, 1969) in order to stop the threatened closures. The tide of public opinion has now swung very much in favour of the smaller hospital, and there was a *volte-face* on the part of the government when, in 1973, they announced their intention of building and developing community hospitals mainly staffed by family doctors (Israel & Draper, 1971; DHSS, 1974c; Kernick & Davies, 1977). A few isolated general practitioner units have also been set up in large general hospitals (Wilkinson, 1968), but for a variety of reasons they are not entirely satisfactory.

3. Maternity hospitals or general practitioner beds within a specialist obstetric unit are spread fairly evenly throughout the country. These facilities are becoming less common and less desired by family doctors as the actual confinement is now more and more the responsibility of specialist obstetricians.

Medical education and primary care

A report on the state of general practice in the UK (Collings, 1950) suddenly brought to light what many people suspected, some doctors knew and nobody wanted to admit. It has been said that the report overstated its case and the descriptions applied only to a small minority of practitioners rather than to the majority. Certainly what was described gave the impression of extremely poor standards of education, lack of facilities and even the basic needs for simple examination (no auriscope, ophthalmoscope or sphygmomanometer); thus morale was at a very low ebb. The profession was shocked into realising that even if the report was exaggerated in some respects, there was enough truth in it to give rise to anxiety. In 1952, whether irritated, stimulated, provoked or merely concerned that the standards of general practice should be raised, a small number of like-minded family doctors founded the College of General Practitioners. Within two years the membership was 5000, and this has risen only slowly over the years until in 1978 it has reached just under 8000. The immediate aim was to initiate thought and action on undergraduate and postgraduate medical education, to stimulate the development of general practice and to organise research. From this small beginning, the College of General Practitioners has flourished and become a major influence on the development of primary care in the UK and on education throughout the world.

Initially, the college concentrated on the undergraduate curriculum, and so successful has it been that most medical schools have either departments of community and family medicine or general practice staffed by family doctors, who are thus able to influence the content of the medical curriculum and, it is hoped, influence the students away from the strait-jacket of hospital medicine. Although special postgraduate training had been thought about for some years, it was not until 1965 that the first official report was published (*JRCGP*, 1965) in which it was recommended that doctors should have at least five years' postgraduate training before becoming established in general practice. In 1968, the Royal Commission on Medical Education reaffirmed this principle, and gradually it has become accepted by almost the entire profession, although the five-year period has been reduced to three. It is anticipated that from 1981, it will be mandatory for any new entrant to general practice to have completed a three-year vocational training course. Meanwhile the number of young doctors following a planned programme of vocational training has continued to increase from about 130 in 1968 to 541 in October 1974 and 667 in October 1975, while the number of appointed general practitioner trainers is now greater than the current intake of doctors into general practice (DHSS, 1975).

Personal assessment

In theory at least, the organisation of primary care in the UK has much to recommend it. Even though it is not as comprehensive as in the USSR or Eastern Europe, it is certainly more readily available than in many other countries. But its particular strength is continuity. Patients register with a doctor who is then responsible for their day-to-day care: such a situation is unique in any health service. By the act of registration there is also the guarantee that the patients' clinical notes will follow them should they move from one part of the country to another and change their doctor. This quite obviously increases the likelihood of continuity and saves an enormous amount of time (and unnecessary investigation) for all concerned.

If it is accepted that much illness, both organic and psychiatric, originates in the family or affects the family, then the insistence on leaving primary care in the hands of family doctors is not only logical but an absolute necessity. Furthermore, the fact that the family doctor has a virtual monopoly of primary care acts in two directions. First, it guards the specialists from unnecessary consultations, thus enabling them to concentrate on their own particular specialty and relieving them of the irksome business of acting as primary care physicians for which they are untrained. Second, it protects the patient from an enormous amount of totally unnecessary investigation which is the inevitable result of considering illness in an episodic, and disease-orientated fashion, without knowing the background of the patient.

But there are various warning clouds appearing on the horizon which some do not see and others wistfully hope will disappear. Basically their origin is the same. At the present time it is apparent that some family doctors are no longer caring for the whole family or providing continuity of care. No night work and no weekend work facilitated by the increasing use of emergency services produces the '9 a.m. to 5 p.m. attitude' which is surely incompatible with good general practice. The problem of deputising arrangements has been carefully studied (DHSS, 1974b) and the committee concluded that some form of deputising arrangement is obviously essential, but that it should be organised in the way least harmful to continuity of care. It is accepted that personal care and the availability of patients' records is important and that there is no excuse for group practices or health centre partnerships routinely using a deputising service: off-duty is best arranged within the partnership so that continuity is maintained. In some partnerships it is common practice for patients not to have 'their own doctor' but to be registered with the whole group. This is surely a negation of all that is so assiduously taught by enthusiasts for the family doctor and this particular concept of primary care. It is the intention of all sections of society to make the working day shorter. This is undeniable and doctors are no exception as is apparent from the changing work patterns, both in hospital and general practice. But if this trend continues, is there any possibility that general practice in twenty years' time can possibly survive as a personal family doctor service? Such questions must be faced and answered honestly, because unless doctors actually do what they say they are doing, they are in danger of believing their own propaganda and deceiving both themselves and their patients. Continuity of care is appreciated both by the patient and the doctor, and if it is to continue then two things must happen: first, patients must not abuse the service and second, family doctors must not abuse their monopoly of primary care.

With the growth of the health team and group/health centre practice, a number of potentially serious difficulties are beginning to appear. Patients are worried that confidentiality, which until now has been so assured by a close doctor/patient relationship, can no longer be guaranteed. Furthermore, it is feared that the delegation of responsibility between the various members of the team may lead to no-one being prepared to accept the final responsibility. In some areas, where nurse/health visitor attachment or the team concept of care has been hastily introduced, a number of undesirable things have occurred. Patients have felt that if they saw anyone but the doctor, they were getting 'second best'. This is untrue, but understandable, and is the result of inadequate preparation and education of the patients about the aims of the team. There have also been a number of reports (Hawthorn, 1971) in which nurses have expressed the view that doctors were merely using them as a 'dogs-body', and were unaware of the real value of attachment schemes. This attitude is much more likely with older practitioners and appears to be diminishing with the newer entrants into general practice. Such problems are not a serious obstacle, provided everyone is aware of the potential hazards.

One of the worst features of general practice in the UK has been the lack of direct access to diagnostic facilities (X-ray, pathology, electrocardiography and physiotherapy). In recent years, there have been great improvements, although the position is far from satisfactory. To any reader from outside the UK it is merely stating the obvious to say that easy access to these services is essential for good primary care. If such organisation is not available, then two things happen: first, the hospital service is overburdened with unnecessary referrals, while the patient is subjected to a great deal of inconvenience and delay in investigation and treatment; second, family doctors merely become signposts to the nearest hospital, which gives rise to feelings of intense frustration and a serious lowering of morale.

Finally, the implications of the 'five-minute consultation', which is a feature and a criticism of general practice in the UK, must be faced: to deny that such a situation does exist is a form of self-deception. Certainly the complaints from patients that doctors never have time to listen to them and are always in a hurry must be related in some way to the brevity of the consultation, and yet it is not the whole story since the same complaints are also levelled at the medical profession in those countries where the consultation time is considerably longer. Furthermore, the continuity of care associated with the registration of patients should lead to a quicker understanding between patient and doctor without necessarily leading to a lowering of standards. However, the reasons and effects of this rapid turnover must be studied and the pattern of work should be flexible enough to meet the changing needs of patients.

Note. While this book was being written, the general economic situation in the UK deteriorated quite markedly and public spending was reduced. Primary care no longer remains one of the government's priorities within the health service, and hopes of the expansion of health centres and the growth of community hospitals (staffed by general practitioners) appears to be fading rapidly.

4

The European Economic Community (EEC) was founded in 1958 through the Treaty of Rome. Six countries – Belgium, France, the Federal Republic of Germany, Italy, Luxemburg and the Netherlands – joined together to form an alliance of cooperation, initially in the field of economics and trade, later to be followed by an attempt to provide a common agricultural and monetary policy. To many this was only the beginning, the ultimate aim being some form of political union so that Europe would never again be in a position to tear itself apart, as has happened with such terrible consequences on two occasions during this century. Whether this aspiration is merely the hope and dream of a few idealists, or is in fact a political reality remains uncertain. At any rate, in spite of gloomy prognostications about its survival, even in a limited economic sense, by 1974 another three nations – Denmark, the Republic of Ireland and the UK – had applied for, and were eventually granted, membership.

Under the Treaty of Rome, there is no obligation to unify the social or health policies of the member countries. The intention rather is to cooperate and learn from each other, so that ultimately there may be harmonisation of these services in an endeavour to raise standards throughout the Community. In fact the achievements of the EEC in the field of health care have been limited to the principle that people moving between nations are now able to receive the same medical care as resident nationals. The ultimate aim of the completely free movement of health workers depends on the recognition of qualifications which can take place only when there are mutually acceptable standards of education and training. From December 1976, all physicians

54

have the right to migrate from one member country to another, provided their qualification is recognised by the member country. In fact most specialties are mutually acceptable, but for those that are not, it is required that the doctor concerned should take a further examination. It remains to be seen how successful these regulations will be.

General practitioners are not yet recognised as specialists, and within the nine countries there are widely differing requirements, both in undergraduate and postgraduate education, as well as in vocational training. Theoretically there will be a free flow of general practitioners, but any country is at liberty to insist on a further examination before permission to set up practice is given. Until there are generally acceptable training programmes for general practitioners, this safeguard is likely to remain. In January 1978, the tenth anniversary meeting of the European Union of General Practice (UEMO) passed a resolution which stated that by 1985 all general practitioners should carry out a period of specific vocational training before being given permission to practise. The resolution was vague and lacked specific details on implementation and financing. It remains uncertain whether the commission of the EEC has the desire or the ability to carry through this resolution.

The population of the EEC is about 255 million and, except for immigrant workers from Turkey, Cyprus, Greece and Yugoslavia, and a small proportion of Asian, African and Caribbean immigrants, it is largely homogeneous, with a common historical background, although it shows different traditions, customs and cultural heritages. Six languages are spoken, as well as a number of dialects, and although English, since the Second World War, has become the common international language, it is by no means the common language of the community.

To draw any reliable direct comparisons between the health services of the member countries is fraught with difficulties. First, the complexities of the social security systems associated with differences in sickness benefits, income levels and taxation make it an almost impossible task. Second, the degree of urbanisation and industrialisation, and the extent of differing social and economic policies have a direct impact on the expectations of people and the pattern of the health services. But perhaps the greatest obstacle to a study is the basic lack of information and statistical data on the organisation of health care, morbidity patterns and the type of work carried out in the field of primary care (exceptions to this criticism are Denmark, the Netherlands and the UK).

There are many misconceptions and much ignorance about medical care in the EEC. In Eastern Europe and the USSR, the health services in Western Europe (including the EEC) are assumed to be very similar to those in the USA, but not quite as bad, while in the North American continent they are also grouped together as providing some sort of national health service, in many ways similar to that of the UK, but again probably not quite as bad! This latter misunderstanding is in part caused by the principle of compulsory health insurance for a large proportion of the population, which is confused with complete coverage regardless of any health insurance. In fact, since 1973, Denmark has been the only other European country besides the UK to pay for its health service out of direct taxation, although the Republic of Ireland and Italy may well follow suit.*

General background

There are some common traditions which apply to all countries within the EEC. Since the Middle Ages, the Church has provided care for the sick and needy, and hospitals have almost always been included within the confines of a religious institution. This religious association has persisted, so that even now many hospitals are owned and run, particularly in Belgium, France and the Netherlands, by various religious orders. At the end of the nineteenth century, voluntary insurance against illness became accepted, and by the end of the Second World War it was decided that the provision of medical care was the responsibility of the state as well as the individual. But this did not take the form of a totally government-financed health service (as in Eastern Europe or the UK), but rather a pluralistic method involving compulsory health insurance, supported by government taxes, private insurance and direct private payments by the patient. This situation exists throughout the Community (with the exception of Denmark and the UK), although the proportions vary considerably from country to country. Government support for the total cost of health care varies from 39.9 per cent in Belgium to 100 per cent in Denmark while direct payment by the patient is determined by two factors. First, how much

---

* Since January 1978, the health service in Italy has been financed through direct taxation by the central government.

patients must contribute directly out of their own pockets, even if they are covered by compulsory insurance and, second, what percentage of the population has compulsory insurance. Initially, insurance was only compulsory for employees (and dependants) earning less than the average income of the country, plus some 'high risk' medical categories, though gradually in all countries it has spread to include the more highly paid workers, the self-employed and professional people. In 1975, it was estimated that the figure varied from 100 per cent in Denmark, 99 per cent in Belgium (although the self-employed only for 'heavy risk' categories) and France to 90 per cent in Italy, 88 per cent in the Federal Republic of Germany and 70 per cent in the Netherlands.

Further complications exist if direct comparisons are attempted even in the limited field of social and health insurance. The proportion paid by the employee and the employer differs widely: from 98 per cent paid by the employer in Italy to 78 per cent in France, 66 per cent in Luxemburg, 65 per cent in Belgium, 50 per cent in the Federal Republic of Germany and the Netherlands, while in the Republic of Ireland (as in the UK) there is only a very small token payment. In Denmark there is no contribution at all through social insurance. In all countries, except Denmark, the Republic of Ireland and the UK, employee contributions are graduated according to income: in the Republic of Ireland and the UK flat-rate payments are made. Furthermore, it is often difficult to be certain about what proportion of social security payments are devoted to actual health care and what proportion to cash benefits received during an episode of illness. Benefits are not uniform, with a tendency for higher income groups to be covered only for 'high risk' diseases. In addition, there are different time limits and waiting periods before claims can be made, while the actual method of payment also varies – whether direct payment by the patient with reimbursement at a later date, or only a percentage payment by the patient and reimbursement by the insurance agency.

Health statistics

The EEC comes high in the international league table of health statistics as would be expected from so-called 'advanced' societies (Table 1).

The chief causes of death are cardiovascular disease and neoplasms, coming first and second, and respiratory diseases and accidents occupying third and fourth place. An exception to this picture is the problem of alcoholism in France, where cirrhosis of the liver comes ahead of respiratory diseases (pneumonia, bronchitis, emphysema and asthma). Morbidity reflects the problems of industrialised, urbanised societies with degenerative diseases of the elderly and middle aged, and psychosomatic disorders in all age groups producing the main bulk of work for the primary care physician.

TABLE 1   *Health indices*

Country	Infant mortality (per 1000 live births)	Maternal mortality (per 1000 live births)	Life expectancy M	F
Belgium	18.1	0.2	67.9	74.4
Denmark	13.5	0.1	70.8	76.3
France	16.0	0.3	69.1	77.1
Federal Republic of Germany	22.8	not available	67.6	74.2
Republic of Ireland	17.8	0.3	68.5	73.4
Italy	27.0	0.4	68.9	75.2
Luxemburg	14.0	not available	67.6	74.3
Netherlands	11.5	0.1	70.9	76.9
UK:				
England and Wales	17.3	0.1	69.0	75.3
Scotland	18.8	0.2	67.2	73.7
N. Ireland	21.0	0.1	67.3	73.6

Source: WHO Statistics and *Fifth Report on the World Health Situation, 1969–72*. Geneva, 1975

The ratio of doctors to population is high (Table 2) as in all developed countries, but again these statistics are misleading and do not reflect the actual situation, as they take no account of the uneven distribution of doctors, nor the numbers who are actually concerned with primary care.

There are no accurate figures about the number of general practitioners and similarly the total number of physicians concerned with primary care is almost impossible to determine, as it is common practice for specialists to work in this field. Again the differences between countries are considerable, with a virtual general practitioner monopoly of primary care in Denmark, the Republic of Ireland, and the Netherlands, while in the Federal Republic of Germany, Italy, France and Belgium there is considerable specialist involvement. It is also important to appreciate that the scope and type of work varies and may only include curative work, while inoculation programmes and preventive measures such as cervical smears and screening for hypertension or diabetes are largely ignored. In addition, some primary care physicians may look after their own patients in hospitals, while others may be concerned with public or industrial health.

TABLE 2 *Distribution of doctors and nurses*

	Doctors per 10 000 population	Habitants per doctors	Nurses per 10 000 population	Habitants per nurse
Belgium	15.9	630	not available	
Denmark	14.4	690	48.7	210
France	13.9	720	29.8	340
Federal Republic of Germany	17.8	560	30.6	330
Republic of Ireland	12.0	830	not available	
Italy	18.4	540	23.6	420
Luxemburg	10.8	930	24.4	410
Netherlands	13.2	760	25.2	400
UK:				
England and Wales	12.7	790 }	33.9	300
N. Ireland	12.4	810		
Scotland	15.6	640	42.6	230

Source: *Fifth Report on the World Health Situation, 1969–72*. Geneva, 1975

The hospital service is also far from uniform and, again, any direct comparisons are almost without value. There are differences in ownership – private (profit-making and non-profit-making) or public – size and nomenclature; nursing homes and old peoples' homes having different meanings and different uses, psychiatric and geriatric hospitals being included in some statistics and excluded from other. No account is taken of maldistribution, with the consequent gaps and overlapping in the service.

It is, therefore, quite clear that the coverage for health care and the benefits provided are uneven; that the methods of financing services are different; that the organisation of primary care is a varying mixture of general practitioner and specialist services – in fact there is no possibility of a homogeneous pattern of health care in the foreseeable future, even if this were felt to be desirable.

BELGIUM

Belgium has a constitutional monarchy with a two-chamber system of government. At the last census, in 1970, the population was 9 650 944 making her one of the most densely populated countries in Europe. During the First and Second World Wars, she suffered severe damage, both through fighting and the general effects of foreign occupation. In spite of this, her economic recovery has been excellent, owing in large measure to intensive industrialisation in iron and steel, engineering and textiles. One of the main problems is internal in character, and stems from the fact that the country is divided into two separate regions with different languages – Flemish and French. Inevitably this has affected education, business and political life, and is directly related to the differing social and economic backgrounds of the two communities. It has a direct influence on the selection of medical students: four universities out of seven are Flemish-speaking only.

As in many European countries, 'sick clubs' sprang up during the nineteenth century to cover the cost of medical care.* There has been steady government support for these funds, by an increasing and considerable subsidy of members' contributions. The insistence on compulsory coverage, paid for by compulsory health insurance, was introduced by law in 1945. Initially this was only for certain categories (low-paid workers, widows, pensioners), but by 1964 it had been extended to cover the self-employed ('heavy risk' only, which included hospital care, certain surgical operations, confinements, X-rays and radiotherapy, certain diseases – for example cancer and tuberculosis – mental and physical handicaps). Finally, in 1969, almost

---

* 'Sick clubs' or 'doctors clubs' were organised by individual patients or groups of workers (such as railway workers or coal miners) with doctors who contracted to look after these individual patients or groups at the time of illness on payment of a small retention fee. These were the predecessors of organised health insurance.

the entire population was included, although the benefits provided varied.

Health insurance

There are six organisations concerned with health and social insurance, with differing religious, political and trade union affiliations. They are supervised by the National Sickness and Invalidity Fund (NSIF), which in turn is the responsibility of the Ministry of Social Affairs.

In 1972, official figures issued by the NSIF stated that 99.3 per cent of the population were compulsorily insured. Such claims must be treated with caution. To a reader from Eastern Europe, the USSR, Denmark or the UK, it may be assumed that coverage equals a full range of medical care (both curative and preventive) both in and outside hospital, even if it is recognised that some direct payment by the patient may be necessary. But this is not the case, and at the present time the self-employed (representing 1.5 million people, or just over 15 per cent of the total population) are only covered for 'heavy risk' medical care. Therefore these people must supplement their compulsory cover, either by additional voluntary insurance arranged through one of the many sickness funds supervised by the NSIF, or directly through a private insurance company.

Revenue for health insurance is basically drawn from two sources:

(*a*) (i) Contribution by employees is 2 per cent per month of monthly income on a sliding scale up to a certain level of monthly income. (ii) Contribution by employer is 3.75 per cent per month of monthly income. This applies to the basic contribution, and additional amounts (1–2 per cent for employee and 2.8 per cent for employer) apply to the self-employed.

(*b*) Central government supplement through direct taxation. The most recent figures for 1971 show that the government's contribution to the total revenue was 33.9 per cent. The remaining 66.1 per cent came from (i) and (ii).

There are no figures about contributions or revenue from private insurance or direct payment by the patient.

All primary care services are paid on an item-of-service basis at an agreed rate between the NSIF and the medical profession. One cause of grievance and dissatisfaction amongst general practitioners is that specialist consultations are refunded at a higher rate than general practitioner consultations, even when the patient uses the specialist as a primary care physician. In 1973 there was some redress, as an agreement was reached between the profession and the government that if general practitioners carried out 100 hours' postgraduate training during the next two years they should then be paid at a higher rate: in fact it amounted to an increase of 19 per cent in their income. A grievance from the patient's point of view is that some doctors charge over and above the agreed rate, and this additional amount is not covered by their normal insurance. Fees are paid directly to the doctor by the patient, who then reclaims 75 per cent from the NSIF. Old-age pensioners, widows, orphans and chronic invalids receive 100 per cent reimbursement. With regard to drugs, patients must pay a small contribution for those on an agreed list, and in the case of some proprietary preparations the contribution is double. All hospital treatment in a public ward is free.

Primary medical care

Primary care is provided by both general practitioner and specialists (Table 3) including medical and surgical disciplines.

TABLE 3 *Number of general practitioners and specialists involved in primary care on 1 January 1975*

	General practitioner	Specialist
Flemish	2950	3130
French	3350	5300
Total	6300 (42.7%)	8430 (57.3%)

Source: *Janssen Pharmaceutica 1975*

Patients have a choice of doctor and need no referral in order to consult a specialist. There is no registration of patients (as in Denmark, the Netherlands and the UK) and in the very competitive atmosphere amongst all doctors, patients may consult as many doctors as they wish during the year, and may even change doctors in the midst of one episode of illness.

The pattern of work is usually that of a single-handed physician (general practitioner or specialist) working from his own home, helped by his wife and occasionally by a part-time nursing assistant. Small partnerships are becoming more popular, particularly amongst younger doctors, and there has been some interest in the concept of group practice (as organised in the UK), although it will be many years before this idea becomes a reality (Boelaert, 1976). In January 1977, there were only six group practices in operation throughout the country. Similarly, the primary health care team is only just beginning as a viable concept, and certainly it will need a great deal more understanding and trust between doctors, nurses, health visitors and social workers before it comes a reality.

> As far as cooperation with paramedical staff is concerned, the Belgians are still in the experimental stage. Our greatest difficulty is in deciding each one's role and field of action. At present, team work in primary care leads to greater difficulties rather than to any reduction in, or alteration of the total volume of work. Much more study and experiment is required to create a better understanding of each-other's potential and role. The general practitioner should always ask himself whether the nurse could not handle this or that particular situation better than himself. Cooperation between the general practitioner and the social worker represents a direct attack on the classical, exclusively biological way of thinking and functioning. The form of cooperation is a fundamental challenge to the physician. (Janssens, 1974)

There are a few exceptions; in 1974, the Christian 'sick funds' and the Scientific Society of Flemish General Practitioners (Wetenschoppelijke Vereniging der Vlaamse Huisartsen) started a feasibility study involving closer cooperation between social workers and general practitioners. Admittedly only seven doctors are involved at the moment but, if the scheme is successful, its influence will almost certainly spread.

Facilities

Some older doctors have their own simple X-ray equipment and laboratory facilities as a number of investigations are paid for by the insurance organisations. But the majority of doctors, and particularly the younger ones, do not feel that such a large capital outlay is reasonable, and they refer most radiological and pathological examinations to the nearest hospital. There is usually no waiting time for investigations although in some areas the facilities are not as satisfactory (for example if the hospital is some distance away) as the patient and general practitioner would like, and so, in this situation, diagnostic (pathology) centres have been set up and organised by groups of local practitioners. These centres have further improved the service both for patients and doctors.

Emergency work

Emergency work at night and at weekends is arranged in two ways. First, through a rota system agreed amongst doctors themselves, although this usually applies to weekends and holidays. Most doctors still prefer to do their own night work, as they fear competition from colleagues, and also that their colleagues' patients may not be as well disciplined as their own. Second, a patient may telephone '900', whereupon an ambulance is sent to collect the patient and transfer him to the nearest hospital.

Maternal and child health services

These services are entrusted to the Oeuvre Nationale de l'Enfance, a body set up under the Act of 5 September 1919 and financed by the Ministry of Public Health and Family Welfare. In 1971, there were 343 ante-natal clinics and 1167 infant welfare clinics staffed by public health nurses, midwives, gynaecologists, paediatricians and general practitioners working part-time.

Until about ten years ago the majority of ante-natal work was carried out by general practitioners who also confined the patient at home or in the local maternity clinic. But this is changing as most of the ante-natal clinics are now staffed by gynaecologists who not only supervise the woman's confinement but often try to continue her medical care throughout her pre-menopausal life.

Likewise the care of children – at least up to a year old – is being gradually taken over by paediatricians staffing the infant welfare clinics. The pattern of work for the general practitioner has certainly changed in recent years.

Hospital service and primary care

General practitioners have almost no influence on the hospital service and are totally excluded from it. As elsewhere, there is a feeling that this complete separation is to the benefit neither of the patient, the hospital service nor the general practitioner. But there are two main schools of thought about how this should be rectified. Some feel that the general practitioner should have access to hospital beds so that he can look after his own medical, geriatric and perhaps normal maternity cases, while others consider that he would be better employed if he worked in his local hospital in a consultative role, giving advice on the family and social background of the patients, and also acting as an 'interpreter' for the patient in the frightening *milieu* of a modern hospital. At the present time, neither possibility seems very likely.

The relationship between specialist and general practitioner is poor, particularly in a large town. If a patient sees a specialist without first being referred by the general practitioner, it is almost axiomatic that there will be no cooperation, and it is most unlikely that the patient will be sent back to the general practitioner for follow-up or continuing treatment. At the hospital level, the specialist complains that the general practitioner's letter is inadequate, while the general practitioner feels he is often 'kept in the dark' and denigrated by his hospital colleagues. The majority of specialists work both in hospital and as primary care physicians.

Clearly this situation needs to be improved, and this has begun in a number of centres where doctors are getting together for regular meetings, learning about each other's problems and benefiting from this experience.

Medical education and primary care

There are seven universities in Belgium, all of which have a faculty of medicine. There are the usual arguments about student selection, and the folly of persisting with selection based solely on examination results in physics, chemistry, mathematics and biology. As in most other countries, it is recognised that such a policy often ensures that pure science students become technically orientated doctors.

The medical course lasts seven years – three pre-clinical, four clinical. Only in two universities – Leuven, since 1968, and Antwerp, since 1972 – has there been any attempt to provide special training for general practice. In Antwerp this occurs throughout the clinical training, and students are attached for short periods to individual practitioners who supervise their day-to-day involvement with families in order to assess the effects of illness and social problems. Finally there are meetings specifically related to the problems of primary care. In Leuven the general practice involvement is restricted to the final year of training even after the internship year. By 1978 the teaching of general practice should have started in the remaining five universities: by 1980 it will be mandatory. The effect of this continuing contact with general practitioners will be watched with interest and hope in the years to come.

Vocational training has not yet started, although it is recognised that postgraduate training is necessary. A beginning has been made in a 100-hour additional training over a period of two years, which will qualify a doctor as a Certificated General Practitioner (Boelaert, 1976).

Personal assessment

The tradition of self-referral by patients to both specialists and general practitioners; the idea of wanting the security of a family doctor and yet never abiding by his advice, or being willing to accept his opinions; of playing one doctor off against another: such practices are the very essence of an inappropriate, ineffective, time-wasting and expensive way of organising primary care. It leads inevitably, particularly with an item-of-service method of payment, to over-investigation and over-treatment for often quite trivial complaints. Patients become confused, bewildered and insecure, while doctors become frustrated and angry about their inability to cope with the situation.

The development of group practice will take a long time to evolve for a variety of reasons: because of the pressures of competition, because the medical profession remains independent and reluctant to change, and because there is a financial disincentive to delegate work to nurses, health visitors and social workers. Certainly the team philosophy is really only a talking point as yet. Perhaps also doctors remain unconvinced that the quality of care will be improved by group practice as compared with the individual attention of a solo practitioner. On the other hand, partnerships are increasing slowly although definite figures are not available.

Is there anything, therefore, that might be done to improve the organisation and efficiency of general practice? The answer is yes: patients should receive a refund of fees from the insurance organisation only if the following conditions are fulfilled. First, patients must only attend a general practitioner in the first-contact situation, and charges for specialist care will be refunded only if the patient is referred initially by a general practitioner. This would be relatively simple to implement, as it is only an extension of the principle already in operation, where no payments are made for home visits by specialists. Such a measure would strengthen primary care and allow specialists to perform tasks for which they have been trained. Second, a patient must register with a general practitioner for at least a year in order to qualify for a refund. This would help to prevent the frequent and aimless changing of doctors, and at least produce some continuity of care and treatment (Denmark, p. 68).

The continuation of home visits by doctors is appreciated by patients. Again there are no exact figures, but a consultation: home-visit ratio of 2:1 is usually quoted. Patients and doctors appear to accept this as satisfactory within their system of primary care. A reasonable compromise has been reached since patients must pay considerably more for a home visit than a consultation while doctors are happy to carry out more visits than in many countries because they are financially rewarded.

DENMARK

Denmark is a small country with a population of 4 950 598 and has a constitutional monarchy and a one-chamber parliamentary system of government. It has a high standard of living, and its prosperity depends on well-organised and productive farming, fishing, some shipbuilding and a variety of minor industries. The population is fairly evenly spread, in spite of the increasing urbanisation and industrialisation which has taken people away from agriculture. It is estimated that between 1930 and 1960, the working population in urban areas increased by 50 per cent, while agricultural workers decreased by 26 per cent. Unlike many countries experiencing the same drift away from the countryside during the years 1960–75, the increased growth has not been concentrated in the capital, Copenhagen, but has taken place in the larger provincial towns, where there is easier access to space for one-storey factory building and parking space (Koch, 1974). Partly on account of this, maldistribution of doctors is no problem.

All the evidence points to a highly developed society with an excellent standard of living and a well-organised, successful health service. In all relevant health statistics – life expectancy and infant and maternal mortality – Denmark comes among the top four countries of the world. The main causes of death are heart disease, neoplasms, cerebrovascular disease and accidents, with respiratory problems much lower than in either the UK or the Republic of Ireland.

Health insurance

The provision of health care on an insurance basis was started in 1857, with the foundation of the first 'sick club'. Initially 'sick clubs' were private organisations, but by the end of the nineteenth century the government had started to supervise and register such funds. In 1961 there was a major reform of health and social insurance, to provide more uniformity in coverage and benefits. Basically, patients were divided into two groups according to their level of income. Group A type, with incomes below an agreed level, paid a fixed contribution which fully covered the cost of all medical care. In fact the level chosen was so high that 80 per cent of the population belonged to this group. The fees charged by doctors, dentists and paramedical workers (for example physiotherapists, speech therapists) were agreed by the insurance schemes and the health professions. There were certain stipulations for the patients. In order to receive the benefits of virtually free medical care, a patient must register with a general practitioner for at least a year, and payment for specialist consultations and treatment would be honoured only if he were referred initially by his general practitioner. Group B type members received full reimbursement for hospital treatment, but were under no obligation to register with a general practitioner for the period of one year. The price paid for this advantage was the fact that doctors need not abide by the agreed fees as negotiated for Group A, and the difference was paid by the patient: on average, the difference was between 25 and 40 per cent.

In April 1973, there was a further fundamental change in the organisation of health insurance. All contributions – both for employee and employer – ceased, and the health service became totally dependent on general taxation levied at the county level. Denmark is only the second country in the EEC (or Western Europe) to decide on this method of financing its health service. The entire population is now automatically insured for almost free health care at the time of use. In 1973, 80 per cent of the population were still in Group A according to their income level. Since April 1976 there has been freedom of choice for the patient between the two groups. It is extremely interesting to note that the majority of former Group B patients have chosen Group A status and accordingly have registered with a general practitioner: more than 90 per cent of the population are now covered by Group A status. All patients must still pay a percentage of the cost of prescribed drugs. There are now three categories – Group A contains all expensive drugs (i.e. antibiotics, cortico-steroids, anti-hypertensives, diuretics) with 75 per cent reimbursement; Group B with 'the less important drugs' (most tranquillisers, sedatives, sleeping tablets) with 50 per cent reimbursement and Group C, where the therapeutic effect is doubtful or non-existent, with no reimbursement at all (Fog, 1976). General practitioner remuneration is a combination of capitation fee and fee per item of service: in central Copenhagen they only receive a capitation fee.

General introduction

Cynics may well say that the success of the Danish Health Service and reasonable contentment of patients, doctors and other health workers is directly related to the fact that there is no ministry or department of health in the government.

> At the national level almost all the major ministries are concerned with some aspect of the public health service, so that none can be regarded as having general responsibility in matters of health, although the Ministry of the Interior is generally considered to be the supreme health authority. The Ministry of Social Affairs is responsible for the social security benefits, primary health care, care of the old, the mentally and physically disabled. The ministries dealing with health questions in their respective fields are Education, Agriculture, Housing and Finance. (WHO, 1975)

The national government has set up a central agency, totally independent of the government, to advise the government and county authorities on all health matters, particularly in relation to planning, organisation and the management of primary care and hospital services. It is also responsible for advising on the postgraduate training of doctors – both specialists and general practitioners – and for issuing full registration certificates for all doctors (and other health personnel). This body is known variously as the 'National Health Service of Denmark' or the 'Board of Health' and is staffed mainly by members of the medical, dental, nursing and pharmaceutical professions. It is of great interest that, by law, if any changes are planned at national government level, there is a statutory obligation to consult the Board of Health. There is a refreshing air about this situation, with at least an attempt to remove health care from party politics (although not, of course, from politics) as the national government, through the Ministry of the Interior, has the ultimate responsibility and right to decide what percentage of the GNP should be spent on health.

In 1970, there was a radical change in the organisation of local government. Prior to this date, Denmark was divided into 23 *amtskommuner* (or counties) and further subdivided into 1200 rural and 90 urban *kommuner* (or municipalities). This has now been reduced to 14 *amtskommuner* (with populations varying from 250 000 to 500 000) and 217 *kommuner* (with populations varying according to the rural or urban situation). Copenhagen and neighbouring Frederiksberg remain unchanged and continue to have special status. The responsibility for providing various aspects of the health service has been delegated to the *amtskommune* or the *kommune* level of government: for instance general and psychiatric hospitals and most public health and prophylactic services to the former and the provision of nurses and health visitors (particularly concerned with child health) to the latter. Institutions for mental defectives remain the responsibility of the national government until 1978 when the *amtskommuner* will take over.

General practitioners are also the responsibility of the *amtskommuner* but remain independent contractors. The contract is negotiated centrally between the Danish Medical Association and the Association of County Councils.

Primary medical care

The general practitioner is still the central figure in the provision and organisation of primary care, and is likely to remain so as long as payments for specialist services are only reimbursed to the patient provided he has been referred first by the general practitioner. There is considerable continuity of care as well, which is again related directly to the insurance regulations and rules of reimbursement.

In 1975, there were about 2600 general practitioners, with average lists of 2400 patients, and 3046 specialists. Since the Second World War, the increase in the number of hospital physicians has been greater than that of general practitioners. During the period 1956–70, there was a 75 per cent increase in all hospital doctors, while the number of general practitioners remained almost static. The reasons for this trend are well known, and are directly related to the problems of medical education (Conclusions, p. 362). It appears though, that since 1970/71 young doctors are showing more interest in general practice: whether this will continue or is merely a temporary phenomenon is uncertain.

The move away from single-handed practice (Table 4) has occurred in Denmark more than any other country in the EEC (except the UK). This has been particularly noticeable during the last ten years, and is associated partly with the building of purpose-built premises and the employment of nurses, secretaries and laboratory technicians. The actual number of district nurses and health visitors employed by the *kommuner* is uncertain. In 1975, more than 50 per cent were working in practices with two or more doctors (Fog, 1976).

TABLE 4 *Physicians in single-handed and partnership practice – comparison between 1968 and 1971*

	Single-handed	2 doctors	3 or more doctors
1968	67.8% (1369)	24.4% (492)	7.8% (158)
1971	61.5% (1256)	23.4% (478)	15.2% (311)

Source: Juel (1972)

Facilities

All general practitioners have open access at the local hospital to full diagnostic radiology and the complete spectrum of pathological investigations. The requests of specialist and general practitioner are treated alike, and no preference is shown to the hospital doctor. In Denmark, the oft-quoted figure of only 10–20 per cent of the population really requiring hospital and specialist treatment is in fact a reality, since general practitioners are given the facilities by which they can fully investigate and diagnose their patients' problems. In Copenhagen, a large central pathology laboratory (originally set up in 1932) is used by general practitioners in preference to neighbouring hospitals. The service is of the very highest quality, with emphasis being placed on organisation, so that a good service is provided both for the patient and doctor. It must be understood that, as there are no specialist out-patient departments in any hospitals, it is essential for general practitioners to have complete and open access to radiological and pathological services.

Workload

It is recognised that there are variations in workload between different doctors within the same partnership, not to mention doctors working in urban and rural areas, but a survey has shown that, on average, a physician has 37 patient contacts per day. Table 5 shows the place and mode of patient contact (Juel, 1972). The importance of the telephone consultation, which is strongly encouraged, can be readily seen.

It is interesting to note that, in a survey carried out in 1962, home visits accounted for 21 per cent of all patient contacts (Eimerl, 1967). This merely confirms that home visiting has declined in Denmark, as in most countries of the world.

TABLE 5   *Patient contacts*

Consultation in the surgery	62%
Telephone calls	32%
Home visits	6%

Source: Juel (1972)

Emergency care

This aspect of the service is a subject of some debate. General practitioners in the large towns have virtually opted out of night work, weekends and holidays, by availing themselves of a quite separate emergency deputising service, staffed mainly by junior hospital doctors. In Copenhagen the Laegevagt now provides a 24-hour emergency service.* By 1970, this had also spread to most towns with a population of 30 000 or more (Hornuil & Poulsen, 1971).

The use of such deputising services has increased since 1973, when health services financing by national insurance was replaced by general taxation and all charges were abolished. A disproportionate reliance on a deputising service or, to put it another way, the request for a large number of 'out of hours' visits, is often the result of inadequate or unavailable primary care. This would seem to be the case in Denmark where general practitioners carry out late afternoon or early evening

---

* Laegevagt is a 24-hour emergency service which is operated separately and is indepedent of both the hospital service and the general practitioners. It is similar to the emergency services found in large cities in the USSR.

consultation sessions only once per week. A further important factor is that some patients deliberately delay a request for a visit until the emergency service is in operation so that they can be guaranteed a home visit (Norway, p. 149; Sweden, p. 162). Most doctors working for deputising services are young hospital doctors, and they are paid for each visit they make, so there is a considerable vested interest in carrying out such a visit (Bentzen *et al.*, 1976).

In rural areas, emergency services are run on a mutually agreed rota basis between neighbouring practitioners, which is much more time-consuming and probably more stressful for the doctor, but undoubtedly appreciated by the patients.

Maternity and child health service

About 80 per cent of all confinements take place in hospital: almost 100 per cent in all large towns. Ante-natal care is provided by general practitioners and midwives working in cooperation and every expectant woman is entitled by law to receive at least three examinations by a doctor, and six by a midwife. Those births which take place at home are always attended by the midwife and by the doctor if any complications arise. Post-natal care is supervised both by the doctor and the midwife.

Children up to the age of one year receive three medical examinations, and thereafter one per year. These are carried out by the general practitioner who receives a fee for each examination. The public health nurse is very intimately connected with the overall care of young mothers and their babies, and this type of work – health education, general advice and reassurance – is increasing and being extended.

Hospital service and primary care

The great majority of hospitals are owned by the *amtskommuner* and they are licensed by the Ministry of the Interior. Only the University Hospital of Copenhagen is owned by the central government. Apart from emergency accident departments, which incidentally are allowed to refuse to see and treat non-emergency cases, general hospitals do not have out-patient departments. Private beds have virtually disappeared as there are now less than ten private hospitals in the country. Single rooms (amenity) are available for purely medical reasons. All doctors working in the hospital service are full-time and salaried.

General practitioners have no access to hospital beds to look after their own patients, nor are they involved in any hospital work. There is criticism between general practitioners and hospital doctors of poor-quality letters of referral by the general practitioner, and of unreasonably long delays with information about patients discharged from hospital.

Medical education and primary care

There are three medical schools at the universities of Copenhagen (founded 1479), Aarhus (1928) and Odense (1966). Any student who has finished the course of compulsory general education at a 'gymnasium' was until 1976 entitled to university education and about 10 per cent of the total university entrants chose medicine. There was therefore, no selection or limitation on the number of students (Italy, p. 110). But this policy eventually caused an overproduction of doctors with some unemployment, and so from 1976 *'numerus clausus'* has been introduced for entry into medicine with the aim of restricting the output of doctors to 600 per year at the most.

The aim of the medical curriculum is to train the student so that at the end of his six and a half year course he becomes a 'basic doctor'. During the undergraduate course, all three universities involve general practitioners in teaching students. The main emphasis is placed on a three- to four-week period working with a general practitioner, although there are formal lectures about available services (social and financial aids) provided in the community, which give an insight into the differing problems of primary care as compared with hospital medicine. The degree to which general practitioners are involved differs in the three universities, and unfortunately their participation is still limited and sporadic: the most in Copenhagen and the least in Odense (Bentzen, 1976). In 1977 a department of general practice was introduced into each university.

Following graduation, an obligatory minimum two years of training in medical, surgical, gynaecological and psychiatric hospital departments is required, plus one year in general practice in order to obtain full registration as a general practitioner (introduced by law on 1 January 1977). The average length of time spent in hospital before entering general practice is four to five years. In 1972, a 120-hour course (emphasising dermatology, ENT and paediatrics) was initiated to supplement the minimum three-year training before a doctor could enter general practice. The National Health Service of Denmark and the Danish Medical Association feels that this is not sufficient, but with the recent policy of unlimited medical graduates, there is considerable difficulty for young doctors in finding even the minimum postgraduate training.

Personal assessment

The Danish Health Service appears to be basically sound and effective. Patients, doctors and other health workers appear to be relatively satisfied, both as consumers and providers of the service. Conflicts between the government and the medical profession are kept within manageable proportions.* It is tempting to ascribe this comparative peace to the absence of party-political intervention, since the actual running of the service, as well as all organisation and planning, is in the hands of the independent National Health Service of Denmark to which parliament, by statute, must refer in all health matters. The wisdom of this interesting relationship is beyond dispute, and removes the health service from the party-political arena which is its fate in the UK. The organisation of primary care allows general practitioners to fulfil their true potential. As there are virtually no out-patient departments, general practitioners investigate their patients as fully as possible before referral to the hospital service: this gives considerable job satisfaction and benefits the patient by reducing unnecessary hospital admissions for investigation. One aspect about which there is some cause for concern is the organisation of the deputising service as doctors appear to feel little commitment beyond the normal

---

* On 1 December 1975, all general practitioners working outside Copenhagen resigned from the health service (Sygesikring). The fundamental issue at stake was the fact that, owing to the overproduction of doctors, the Sygesikring wanted to restrict the maximum practice size to a different level from that proposed by the general practitioners themselves. For years it had been realised by general practitioners that they must try to maintain a reasonably even distribution of doctors throughout the country, and it was felt that government intervention was unnecessary. In addition, the Sygesikring wanted to freeze doctors' income by extending their work (cooperation with social services and free family planning service) without any additional payments. The dispute has now been resolved so that general practitioners are paid for the family planning service, and a committee composed of doctors and health service officials has been set up to decide when a particular area of the county is 'saturated' with general practitioners. The strike ended on 31 March 1976 (Frølund, 1976).

8-hour day. Such services have been set up in most urban areas to cover the 'out of hours', weekends and public holidays. Doctors seem satisfied but what is less certain is the attitude of patients – whether they are happy with this arrangement, or whether they would prefer to be seen by their own doctor or one of a group whom they know. Certainly such deputising services, staffed not by experienced general practitioners, but by young inexperienced hospital doctors, are felt by some to be a complete negation of this important aspect of primary care and in the end are liable to be counterproductive by causing fragmentation and lack of continuity both for the patient and doctor. Particularly in Copenhagen, the emergency service has become a parallel system of primary care, and if this alternative is allowed to extend, the standard of general practice in Denmark will decline. The solution of this problem lies in the hands of patients, politicians and doctors, who must decide what type of service is required. (Conclusions, p. 370.)

FRANCE

France is one of the largest countries in Western Europe. She is a republic, with a presidential head of state, and has a two-chamber system of government – the Senate and the National Assembly, which is an elected body. Farming, forestry, viniculture and industry have enabled her to become one of the most prosperous nations in Europe, although this could never have been achieved without the leadership and resolution of the Fifth Republic.

The population is 51 million, and she has the lowest population density and the highest percentage over 65 years (13.4 per cent) in the EEC. Between 1964 and 1970, the birth rate fell from 18.1 to 16.7 per 1000, in 1971 it rose to 17.1, at which level it appears to have stabilised. In economic terms, the large number of old people who are unproductive, puts a strain on the social security and pension schemes. They also use the medical services to an even greater extent than the very young.

The mortality and morbidity statistics show a number of interesting features: industrial and road-traffic accidents are the third most important causes of death, while cirrhosis, almost certainly brought about by alcoholism, comes fourth. The implications of these statistics are being considered seriously in future health planning priority programmes.

Although there is one doctor per 730 inhabitants (which is higher than the Republic of Ireland, Luxemburg, the Netherlands, England,

Wales and Northern Ireland), the overall situation is very unsatisfactory, with tremendous variations in distribution between different parts of the country. 'In 1968, 12 per cent of doctors were practising in rural areas (34.6 per cent of the population) and 28 per cent in the Paris region (17 per cent of the population). These disparities are even greater in many specialties. In 1970, medical density was more than 120 doctors per 100 000 inhabitants in 6 regions (including Paris), 90 to 120 in 13 regions, and less than 90 in 3 regions.' (Cornillot & Bonamour, 1973). Or, to put it even more graphically, Paris has 367 doctors per 100 000 inhabitants, while provincial areas have only between 60 and 70.

The same problem of maldistribution arises with nurses and midwives, and although there is not an overall shortage, the situation is further complicated by the high proportion who leave nursing soon after completing their training.

Organisation of the medical profession

In 1945, the Conseil de l'Ordre des Médecins (Order of Doctors) was established, and it concerned itself with professional standards and the absolute inviolability of the independent French medical tradition. Until 1973 no doctor could practise in France unless he had a French medical qualification, was a French national and was a member of the Conseil de l'Ordre des Médicins.

Since then a doctor has been able to apply to a special commission which would scrutinise his credentials and give him a certificate to practise. It is estimated that 300–400 foreign nationals are now practising in France.

What is this unique French tradition? It encourages the 'liberal' system of practising medicine, the principles of which are embodied in the Code of the Medical Profession, drawn up by the Conseil de l'Ordre des Médecins. There are five principles: free choice of doctor by patient; the doctor's freedom to prescribe any treatment; direct payment of fees by the patient; professional secrecy; and the doctor's freedom to choose where he practises. How essential these principles are for a good standard of general practice remains a matter for debate.

Health insurance

Compared with other countries in the EEC, France was relatively slow to initiate any form of insurance against the cost of medical care: this comes as something of a surprise in view of the egalitarian principles of the French Revolution. Not until 1928 was any initiative taken in organising even limited coverage for the very poor. In 1945, all wage earners were included, and the coverage was further extended in 1967 to cover 70 per cent of the population under a general scheme of insurance. The present social security system is complex with variations in payments, coverage and benefits. There is no uniform plan, so that patients' contributions vary according to the category of worker (industrial, commercial or agricultural), and the degree of illness (acute, chronic or maternity) or the risk involved (whether prone to industrial accidents). Patients spend more on health care 'out of their own pockets' than in any other country in the EEC. 'It is estimated that, in 1965, 10 per cent of total expenditure by private individuals was on health care.' (Groot, 1972), and there is every reason to believe that it has continued to rise. By 1972, 27 per cent of heath expenditure, on average, came directly from the patient.

Patients may be insured in the following ways:

(*a*) Compulsory insurance through the general scheme (*régime général*) for about 70 per cent of the population, including all employees, pensioners, unemployed persons and their dependants. This has been the situation since 1966, when the self-employed were included.

(*b*) Special schemes for miners, agricultural workers, seamen, civil servants and railway employees – accounting for nearly 25 per cent of the population.

(*c*) Mutual Societies (private insurance) by which many people supplement their insurance. It is estimated that 30 million people (nearly 59 per cent of the population) are members of these private insurance organisations.

(*d*) Social aid programmes financed by central and local government. These support about 1 per cent of the population, enabling them to have completely free medical care.

Contributions to the general and special schemes are based on the same principle, and are graded according to earnings, with the employer paying 78 per cent and the employee 22 per cent. These contributions account for 63 per cent of health service financing. Central government pays less than 5 per cent (i.e. there is virtually no state subsidy), and therefore, in periods of high inflation and increasing medical costs, the contributions are constantly rising.

Approximately 99 per cent of the population are covered, and qualify for medical care provided they have been employed and insured for either 200 hours in the three months or 120 hours in the month prior to the onset of illness. There is no time limit on the benefits, provided the insurance is up to date.

The *régime général* is administered through the National Sickness Insurance Fund (La Caisse Nationale d'Assurance Maladie) which is under the supervision of the Ministry of Labour and Social Security. Doctors' fees in most countries are a matter for argument, and France is no exception. In 1971, the Act of 3 July was passed. This was an agreement between the medical profession and the National Sickness Insurance Fund, whereby an agreed tariff of fees was negotiated. After much discussion, most doctors accepted the negotiated fees and, 'by March 1972, out of 52 499 practising doctors, 50 315 (96 per cent) had accepted the convention'(Caylon, 1975).

Doctors working in primary care, are paid on an item-of-service basis. The patients pay directly and then claim a refund. Although there are slight differences, in general terms the patient must pay 20 per cent of all hospital costs for up to 30 days' in-patient treatment (thereafter all payments are waived), 25 per cent of general practition- ers' services and 30 per cent of most drugs (for certain expensive preparations, only 10 per cent). The general and special schemes will only reimburse the patient if he is attending a doctor who has already agreed to the *'tarif d'autorité'* and will therefore keep to the agreed schedule of fees. In addition, a proportion of doctors are considered to be so excellent and outstanding, either by way of qualification or general talent, that they are at liberty to charge even higher fees. The list of such doctors is organised and drawn up through a special commission composed of doctors and social security administrators. It is estimated that 17 per cent of all doctors are on this list, of whom 35 per cent are general practitioners and 65 per cent are specialists.

Primary medical care*

In 1975, approximately 70 000 physicians were on the official list of the Conseil de l'Ordre des Médecins; 50 000 were engaged in

* I was informed that there is a serious objection amongst many French doctors to the phrase 'primary medical care'. To them it is meaningless and it is even suggested that it cannot be translated into the French language! 'Everyone in France knows what general practice means and therefore it is unnecessary to introduce another term.' I feel that, to these doctors, primary medical care is a distortion of the concept of general practice and it dilutes and changes the

general practice and, of those, 27 500 were general practitioners working full-time, and 22 500 were specialists who, in addition, held either salaried (28 per cent) or private part-time appointments (35 per cent) in hospitals or clinics.

There is no registration of patients, although there is an unwritten loyalty between patient and doctor. Patients are free to choose their doctor – either specialist or general practitioner – and doctors are free to refuse patients. In theory and in reality, patients can 'shop around' and see as many doctors as they wish, even for one episode of illness, and can change their doctor as often as they like.

Between 80 and 90 per cent of doctors are in single-handed practice, often working from their private houses, with the help of a part-time secretary/nurse, who is often the doctor's wife. 'L'Association Syndicale Nationale des Médecins exerçant en Groupe' is trying to encourage partnership and group practice, which seems to be more popular, particularly amongst younger doctors, but there is little evidence to indicate whether or not patients are pressing for such changes. Originally group practice started in rural areas and small towns by providing better facilities which could be shared, and also by helping the doctor and his family to feel less professionally and geographically isolated. Recently an attempt has been made to interest general practitioners and specialists working in the larger cities, but it is too early to decide if these ideas will spread.

For the moment inflation and the very high cost of producing suitable accommodation have stopped the growth of group practice. In the Départment Seine et Marne there are 650 doctors of which 150 are working in groups. In France, as a whole, L'Association Syndicale Nationale des Médecins exerçant en Groupe estimate that 30 per cent are working in groups (Grunberg, 1976).

The ultimate aim is to provide adequate facilities in an area by: (*a*) ensuring a reasonable distribution of general practitioners throughout the country; (*b*) trying to persuade specialists to practise away from the large cities. It is felt and hoped that the stimulus of grouping and the expectation of good facilities may help with this problem. At the

doctor/patient relationship by introducing a different approach to health care usually involving cooperation with nurses, health visitors, midwives, social workers and other paramedical workers eventually leading to a 'team approach'. This is a complete anathema to the French tradition of medicine. The highly developed Industrial Health Service has likewise not been considered as French doctors do not consider it to be part of general practice.

present time, success is elusive as the maldistribution of both general practitioners and specialists continues.

It must be emphasised that the French idea of group practice does not involve increased cooperation between doctors and nurses, midwives, health visitors or social workers; only cooperation amongst doctors themselves. It is limited in concept and does not involve the team approach to general practice. It is intended to form multispecialty groups similar to those in the USA (p. 247).

The paramedical staff – receptionist, nurse, midwife – attached to any doctor depends on a number of factors: whether he is single-handed or in group practice, or whether he lives in town or country. Obviously the variations are considerable, but few doctors collaborate closely with nurses, health visitors and social workers employed through the local health services. Equipment in the consulting room also varies, depending on whether the doctor is a general practitioner or specialist (i.e. surgeon, internist, gynaecologist, ENT specialist, ophthalmologist) (Simon, 1975).

Information about the type and scope of work in primary care, including morbidity patterns, is very scanty, but two reports suggest that there is nothing unexpected or unusual in the general day-to-day problems presented to French general practitioners compared with their colleagues in the rest of the EEC (Jones, 1974; Wright, 1975). Home visiting is still very much more common than in most countries, and undoubtedly patients appreciate this aspect of medical care. It is estimated that for the whole of France, 40 per cent of a general practitioner's time is spent on home visits and this rises to 60 per cent in many rural areas.

Facilities

Both radiology and pathology are usually provided at the local hospital or private clinic, and occasionally in diagnostic centres. In isolated rural areas over the last few years, general practitioners have been installing simple X-ray equipment for skeletal and chest films. Referral to physiotherapists is a private arrangement with reimbursement to the patient of 65 per cent of the fees. There are 20 500 physiotherapists which is considerably more than in the UK (7687) with a similar population.

Emergency care

This varies a great deal. In towns doctors may be 'on call' individually, or have a 'gentlemen's agreement' with neighbouring doctors. Hospital emergency departments are widely used by patients, as well as direct assistance from the ambulance service. In isolated rural areas, doctors are on call for more hours than their urban counterparts but, in country towns, rota arrangements are the usual method.

There are no separate emergency call or deputising services for general practice as in Scandinavia and the UK.

Maternity and child care service

The government organises and finances the Protection Maternelle et Infantile (PMI), whose clinics are staffed by 7000 doctors, a number of whom are employed full-time, the rest being either part-time obstetricians or general practitioners. The maternal clinics, of which there are about 600, each cover a population of approximately 20 000, and provide free ante-natal supervision at the fourth, sixth, eighth and ninth months of pregnancy: in other words they are covered by the general and special insurance scheme. There is a 97 per cent hospital and private clinic confinement rate, with a maximum of 12 days' in-patient care and a post-natal examination, also covered by the insurance schemes.

Infant and child clinics each cover a population of 8000, and in 1972 there were 8000 infant welfare clinics and 2000 welfare clinics for children aged 3–5 years. These clinics are organised and run by *'puéricultrices'* or health visitors specialising in the problems of children, but it is stipulated that free examination by a doctor should take place on the eighth day, at nine months and at two years.

The recent concentration on maternal and child health has brought great benefits to the standard of care, and is one of the factors which has reduced the infant mortality rate from 29.2 per 1000 live births in 1957 to 16.0 per 1000 live births in 1972.

Hospital service and primary care

The French system is notable for the high percentage of private hospital and clinic beds: 33 per cent of general hospital beds, 10 per cent of psychiatric beds and 51 per cent of convalescent and chronic sick beds are privately owned; or, to put it another way, in 1968 private hospitals accounted for more than 28 per cent of the total capacity and more than 41 per cent of the number of admissions (Caylon, 1975).

A problem has been the rational integration of the public and private sectors in order to encourage the proper distribution of hospitals, as well as grading them to specific objectives, for example super-specialist, specialist and rural at regional, area and district levels. If this is not accomplished, the present unevenness in the hospital service will persist, with the consequent reduplication or gaps in the service.

In an effort to reform the situation, the Act of 31 December 1970 (Hospital Law) was passed. Its basic aim was to coordinate hospital planning, and to integrate the best of both the private and public sector ideas in any future plans. The initial emphasis has been placed on redressing the uneven distribution, both quantitatively and qualitatively, of all types of hospital. At present, those areas of the country with the highest standard of living have the best equipped and staffed hospitals: a situation familiar to most countries.

General practitioners use the hospital service for referral purposes (for example radiology and pathology) and to a more limited extent for out-patient referrals to specialists. These are kept to a minimum, as most investigations have already been carried out by either the general practitioner or specialist working in primary care. Urban general practitioners are allowed, but not encouraged, to visit their patients in hospital and, theoretically, to discuss the treatment with the appropriate specialist, but few avail themselves of this opportunity, partly due to lack of time, and partly because the relationship between specialist and general practitioner is far from satisfactory.

Rural hospitals, occasionally with as many as 100 beds, providing general medical, paediatric and obstetric care, are staffed on a part-time basis by local general practitioners, who are responsible for the daily management and care of patients. Surgical cases are not accepted. Usually these hospitals have radiological and pathological facilities, and in 1972 there were nearly 400 rural hospitals.

Medical education and primary care

Doctors undergo a six-year period of training at 24 university hospital centres in Paris and the provinces. Medical education has remained formal, stereotyped and almost entirely hospital-orientated. The undergraduate course has a two-year preclinical and a four-year clinical component. On qualification there is a compulsory one-year internship.

How involved are general practitioners in teaching, and how orientated is the medical curriculum to the particular problems and opportunities of primary care? The answer is not very much. So far only one university has incorporated general practitioners in their undergraduate teaching: the University of Bobigny, Paris, although a further four universities in Paris are making tentative experiments in incorporating general practitioners in the teaching of final-year students (Reynolds, 1976).

Postgraduate and continuing education are far from satisfactory and at present only the University of Nancy is involving general practitioners in these activities. For the most part they are confined to formal lectures and meetings, but so often it is difficult, almost impossible, for a single-handed doctor to find the time to attend. Of course there are some enthusiasts – perhaps 10–15 per cent – but even the conscientious physician finds it impossible to get a locum, and there is no incentive or encouragement for him to keep up to date.

Personal assessment

The 'liberal tradition' in medicine, with its insistence on allowing doctors to practise where they like, is directly responsible for the maldistribution and apparent shortage of doctors. Whether using specialists as first-contact doctors is a sound and efficient way to organise general practice, remains a matter for discussion (Conclusions, p. 372). The cherished ideal of the freedom to change doctors at the slightest pretext, or for no pretext at all, can lead to confusion and a feeling of frustration on the part of both doctor and patient. Doctors do not appear to recognise this as a problem, but rather as an essential part of a totally independent doctor/patient relationship.

The professional status and prestige of the general practitioner compared with his specialist colleague is poor. This is encouraged right from the undergraduate stage, and until there is a radical change in medical education, students are unlikely to believe otherwise. This idea is reinforced by the fact that specialists are able to charge higher fees than general practitioners, so it is hardly surprising that the number of specialists is steadily rising: from 33 per cent of 1966 to 42 per cent in 1969. How to alter this imbalance should be one of the main points for discussion over the next few years, but this will certainly never take place until general practice is fully integrated into the undergraduate curriculum and postgraduate training.

Rising costs in health care are common to all countries, but in France expenditure on drugs (excluding hospital treatment) has risen at a greater rate than other aspects of the health service. 'Between 1960 and 1970 expenditure on health increased by 10 per cent per annum. Expenditure on medical and nursing activities increased by only 6.5 per cent: hospital expenditure by only 9 per cent, whereas expenditure on drugs increased by 14.6 per cent. Thus the increased expenditure on drugs is one of the main factors in the general increase in medical expenditure! (Cornillot & Bonamour, 1973). The present arrangement of social security reimbursement of payments for drugs puts pressure on the primary care physician to prescribe the most expensive drugs, so that the patient receives 90 per cent reimbursement, instead of the usual 70 per cent for the normally listed preparations. It is anticipated that changes will have been introduced by 1978: the new rate of reimbursement being as little as 10 per cent for the cheaper drugs. In this way it is hoped to reduce the drug bill but, in fact, it may prove counter-productive and only increase the pressure on the general practitioner to prescribe expensive preparations.

Individuality in medical practice is highly prized, and the majority of the medical profession in France would insist that without it there can be no satisfaction or effective doctor/patient relationship. Furthermore, it would seem that most doctors maintain that only by safeguarding all the principles of 'liberal medicine' can the doctor/patient relationship be safeguarded, and that such medicine can only be practised in a 'free market' system. Many doctors would hotly contest this view, and, in France itself, some patients and politicians are beginning to have doubts.

General practice in France demonstrates very clearly one of the seemingly insoluble dilemmas facing medicine. Patients appreciate the personal and individual attention they are able to receive in those parts of the country which have an excess of doctors – Paris and many large towns – but what about those patients who, because of the maldistribution of doctors, do not receive such excellent care? Is 'liberal medicine' incompatible with the egalitarian principle in medicine?

THE FEDERAL REPUBLIC OF GERMANY

The remarkable post-war economic and political recovery of the Federal Republic of Germany is well known throughout the world. With a sound coal, iron and steel industry, with adequate farmland, with effective management and hard work it has become one of the most prosperous nations in the world. The population is 61 500 000, with 36.2 per cent either under the age of 15 years or over 65 years. As in all other industrialised countries, the proportion of the gross national product devoted to health care is rising steadily: 6.84 per cent in 1965, 7.64 per cent in 1970 and 8.09 per cent in 1972. The health statistics are unremarkable except for an infant mortality rate of 23.2 per 1000 live births (1971), which is higher than any other country in the EEC, except Italy.

In 1973, there were 125 000 doctors in the Federal Republic of Germany and the west zone of Berlin. Although the number of doctors in the last 15 years has increased each year by about 4000, the number of those working in primary care has remained almost constant (Waldman, 1973). Obviously the hospital service has benefited most from this tremendous output of doctors. In fact, between 1960 and 1970, there was an increase of 31 000 physicians, 68 per cent of whom were working in hospital. The situation is, therefore, serious if there is to be any hope of a rational approach to the organisation of primary care. In addition, although the number of primary care physicians (general practitioners and part-time specialists) has remained almost constant, the number of general practitioners (as opposed to specialists) has actually declined.

Health insurance

Germany was really the initiator of 'sick funds' to protect people against the cost of medical care. The original concept began in Prussia in 1854, even before the creation of the German State, but, in 1881, a Social Insurance Act was passed by the Bismarck administration, whereby there was compulsory insurance for low-paid industrial workers. By 1903, 10 million people were insured and gradually over the next seventy years the coverage has been extended until, by 1971, 88 per cent of the population were covered by compulsory health insurance (*Krankenkasse*).

Labour and social welfare is concerned with general health policy but the actual administration is the responsibility of the state (*Länder*) governments with the Ministry of Labour and Social Welfare. The day-to-day administration is organised through local Health Boards and it is at this level that the *Krankenkasse* is arranged. There are seven basic categories of compulsory health insurance (farmworkers, seamen, miners, white- and blue-collar workers, professional and general non-specific group) with 1850 separate sickness funds.

Of the remaining population, 10 per cent are involved in private insurance, and a small proportion of those insured through the *Krankenkasse* also insure privately in order to supplement their normal benefits. This only applies to the hospital service where such additional insurance will guarantee single- or two-bedded rooms. The social aid programme cares for the remaining 2 per cent, providing totally free medical care in hospital, general practice and with regard to drugs.

Contributions, which are paid by the employee (50 per cent) and employer (50 per cent), are graduated according to income. There are some variations, with employers in some circumstances (very low-paid workers) providing 100 per cent contributions, and since 1970 pensioners make no contribution at all. *Krankenkasse* receives almost no support from the *Länder* (or state) governments, and must therefore be self-sufficient. Such a statement is rather misleading for, although since 1972 all general practice, pharmaceutical services and certain hospital costs (food, medical care and staffing) are the responsibility of the *Krankenkasse*, all hospital capital costs (building and equipment) are provided by taxes from the federal and *Länder* governments. It is estimated that these investment costs amount to 15 per cent, so the *Krankenkasse* is responsible for the other 85 per cent of hospital expenditure.

Benefits consist of totally free general practice services and 20 per cent of the cost of drugs, up to a certain maximum. Pensioners, the chronic sick and those who have been sick for over six weeks pay nothing. Hospital costs are free up to a maximum of 78 weeks in any three-year period. Patients are free to choose any doctor, either general practitioner or specialist, provided he is registered as a 'sick fund' doctor (*Kassenarzt*).

The relationship between the *Krankenkasse* and the medical profession shows several interesting features. All doctors are members of general medical councils (*Ärztekammern*) with compulsory membership and contributions. They are organised on a state basis, and are responsible for professional standards, ethics, education and negotiating with the local 'sick funds'. Doctors apply to the 'sick fund' for membership of their 'panel': there are various stipulations and minimum requirements concerning vocational training before they are accepted by the 'sick fund' – in general 4–6 years' training (depending on the specialty) must have been completed. Payment of the doctor and the scale of fees allowed has often been the cause of considerable friction between the various *Krankenkassen*, the medical profession and the government. Each fund pays the local doctors' association a lump sum of money (determined locally and in a variety of ways) which is then distributed on a fee for item-of-service basis. This lump sum is negotiated every year. By 1969, 99 per cent of all doctors working outside hospital were registered with a panel.

The 'sick funds' have attempted, with only slight success, to control primary care physicians in a variety of ways. First, although a doctor is free to practise where he likes, he must first be accepted on the panel of the local 'sick fund', and if the area is over-doctored, in theory they can refuse to register him. Unfortunately from the patient's point of view, it would appear that this right is rarely applied, as can be seen from the fact that in 1970 Hamburg had 56 per cent above average, and Lower Saxony had 14 per cent below average distribution of doctors (Wolff, 1970). Second, any doctor who appears to be making too many claims or using too high a proportion of expensive drugs may be asked by the board of the panel to explain his actions. How often this happens is open to conjecture. Finally, the *Krankenkassen* tried an interesting scheme several years ago in an attempt to curb consumption. Patients were given a refund of money each quarter if they had not attended their local general practitioners during that time. The scheme quickly foundered, as it had no effect on the consultation rate.

Payment of doctors is on an item-of-service basis: all payments are arranged through the *Krankenkasse* and patients pay nothing directly to the doctor. Specialists are paid at a higher rate than general practitioners. At the present time a doctor will receive more money for giving an intravenous injection than for carrying out an examination or consultation or just giving advice (Häussler, 1973). The absurdity of this arrangement needs no further comment and is similar to the situation in Japan (p. 306).

Primary medical care

Primary care is still very much the province of single-handed doctors, both specialists and general practitioners. In 1970, the total number of physicians was 99 654 of which 43 876 (about 44 per cent) were involved in primary care. Of this 43 876, 66 per cent (28 958) were general practitioners and 34 per cent (14 918) were specialists. A further 6855 specialists, comprising the *élite* group of department chiefs (*Chefärzte*) work part-time as primary care physicians. It is estimated that 54 per cent of all specialists are involved in some form of primary care (Eichhorn, 1973), and that this percentage is rising.

There is no formal registration of patients, who tend, in any case, to keep to the same doctor, as one of the stipulations of the *Krankenkasse* is that, in order to qualify for reimbursement of medical fees, the patient must remain with the same doctor for a minimum of three months. Patients are free to choose any doctor, and they have direct access to specialists without any need for referral by the general practitioner.

Group practice has not really developed for a variety of reasons. Probably the main obstacle originated in restrictive regulations affecting the cooperation of doctors in private practice. It was not until 1969 that the Federal Medical Council (representing the *Länder Ärztekammern*), after constant pressure from the Hartmann and Marburger Bund (associations of leading physicians), finally agreed to abolish all such restrictions. At the moment, out of 51 000 primary care physicians, there are about 300 'communal practices' (*gemeinschafte Praxen*) which is a technical term to describe what is in fact a partnership between two doctors. In addition to these 'communal practices', there are about 30 'shared equipment practices', which involve 15–20 physicians collaborating in order to centralise diagnostic and therapeutic equipment. The new generation of primary care physicians has not shown any great enthusiasm for 'communal practices' and the position in 1976 remains much the same as in 1970 (Nusche, 1976).

Facilities

Doctors almost always practise from their private houses, and usually they have available all the necessary facilities for diagnosis and treatment: the amount of equipment depending on the local situation – urban or rural – and the ease of access to local hospitals. 'Most general practitioners possess their own X-ray equipment and have an ECG machine. From 1 January 1974, general practitioners and specialists have been subjected to quality controls of their laboratory tests and X-ray examinations, and in the future this will also apply to cytology examinations: if they fail these tests, they will lose the right to carry out these examinations in their own practices'. (Häussler, 1973) The capital expenditure is enormous, the duplication of equipment is wasteful and unnecessary, and the standard of reporting and the quality of work cannot compare with that provided by a specialist radiologist or pathologist. Practitioners in recent years have acknowledged these difficulties and, perhaps catalysed by rapidly rising costs, have embarked on forming their own local diagnostic and treatment centres (Japan, p. 312). This, of course, is a much more rational way to organise things and, in the long run, improves the quality of care and the standard of medical practice. Most large towns now have such centres, usually containing X-ray, pathology and physiotherapy departments.

To summarise, the team concept of care has not evolved to any great extent, and doctors continue to work individually, with secretarial/ nursing help in the consulting room but very little direct liaison with the district nurses or midwives.

Emergency care

To ensure that there is medical care at night and at weekend, emergency 'on call' rota systems exist. Every general practitioner who is on the panel of the local 'sick fund', is compelled to take part in such schemes, as this is part of the contract between doctor and 'sick fund'. The actual day-to-day rota of 'on call' arrangements is drawn up by the local medical councils (*Ärztekammern*).

Hospital service and primary care

The hospital service of the Federal Republic has a number of anachronisms and anomalies which have a direct bearing on general practitioners and the service that they can provide for their patients. With few exceptions, hospitals are not licensed institutions to treat out-patients. The present system whereby the work of the hospital is limited almost exclusively to in-patient diagnosis, treatment and care, has developed mainly out of the arrangements for financing the various stages of medical care.

(a) It results in excessive concentration of personnel and equipment both in hospital and in private practice. The joint use of hospital diagnostic and therapeutic resources for out-patients and in-patients would enable existing equipment to be paid for more quickly and new equipment to be obtained at shorter intervals without any increase in cost.

(b) Despite a shortage of hospital specialists, the services of those in private practice are commonly unavailable to the hospital. Yet with increasing specialisation, the number of patients referred to each specialist or super-specialist will become smaller. It is unreasonable to have two specialists working in proximity but separately, one in private practice and the other on the hospital staff. Furthermore, to obtain enough experience, each doctor should treat a large enough group of patients, and under present conditions this cannot be guaranteed.

(c) The separation of in-patients from patients not admitted to hospitals tends to increase the number of in-patients and extend their stay in hospital. At present patients must be admitted to hospital for diagnosis and treatment and put to bed, even where out-patient or semi-hospitalised treatment in day or night hospitals would suffice. (Eichhorn, 1973)

All doctors working in hospitals are on a salary except for the *Chefarzt* (4.4 per cent of the total) who is allowed and does accept private patients. Many full-time hospital doctors are dissatisfied with their situation – both financial, which lags behind private specialists, *Chefärzte* and general practitioners, and the fact that the *Chefarzt* has too much power and influence in the hospital service.

There is almost no opportunity for general practitioners to supervise or share in the care of their patients in hospital. This, of course, is not surprising when even the services of specialists working in the community (in primary care) are debarred from the hospital. This truly absurd position, with specialists working in parallel, also leads to a serious dilution of clinical experience. The isolation of the majority of hospitals from the needs of the community, the absolute and unreasonable power of the *Chefärzte* and the isolation of the general practitioners – all these things are certainly an obstacle to rational and economic health planning.

Medical education and primary care

There are 27 university faculties of medicine in the Federal Republic. The medical training lasts 5½ years, and is almost exclusively hospital-orientated and, as far as general practice is concerned, dominated by departments of internal medicine. After a trial period in 1968, clerkships in general practice have been made a compulsory part of the undergraduate curriculum; usually two 4-week periods. In 1972, the undergraduate curriculum included psychology, social science and psychosomatic medicine for the first time and by 1976/7 37 professors and lecturers in 19 of the faculties of medicine were involved in teaching general practice, although there are no independent departments of general practice.

After completion of the undergraduate course and a further one year's compulsory internship, a recognised vocational training scheme is being started for general practitioners. In order to become a general practitioner recognised by the *Krankenkasse*, it is necessary to complete a further four years' training: one year internal medicine, one year surgery and/or gynaecology, at least three months as an assistant to an approved general practitioner, and the rest of the time either in hospital or general practice according to choice. The Federal Republic of Germany, as much as any other country in the EEC, has tried to rectify the previously inadequate training of general practitioners. Improvements obviously could be made in the content of the vocational training schemes, but it would be unjust to minimise the efforts that are being made. One of the major difficulties is finding enough suitable training practices.

Continuing education is voluntary and is confined to lectures, meetings and hospital seminars.

Personal assessment

With the costs of health care rising as rapidly in the Federal Republic of Germany as anywhere in the Western World, anything which can help to remedy this situation should be looked at closely. In the field of primary care the cost of installing diagnostic facilities, particulary radiological equipment, and carrying out complex laboratory tests is, for individual doctors, of course, very high. The only way by which the physician can recoup this capital expenditure is to use the equipment and charge the patient: the more investigations which are carried out, the quicker the return on the original outlay. Inevitably over-investigation results, so that, until a more rational solution of organising the hospital service is found, the situation will remain unchanged. It is essential that all hospitals combine an in- and out-patient role. First from a cost/benefit point of view so that radiology and the automated facilities of the pathology laboratories can be used more intensively; this, in turn, will reduce the need for individual doctors or groups of doctors to provide their own facilities. Second, as an inevitable and necessary corollary of this integration, the specialists should be allowed to work in both the in- and out-patient departments of the hospital. This would provide continuity of care for the patient and satisfaction for the doctor; it would prevent the present position of two specialists working in parallel, one inside and the other outside the hospital, and it would strengthen the position of the general practitioner in his role as the main provider of primary care.

REPUBLIC OF IRELAND

In 1921, the Republic of Ireland gained independence from the United Kingdom of Great Britain following many hundreds of years of bad government, mismanagement and mistrust. The last census, in 1971, showed the population to be 2 978 000, but, on account of mass emigration over the past century and a persistently high birth rate, the percentage of the population in the working age group is small compared with other countries: or, to put it another way, there is a higher percentage of under 20s and over 65s (Table 6); this directly influences the demands and work patterns of any health service.

TABLE 6 *Age distribution in selected countries*

Country	Population in dependant age group (under 20s and over 65s) (%)
N. Ireland	51.1
USA	47.8
Netherlands	46.0
France	45.7
Scotland	45.7
England and Wales	43.2
Federal Republic of Germany	42.8
Sweden	41.6

Source: Consultation Council (1975)

Compared with other countries in the EEC, her *per capita* income is low and, if a high standard of living is assessed by the number of private cars or television sets per 1000 population, the Republic of Ireland comes bottom of the 'prosperity league'.

Emigration has affected Ireland over the last 150 years, principally due to lack of opportunity at home, although this is gradually slowing down with the increase in industrialisation over the last 25 years. Even so, it is estimated that nearly 30 per cent of the population is working in agriculture and, to a diminishing extent, in fishing. Southern Irishmen, not surprisingly, think very differently from their neighbours across the sea in many political and social matters, but few would disagree with the statement that the UK and the Republic of Ireland are united in rugby football, golf and clinical medicine! No two countries in the EEC are so closely linked in their attitudes to medical education, clinical teaching and the general ethics of medicine. But here the similarity ends, for in matters of organisation and the provision of health care the philosophies of the two countries are entirely different.

The health service for the poor originated in the late eighteenth and early nineteenth centuries. There were great variations in the standard of care, particularly in the more remote rural areas. Dispensaries for the poor were set up by voluntary effort and a 'dispensary doctor' was employed to look after as many as 20 000 people. He provided care for the poor without charge and was permitted to treat the remaining population privately.

To quote from a recent report:

> In 1838 in the face of a large and greatly impoverished population, the workhouse system was established by the government. It was a fundamental part of the original scheme that all care (food, shelter or medicine) required by the poor could only be obtained within the workhouse. Although there was a strong body of opinion that a well registered system of dispensaries should be incorporated into the poor law system, nothing was done until 1851, when the government established the dispensary scheme under the aegis of the local board of guardians who were already responsible for the operation of workhouses. The dispensary doctor was obliged to attend at designated times and to give medical care to any person presenting a ticket which was issued by the board of guardians. It was clear that, in rural Ireland in particular, the dispensing system met a pressing social need.

Payments received by the dispensary doctor, although small, supported him whilst he built up his private practice. While the dispensary system did not alter significantly during the early decades of this century, the authorities responsible for its administration changed with the coming of self government. With the passage of time there was a general acceptance too that the dispensary system itself required to be altered or abolished. In 1954, the issue of tickets was terminated and eligible persons were placed on a register and issued with medical cards. But while the standard of service given by dispensary doctors was recognised as being of a high order, the system still contained basic features which are not in harmony with the egalitarian principles on which modern social policies are based. (Consultative Council, 1975)

In 1972, the dispensary system was finally abolished, and the patients were given as wide a choice of doctors as practicable. By law there was to be no distinction between eligible and private patients, either in treatment or in the consulting room in which they were seen. In practical terms there was probably very little difference between the two systems, but it was an attempt to remove the stigma associated with the poor-law system implicit in the previous organisation.

Provision of health care

After independence, medical care was financed by local taxation, although in 1933 a novel idea with a truly Irish flavour was initiated: all profits from Irish horse-racing sweepstakes were diverted to help hospital capital expenditure, and this has remained to the present day. Over the years, the organisation of medical care has been transferred gradually from local government to health authorities, and financial responsibility is being taken over by central government. By 1970, direct taxation accounted for 56 per cent of the total cost of health care, and by 1972/3 this involvement had increased to 66 per cent, while local taxes accounted for 34 per cent. The intention to finance health care entirely by direct taxation, following the example of Denmark and the UK, has not been pursued. There are no accurate figures regarding private expenditure by patients on general practitioner services.

In 1957, the wealthier sections of the population were encouraged by the government to supplement their own modest coverage by contributions to the Voluntary Health Board. The main benefit from this insurance is to ensure total coverage for hospital care: by 1973, just over 500 000 people were contributing.

Since 1974, about 37 per cent of the population, made up of people in the lower income brackets, known as a 'full eligibility group', receive free medical care, both in hospital and general practice. They also receive free drugs.

The remaining 63 per cent are divided into the middle income or 'limited eligibility group' and the higher income group. The former consists of those whose income exceeds the 'full eligibility group' but is limited to small farmers and to insured workers whose income is under a certain level and to all insured manual workers irrespective of income. Self-employed persons (there is no compulsory insurance for this group) must give proof of their eligibility by presenting a certificate of income issued by the inspector of taxes. This group is now being identified precisely and its members are being issued with medical cards. They are entitled to free hospital treatment in the public wards, free radiology, pathology, out-patient specialist referrals and free maternity services. General practitioner services are not covered and payment is on a private basis. Patients are now being encouraged to insure with the Home Scheme provided through the Voluntary Health Board which covers general practitioner services. Patients avail themselves of this scheme in the cities and larger towns but not to any appreciable extent in rural areas. In addition, welfare services for children up to six years of age are also free for the 'limited eligibility group'.

The rest of the population (i.e. those above a certain income level) are in the higher income group and are responsible for the cost of all hospital (including maternity) and all general practitioner services including drugs. They may, and are encouraged to, insure themselves through private insurance to cover their maintenance and treatment in hospital. There is also an 'optional extra' for general practitioner services although this is not very satisfactory as the patient is responsible for between £80 and £100 per annum before a claim can be made.

General practitioners are paid by the local Health Board on an item-of-service basis for the 'full eligibility group'. Each doctor has to sign an agreement with the Board before he can treat such patients. The fees charged to the 'limited eligibility group' are on a higher scale and are a matter entirely between the doctor and patient.

The mentally ill (if under 16 years), and all patients with specific chronic diseases, receive drugs free of charge irrespective of income.

Furthermore, if a patient belongs to the 'limited eligibility group' and requires long-term drug therapy, part of this cost is defrayed by the health authorities if the cost per month is above a certain figure.

Primary medical care

The administration of health services was in the hands of 27 county councils until 1972. Following the Health Act 1970, which was implemented in 1972, responsibility for the general practitioner and hospital services came under the province of eight newly formed Health Boards, and at the same time the 600 remaining dispensary districts were abolished. It is probably more accurate to say that a change in attitude of mind was accomplished rather than any radical differences in general practice organisation. The intention was to take away the stigma of the poor-law system and to give the greatest possible choice of doctors and the least practicable distinction between the private and the eligible groups of patient. Partnerships are becoming much more popular and a few group practices are developing in the larger cities although accurate data are not available.

But general practitioners remain predominantly single-handed, often working with the minimum of receptionist and secretarial help. They frequently work from their private houses and have only the basic instruments for examination and diagnosis. The old dispensary premises may still be used provided there is no discrimination between private patients and those covered by medical cards. It is obligatory that they both use the same waiting and consulting rooms.

It was estimated in 1975 that there were 1460 general practitioners (O'Connor, 1975), giving an average list size of 2040. There is only registration of patients for the 'eligible groups', and the rest – the 'limited eligibility' and private – can consult and change their general practitioners as often as they wish. Specialists play no part in the provision of primary care, and consultation with a specialist can only take place after referral by a general practitioner. By 1978 the number of general practitioners looking after 'fully eligible' patients had risen to just under 1500 compared with 1000 in 1972. The considerable increase is due to several factors. First, as a direct result of the introduction of the general medical services scheme in 1972, the average general practitioner's income from 'fully eligible' (non-paying) patients has increased by 70 per cent. Before 1972, dispensary doctors received a salary irrespective of how many non-paying patients they were looking after. As a result, it was impossible to provide a good service, and consequently a number of patients sought private treatment. But the situation has now changed radically, so that many private doctors have been encouraged to take on 'fully eligible' patients, who in turn are no longer resorting to private medicine.

Public health nurses and social workers are employed by the local Health Boards and are not directly attached to local general practitioners, although part of their duties involves visiting and caring for patients on request by the general practitioner. In fact, in rural areas they cooperate very well and are 'attached' in everything but name. In the old dispensary system a resident midwife resided in each dispensary district. She was paid a state salary to attend 'poor-law' cases and was also allowed to have private patients. Now the public health nurse stands by for any emergency midwifery.

There are wide differences in the distribution of medical card holders (eligible groups) from 14.6 per cent in Dublin to 50.8 per cent in County Kerry, and an average for the whole country of 37 per cent. Inevitably, the number of private patients varies enormously with the greatest number in Dublin and the larger towns. A restriction of 2000 medical card holders is placed on any doctor, although, in extreme circumstances in isolated areas, this figure may be increased if no other doctor is available.

Type of work

First-contact care is provided both in the consulting room and by home visits. No definite figures are available, but the trend away from home visits is a fact of life, although to a lesser extent in rural areas. Curative medicine and immunisation procedures comprise a large part of the doctor's daily work, although increasingly he is being involved in the psychological and social problems of patients (Tables 7 and 8).

Diagnostic facilities

It is becoming increasingly recognised that if the general practitioner is to work to his full potential, then the undoubted difficulties associated particularly with radiology and physiotherapy must be solved. At the present time, access to radiology for a general practitioner is through the local hospital. As in the UK, it has been found that as soon as a radiology department becomes overloaded, it is the general practitioner service that is first contracted. General agreement has now been reached between Health Boards, hospitals and general practitioners that this should not happen. Furthermore, it has been stated that all practitioners should have direct access for all simple radiological procedures including contrast media examinations.

Pathological investigations do not present such problems and, with increasing automation, laboratories are able to carry on with an expanding workload. From the doctors' and patients' point of view, in rural areas the main difficulty is the actual transport of specimens to the nearest laboratory.

Physiotherapy is not usually available directly to general practitioners and can only be arranged after referral to a specialist colleague,

TABLE 7   *Consultation in 'average' general practice*

Classification	Percentage of total GP consultations
Communicable disease	3.0
Neoplasms	1.6
Allergic, endocrine, etc.	3.2
Disorders of blood etc.	2.5
Mental, psychiatric, etc.	8.4
Disorders of central nervous system	6.2
Disorders of circulatory system	10.5
Disorders of respiratory system	20.9
Disorders of digestive system	7.9
Disorders of genito-urinary system	4.8
Deliveries and complications	6.4
Disorders of skin	5.2
Disorders of bones and joints	6.9
Congenital malformations	0.2
Disorders of early infancy	0.2
Symptoms of ill-defined conditions	1.2
Accidents, etc.	5.8
Prophylactic	4.9
Administration	0.6

Source: Survey by the South of Ireland Faculty of the Royal College of General Practitioners (Recorder, John F. Gowen)

although in some areas it can be provided at the district hospital on request by the general practitioner (United Kingdom, p. 46).

Emergency care

This is still provided to a large extent by the general practitioner, who does all his own night work, but often has a rota arrangement with neighbouring doctors at weekends and on public holidays. Obviously, the more remote the area the less chance there is for such an arrangement. In some small country towns where there may be one or two partnerships, each practice arranges its own off-duty rota, including night work.

TABLE 8   *Persons consulting for chronic illness in a year in a hypothetical average practice of 2500*

Conditions	Consultations per 2500 patients
Chronic rheumatism	100
Rheumatoid arthritis	10
Osteoarthrosis of hips	5
Chronic mental illness	55
Chronic bronchitis	50
Anaemia	
Iron deficiency	40
Pernicious anaemia	3
Chronic heart failure	30
High blood pressure	25
Asthma	25
Peptic ulcer	25
Coronary artery disease	20
Cerebrovascular disease	15
Epilepsy	10
Diabetes	10
Parkinsonism	3
Multiple sclerosis	2
Chronic pyleonephritis	less than 1
Tuberculosis	less than 1

Source: Report from general practice No. 16. *Journal of Royal College of General Practitioners* 1973)

In Dublin, deputising services have grown up in recent years, closely followed by criticism from the patients and an uneasiness on the part of many doctors that perhaps they are 'opting out' of an important aspect of good general practice. It is assumed (perhaps incorrectly) that with the increasing growth of partnerships, the use of deputising services will diminish: certainly the evidence from the UK shows that the increase in partnerships does not necessarily in the end lessen the use made of deputising services (Consultative Council, 1973).

Maternal and child health service

There is a free maternity service for the 'full eligibility' and 'limited eligibility' groups. It provides routine ante-natal care and post-natal care up to six weeks after confinement, both by the general practitioner and midwife. Hospital treatment is free although some 'eligible' patients still prefer to pay for private hospital care. A percentage of confinements still take place at home, and without any charge.

There is a free infant and child welfare service, which was initially restricted to towns with a population of 3000 or more, but by 1975 it had been extended to cover the whole country. Basically this service is run by the public health nurses and general practitioners employed by the Health Board on a part-time basis.

Hospital service and primary care

The general hospital system is organised in three ways. First, hospitals are owned and organised by the eight Health Boards. The county hospital (there is one to each of the 26 counties) is equivalent to a 100–150-bedded general hospital containing medical, surgical and maternity services.

Second, there are voluntary hospitals – owned privately or by various religious orders – which are usually situated in large towns. A number of these larger, voluntary hospitals are associated with the three university centres of Dublin, Cork and Galway. Super-specialist services are provided by regional hospitals – one in each of the eight Health Board areas. At the community level, there are district or rural hospitals with 20–40 beds, providing non-specialised medical and maternity care. Each county has at least one of these hospitals, which are staffed by local general practitioners. In 1970, there were 58 rural hospitals with 2123 beds. The role of the district hospital has become more obscure over recent years. Originally they were intended to cater for minor surgical and acute medical cases but they now deal predominantly with geriatric and long-stay patients.

Thirdly, private hospitals and nursing homes, for the most part in cities and larger towns, provide services for patients in the top income group.

Medical education and primary care

'The principle that the object of the undergraduate curriculum is to produce a doctor equipped to undergo further training (vocational training) in his chosen field, and that it is not until that training is complete that he may be said to be fit to accept unsupervised responsibility for the care of patients is agreed. We are also convinced of the importance of lifelong, continuing education' – such is the recommendation of the Consultative Council on general medical practice.

There are five medical schools – Trinity College, Dublin, National University of Ireland with Colleges in Dublin, Cork and Galway, and the Royal College of Surgeons, Dublin. Cork has led the way in exposing students to general practice. Since the mid-1960s they have been attached to individual practitioners on a weekly basis and practitioners have been involved in lecturing at the university.

Formal vocational training was introduced in 1972 and a general practitioner was attached to the Department of Social Medicine in charge of both the student and vocational schemes. In 1976, another general practitioner was appointed to take complete charge of the vocational trainee scheme which was being run in association with the Royal College of General Practitioners.

Trinity College, Dublin, appointed a general practitioner as Professor of Social Medicine in the early 1970s, and undoubtedly his influence will be felt over the coming years in promoting the status of general practice, particularly at undergraduate level.

Continuing education, once the doctor is established, is by lectures and seminars attended on an entirely voluntary basis. Such courses are arranged mainly in Dublin and Cork, again in collaboration with the Royal College of General Practitioners.

Personal assessment

Medical care in the Republic of Ireland is in a state of flux after the changes of the last few years. Regarding general practice, there is a realisation that the Republic of Ireland cannot remain aloof and separate from the rapid changes which are affecting society itself. Furthermore, there is considerable discussion about such topics as: group and health centre practice; the practice team, with involvement of district nurse, health visitor and social workers; the improvement of practice premises and how this can be accomplished; and the relationship of the general practitioner and the hospital service. There is no lack of ideas or recommendations, but whether they will be implemented in the foreseeable future is doubtful.

Following the lead of Cork, students are now given the opportunity at fourth-year level to attend general practitioners for one week; often living in the doctor's home, especially in rural areas. This has proved increasingly popular with the students and it is hoped to extend the scheme even further.

Vocational training is beginning to expand: Galway has had a scheme in operation since 1975 and Dublin placed their first batch of vocational trainees in selected general practices in 1976. At present there is no intention of making vocational training compulsory before a doctor can enter general practice. For the moment, therefore, many young doctors will still continue to make their own arrangements in preparing themselves for general practice.

Immediate practical problems include the difficulty of providing medical care for some rural and remote areas: the use of paramedical staff or medical auxiliaries has not been considered as a means of solving this difficulty. Excessive consultation rates in some areas and the overburdening of hospital out-patient departments, brought about by the lack of diagnostic facilities available for general practitioners, are also a cause for concern. But, in spite of recognised deficiencies and acknowledged problems, the Republic of Ireland has a basically sound and strong base of general practice from which developments and improvements can take place.

ITALY

The peninsula of Italy, which together with Sicily and Sardinia makes up the Republic of Italy (since 1946), has a parliamentary system of government, the main feature of which, over the last thirty years, has been repeated unstable coalition governments with virtually no power to act decisively. More than any other country in the EEC there are extremes of poverty and wealth, and this situation is reflected in various health statistics. The problems have been identified, and in an official report of the WHO it is stated that 'the various plans for reorganisation of health services include the following provisions: establishment of a national health service to be financed through taxes, and the establishment of a network of local health units in charge of all health activities in a given territory' (WHO, 1975). Unfortunately, there seems little prospect of implementing these plans, and the situation is well summarised as follows:

> The Italian health care system is a heterogenous product of social, political, religious and economic forces. Historically, Italy has existed as a single entity for only a little over one hundred years. During this time her politicians have attempted, with some limited success in the period of rapid economic growth since the last war, to reduce inequality between the relatively affluent North and the relatively poor South. The divergences between the levels of economic development in these two areas continue to be large, and it is not without reason that, for instance, Naples is referred to as the 'Calcutta of Europe'. Many of the problems associated with this inequality are recognised by Italian politicians. However, by and large, they have been unable to adopt radical palliatives due to the basic weaknesses of post-war governments. This failure to reform can be seen clearly in the field of health care. (Maynard, 1975)

With a maternal mortality rate of 0.4 and an infant mortality rate of 27.0 per 1000 live births, Italy has the worst health statistics in the EEC (Table 1).* In fact of all the developed countries under consideration in this book, only Hungary has a worse infant mortality rate. The cause of this gloomy picture is as much concerned with poverty and poor housing as with a poorly organised health service. The argument which is so often put forward, particularly by doctors, that one of the essentials for improving health care is the provision of more doctors, is finally exploded by the situation in Italy: no country in the EEC has more doctors per 10 000 population (Table 2). It is also not without relevance that no country has fewer nurses per 10 000 population (Table 2).

Italy has a population of 55 million, with 97 000 practising doctors of whom it is estimated over 50 per cent work in the field of primary care.

---

* Improvements have been made and statistics for 1975 show a maternal mortality of 0.2 and infant mortality of 20.7 per 1000 live births (varying between 12.7 in Umbria and 30.0 in Campania).

How many are general practitioners and how many are specialists is not known, and some authorities would put the number of doctors involved in some form of first-contact care as high as 70 000: this would include many full-time, salaried hospital physicians as well as a percentage of doctors considered as true specialists.

Italy is divided into 20 regions with populations varying from 100 000 to 8 000 000. There are 94 provinces, and, until the reorganised health service is introduced, it is at the provincial level that all public health matters are administered. Below this there are 8900 municipalities which employ public health officers whose tasks correspond with those of other Western countries – sanitation, immunisation programmes and limited mother and child care clinics. The municipalities also employ 'municipal doctors' whose task is to care for the poor: estimated to be 4 per cent of the population (see below under primary medical care).

Health insurance

Most of the population must have compulsory sickness insurance which is provided by a wide variety of *mutua* or independent health insurance agencies. This provision was not started until the early 1940s, and remains unchanged in basic organisation at the present time, although the proportion of the population covered has been greatly increased. 'The Italian system of comprehensive sickness insurance is, like many of her institutions, very complex in nature. Indeed, some unkind observers might view its nature as chaotic rather than complex.' (Maynard, 1975)

The biggest sickness scheme is operated by the Istituto Nazionale Assicurazione Malattie (INAM) – started in 1943 and covering 53 per cent of the population (agricultural workers, blue- and white-collar workers, old age pensioners, orphans). Ente Nazionale Previdenza Assistenza Dipendenti Statali (ENPAS) and a number of other funds provide cover for a further 35 per cent of the population.* A further 4 per cent are catered for by about two hundred small agencies, so that in fact 92 per cent of the total population have some form of compulsory insurance, even though it may be far from totally comprehensive. The poor and unemployed, making up an additional 4 per cent, are provided with free health care both in hospital and in general practice.

---

* Public services: ENPDEDP, INADEL, ENPAM and a variety of further funds for self-employed farmers, artisans and traders.

It is impossible within the limitations of this book to give an accurate account of the financing and benefits provided because not only are there differences between the different agencies, but also differences within the same agency according to the category of the insured person. What follows broadly applies to the INAM. Contributions are graduated and predominantly paid by the employer – 98 per cent – and the benefits of free hospital care are valid for six months, while general practitioner services are provided free of charge, as are drugs on the presentation of a doctor's prescription. Until recently, ENPAS and other agencies did not provide such benefits, and the patient was responsible for 20 per cent of general practitioner fees and 25 per cent of all drugs. However, in 1976 all insurance agencies joined INAM in providing the same services; there followed a considerable increase in prescriptions and a tremendous rise in medical costs.

General practitioners are paid either by item of service or by capitation fee, or a mixture of both depending on the *mutua* and the part of the country involved. Specialists, working as primary care physicians, are paid an agreed fee worked out on a 'per hour' basis. All general practitioners and specialists are free to undertake private practice, although INAM does impose certain regulations on its full-time, salaried doctors regarding 'on-call' duties at weekends, and arranging satisfactory holiday rotas. Certain administrative duties, immunisation programmes and examinations of school children are also necessary but they rarely occupy more than 1–2 hours per day.

Primary medical care

The delivery of primary care is organised in a variety of ways.

1. General practitioners, specialists working part-time in hospital and specialists without hospital appointments, all work as primary care physicians. They are registered with any of the various insurance agencies (INAM, ENPAS, INADEL, ENPAM) and are free to accept or refuse patients who, in turn, can only register with a doctor employed by the agency to which they belong. If a patient decides to see another doctor with whom he is not registered, then he is treated on private basis.

Accurate figures are not available, but it is thought that nearly 55 000 doctors are working for INAM, the majority being general practitioners. Payment for general practitioners is either by item of service (in 50 per cent of the provinces), by capitation fee, or a combination of both, and is decided by the doctors in each area depending on a variety of factors – the number of doctors and of patients, and the standard of education of the patients (as it is felt that the higher the level of education, the less demands are made on the medical services). It is interesting to note that the average number of visits per patient per year is 15 when a fee for item of service is applicable, as against 8 when the capitation fee is in operation.

2. Municipal doctors – about 10 000 – are paid a small salary by the municipality to treat the poor and unemployed (4 per cent of the population). They work from *condotta medica* – consulting room, simple treatment room and sometimes a dental department. These doctors not only perform curative medicine, but are also responsible for immunisation programmes and the supervision of the local school health service. Working alongside these doctors there are 3000 nurses and midwives. This category of doctor is most important particularly in the poorest rural areas in the southern half of the country. They are able to supplement their income by registering with one of the insurance agencies and treating these patients in the usual way. Depending on the geographical situation and population density, some doctors provide 24-hour cover for six days per week, and for this extra duty they receive a free house or flat.

3. There are a few general practitioners and specialists who work entirely in the private sector: exact numbers are not known. Another group who work privately are university professors and other leading specialists in university or public hospitals who officially work on a full-time salaried basis. Their presence in the private sector is quietly connived at.

4. Primary care is also provided through hospital out-patient departments and *ambulatorii* (polyclinics) in the community (see below).

Facilities

Each insurance agency has built its own polyclinic or *ambulatorio*. In large cities they may cover a catchment area of 90 000: the staff and facilities depending on population size.

The largest contain all necessary specialists with appropriate radiology, pathology and physiotherapy departments. In rural areas they are less comprehensive with only the basic medical, paediatric, gynaecological and surgical departments.

Specialists are employed and paid on an hourly basis by the appropriate insurance agency; full-time university specialists are limited to a maximum of eight hours per week! They are paid at an even higher rate than ordinary specialists which, in any case, is high – it is worth noting that, in October 1976, 16 000 part-time specialists working for INAM were paid more than 55 000 full-time general practitioners!

If investigations or specialist opinions are necessary, then the patient is referred to the appropriate *ambulatorio*. But patients are also allowed direct access to certain specialists without referral (paediatricians, general and orthopaedic surgeons, gynaecologists, ENT specialists, ophthalmologists and dermatologists) and so this constitutes a further point of access for primary care. The same principles also apply to out-patient departments attached to the larger public hospitals. Private hospitals have no out-patient facilities.

The *ambulatorio* service has a number of defects, similar in fact to those of the USSR. Accurate data are not available, but it is estimated that 50 per cent of specialists have no hospital appointments. This has a number of predictable consequences; poor job satisfaction for the doctor in that he is unable to take full clinical charge should the patient require hospitalisation. This is unsatisfactory and time-consuming for the patient, especially as the initial investigations carried out in the *ambulatorio* are rarely acceptable to the hospital specialist. It is no wonder that the costs of investigation are excessively high.

Emergency care

This is arranged through the emergency departments of the public hospitals. There is little screening or referral by general practitioners. It is estimated that at least 30 per cent of patients should first have been seen by a general practitioner. The situation is even worse at night, at weekends and during holidays, when it is almost impossible to find or contact a doctor. Chaotic overcrowding of emergency departments inevitably results and the situation also leads to unnecessary admissions because of the poorly organised medical and nursing services in the community.

At the present time there is a trend for all major hospitals to develop medical and surgical emergency departments, including a number of beds for observation. If the diagnosis is in doubt, patients are kept here before referral to the appropriate specialist department. Unnecessary admissions often occur simply because there is no liaison with the general practitioner and it is impossible for the hospital to know the home circumstances of the patient.

As with out-patient departments, private hospitals provide no emergency care. The lack of cooperation and organisation between the public and private sector leads to enormous gaps in the service, and imposes impossible demands on public hospitals. This, of course, is to the advantage of private hospitals, for the greater the overcrowding, the lower the standard of care; and the longer the waiting time, the greater the demand for private treatment (Muri, 1976).

Maternal and child health services

These were under the supervision of the Ministry of Health and were directed by the 'Opera Nazionale Maternità ed Infanzia' and its services included 2000 child health and 1500 maternity clinics staffed by 300 full-time paediatricians, 1600 public health nurses, 2000 midwives and 3000 social workers. It had been felt for a number of years that the organisation was too centralised – all decisions came from Rome – and too inflexible.

Therefore, since the beginning of 1976, the work has been taken over by the 'municipalities' and at the same time an attempt has been made to reform the actual organisation. The intention is to establish a network of 'family clinics' centred on the old maternal and child health clinics, with much wider family-centred objectives – birth control, contraceptive advice, health education, child guidance and counselling. It is also hoped that decisions can be made locally to serve the needs of a particular community rather than directives descending from Rome.

Hospital service and primary care

The bed: population ratio in 1971 was 10.6 per 1000 population. This compares favourably with England and Wales (9.1 per 1000), France (10.5 per 1000), Denmark (9.0 per 1000) and Belgium (8.3 per 1000). But, in fact, such statistics are misleading because Italy exhibits the typical picture of any health service without any overall planning and with the minimum of cooperation between the public and private sector. At the present time maldistribution of beds is particularly noticeable between the north and the south, and in general there is little coordination in relation to size or function, resulting in the usual gaps and duplication of services. Needless to say, primary care cannot function effectively unless it is supported by well-organised hospital and specialist services. The government has no control over the private sector with its 100 000 beds (public sector 400 000 beds). Private hospitals are usually owned by various religious orders or by groups of doctors. Inevitably, acute, curative medicine wins the day, and the provision of beds for the necessary but less glamorous medicine, particularly geriatrics, is neglected and left for the public sector to provide.

General practitioners are not involved in public hospitals in any way.

Medical education and primary care

Italy has 27 university medical schools which 'have been declining in standard over the last 50 years owing to rigid curricula, a faulty recruiting system for professors and, above all, 20 years of intellectual segregation during the Fascist period followed by too much concern for economic reconstruction after the war' (Zanchetti, 1973).

During the 1960s, along with many countries in the Western World, there was considerable student unrest and dissatisfaction throughout the universities. This ferment, amongst other things, focused attention on the archaic methods of medical education and training: in fact the riots in Paris in 1968 were started by medical students who are not usually noted for their political agitation. In Italy, few disputed that there was a need for radical change, but what in fact emerged was a disaster, even worse than the situation it was trying to change. In 1968, it was decided to allow entry to universities for all students provided they had completed their secondary school course. Furthermore, any course could be chosen, and medicine proved to be the most popular. By 1975, 30 000 students were admitted to medical schools irrespective of ability or suitability. The situation became even more absurd when it was realised that there had been virtually no increase in the number of teachers or facilities. It was (and still is) freely admitted that there was no obligation for students to attend classes – in fact if they had done, the classes could not have been held! Clinical teaching was nothing more than a mockery so that it was possible, and frequently happened, that a student was able to pass through the system with almost no direct patient contact.

It is no surprise that there is no undergraduate introduction to general practice, no vocational training for general practice and very little postgraduate continuing education for the general practitioner.

Personal assessment

The problems underlying both primary care and the hospital service are the direct result of the poor, haphazard planning and an inability to build up a sound primary care sector. At the present time there is a very strong and growing opinion amongst the trade unions that it is necessary to find a different model of health care organisation. The Italian Medical Association and the majority of Italian doctors do not appear to understand the reality of the situation or, if they do, feel unable to deal with it. The political pressures for reform cannot be ignored and unless doctors act quickly and show that they intend to bring about changes, control of their own profession may be taken from them.

Changes have been forecast by the government, and by early 1978 all the health insurance agencies (INAM, ENPAS, etc.) had been dissolved and organised into one National Service (Health).

The intention is to eliminate inequalities between the various agencies and to provide a 'free at the time of use' service similar to the National Health Service in the UK. The service is to be financed by the central government through direct taxation while the administration is to be handed to the 20 regions. Theoretically, this reorganisation should simplify administration and render it less expensive. Whether the service to the patient will improve is far from certain, particularly as there has been no attempt to reorganise the present system of health care and there is no indication that enough money can be found by the government to finance such a service. To introduce a reform of health insurance without at the same time dealing with the deficiencies of both primary care and the hospital service is surely a recipe for even greater chaos. The government is attempting to introduce an element of control over the medical profession by forbidding salaried hospital doctors to practise private medicine and by insisting that all doctors working in the field of primary care provide some emergency care at night and at weekends. In addition, there are plans to rationalise and integrate the hospital out-patient and community *ambulatorio* services.

The status of general practitioners, both in the eyes of the patients and the medical profession itself, is poor. The remedy, involving major reforms in organisation and medical education, is unlikely to occur in the foreseeable future if left in the hands of the medical hierarchy and the universities. Recently groups of young doctors who favour a different approach to health care have started what is called the 'new model of medicine' involving the setting up of 'free clinics' as in the USA (p. 257) The example of these doctors naturally catalyses the discontent many people feel with the present situation, and influences their demands for change.

Whether the majority of the medical profession will continue to oppose the obvious improvements that are being attempted both in the hospital and primary care services, remains to be seen. Nobody knows if the trade unions and the Communist party are strong enough to force through their ideas on health care. But whatever happens, success probably depends on a sound economy and a stable political system. Italy has neither of these assets.

LUXEMBURG

The Grand Duchy of Luxemburg is the smallest country in the EEC, with a population of only 350 000. It is important industrially, particularly in relation to coal and steel. Facts and figures about its health service are almost non-existent, and even up-to-date information about organisation is lacking.

It has had a health insurance scheme since 1901 which has gradually extended, so that, by 1970, 98.9 per cent of the population were compulsorily covered. There are four main sickness funds – Workmen's National Insurance Fund (about 30 per cent), Sickness Funds for Employees (21 per cent), Wage Earners' Central Fund (about 19 per cent) and Employees' Central Funds (9 per cent).

Contributions are based on salary, but unlike any other scheme in the EEC, employees pay more than employers. Each scheme is different, but in general terms the employee pays 4 per cent and the employer 2 per cent. The overall state involvement or subsidy to the insurance schemes is small, being only 4.65 per cent of the total income.

Medical care is provided by the doctors who have an agreement with the various agencies. The benefits provided vary from one agency to another, but generally there is free treatment, both in hospital and general practice – at least for the first six months of illness. Thereafter, the differences depend on the scheme to which the patient belongs. Fees are paid directly by the patient, who then sends in a claim for the refund. Patients never pay more than 25 per cent of the cost of drugs, and very expensive ones are free. Patients are free to choose doctors.

Primary care is carried out by both general practitioners and specialists – usually in single-handed practice with the minimum of paramedical staff. Doctors are paid by capitation fee and item-of-service arrangement.

For the most part doctors are allowed to work in the nearest hospital, and are permitted to look after their own patients. There are no salaried physicians in the hospital service: in other words, most work at both primary and secondary care level. An exception to this rule will be the new hospital being built in the city of Luxemburg where all physicians will be salaried.

There are no medical schools in the country, all doctors being educated abroad. Vocational training for general practice does not exist and continuing education lacks any real organisation.

THE NETHERLANDS

The Netherlands has one of the oldest constitutional monarchies in Europe, and is well recognised for its stable parliamentary democracy. Since the Second World War, the standard of living has been rising steadily and this is reflected in the excellent health statistics. No country in the EEC has a better infant mortality rate (11.5 per 1000 live births), while the maternal mortality (0.1 per 1000 live births) is only equalled by Denmark. With a population of 13 600 000 (1975) the Netherlands has the highest population density in Europe, which so often is synonymous with poor infant and maternal health.

Medicine is still held in high esteem, with a strong tradition stretching back to medieval times. In 1975 there were 20 200 doctors of whom 33 per cent were specialists, 24 per cent were general practitioners and the remaining 43 per cent were either specialists or general practitioners in training or doctors working in public health. As in all countries under consideration, the problem of recruitment to general practice is unsolved, and in the decade from 1960 to 1970, the number of specialists increased by 1603, while the number of general practitioners remained unchanged. Since 1970, however, there has been an increase of general practitioners and it is expected that by 1985 either there will be an increase of 50 per cent in the total number of general practioners or there will be unemployment among young general practitioners (Van Es, 1976).

There is a relative shortage of nurses who average one per 400 population: only Italy and Luxemburg have less favourable figures than this.

The medical profession, whose Central College is organised through the Royal Netherlands' Medical Association (RNM Association), founded around 100 years ago, is responsible for the postgraduate training and registration of all specialists. Half the representatives of this Central College are elected by the RNM Association and half by the university faculties. The college is also responsible for maintaining professional standards. At present, 95 per cent of the Dutch physicians are members. The Ministry of Health and the Ministry of Education and Science have observers at the Central Board and therefore are able to keep a close watch on prevailing training programmes. All formal decisions need the consent of the Minister of Education and the Minister of Health. There is a strong Board of General Practitioners which is responsible for the compulsory postgraduate vocational training in general practice at the eight university medical schools. There is a similar arrangement for training in public health.

Health insurance

As in almost all EEC countries, the organisation of health care began in the middle or towards the end of the nineteenth century, and the first Act was passed in 1865, whereby the state was made responsible for certain aspects of public health. Very little progress was then made until 1913, when another law was passed: this did not involve insurance against medical expenses, but only cash benefits for being off work while ill. The complete separation of health care provision from sickness benefits is a feature of the Dutch system which has persisted to the present day.

In 1942, the Sickness Fund Insurance Act (Ziekenfondswet – ZFw) was made law, and this instituted compulsory health insurance for three categories of people: workers (and their dependants) earning less than an agreed minimum wage (50 per cent), old people (7 per cent) and persons who voluntarily subscribe to the scheme (11 per cent). At the present time there are 91 sickness funds operating under the ZFw, although there is now an increase in the fusion of these funds. The remaining 32 per cent of the population are able to insure with a wide variety of private insurance companies. In the ZFw scheme, contributions per month vary according to the category involved: in 1975, for workers it was 9.2 per cent of daily earnings up to a maximum level, and the employee and employer both paid 50 per cent; the contribution of the elderly depended entirely upon income.

Patients are free to register with a doctor who is listed with one of the sickness funds affiliated to the ZFw, and receive all general practitioner services free. Doctors receive a capitation fee and the patient is not involved in any financial transaction. Drugs are provided either by registered pharmacists, or in some rural areas doctors (1314 in 1975) are allowed to dispense drugs (similar to the situation in the UK). There is again no payment by the patient, the sickness funds being entirely responsible: the Netherlands is the only country in the EEC where drugs are totally free. All hospital care for ZFw members is also free.

It should be understood that the ZFw initially only provided care for comparatively short-term illness lasting under a year. Hence, in 1967, further legislation was passed in the form of the General Special Sickness Expenses Act (Algemene Wet Brjzondere Ziektakosten – AWBZ). This is compulsory insurance for the entire population, providing coverage for long-term illness only – i.e. anything over a year. At present, contribution to the AWBZ is 2.7 per cent of earnings, paid entirely by the employer. It does not provide for short term hospitalisation and general practitioner services for the 32 per cent of the population not covered by ZFw.

Neither the ZFw nor the AWBZ provide any cash benefits while the insured person is off work, these being provided by quite separate legislation: first the Sickness Act 1913 (Ziektewet – ZW) and then the Incapacity Insurance Act 1966 (Wet op Arbeidsongeschiktheidsverzekering – WAO) for long-term benefits lasting more than a year.

Historically, the state has always been involved as little as possible with health care, and even today this policy remains in force. However, owing to rising costs the government is preparing new legislation so that it will have a greater opportunity to influence the various organisations of health care. The private sector is also very strong, as 32 per cent of the population have no compulsory insurance. 'Out of pocket' fees paid by this higher income group through private insurance or direct to the doctor, are higher therefore than in any other comparable group in the EEC. But for the remaining 68 per cent there is, in effect, a totally free health service with no necessity to supplement their coverage by private insurance, thus still leaving France with the biggest private sector (p. 78).

Primary medical care

In 1975, there were 20 000 physicians in active practice, of whom 4809 were general practitioners. As in Denmark, patients in the ZFw scheme must register with a general practitioner who has been appointed by one of the sickness funds. The great majority of general practitioners are accepted by the ZFw scheme, so patients in effect have a free choice of doctor within a specific area. Only those doctors who are registered by the Registration Committee of the Board of General Practitioners are approved. All new general practitioners can be registered only after vocational training in general practice. A general practitioner will not be paid for more than 3000 patients on his list. In exceptional circumstances this proviso can be lifted, for example if there are not enough doctors working in a particular area. In reality the majority of general practitioners have more than 3000 ZFw patients on their lists. Doctors are paid by a capitation fee, agreed each year and geared to inflation and the cost of living, with additional payments for maternity work if a midwife is not available, and mileage allowance in a few remote rural areas. The capitation fee has two separate elements – a basic salary and an amount related to practice expenses: this latter element is not increased if the doctor has more than 1800 ZFw patients. This was intended to act as a disincentive to try to prevent doctors from having too many patients. In 1974, the average list was 2857, of whom 1937 were insured with a sickness fund. This figure is misleading and is due to the fact that it includes a number of elderly, married women and part-time doctors, who have very small lists.

In theory, members of a family can register with different doctors, but, in fact, this rarely happens. The concept of the family doctor or 'house doctor' as he is more familiarly known, is strong. By agreement with the various insurance organisations, patients are permitted to change doctors as frequently as they wish. Doctors themselves often display less loyalty to each other than their patients show to them!

Primary care is carried out only by general practitioners, and there is no direct access by patients to specialists (a similar situation to that in Denmark, the Republic of Ireland and the UK). The family doctor is, therefore, in a key position in the health service.

Single-handed practice remains the commonest method, although amongst the younger generation there is interest in partnership and group practice, as well as the team concept of delivering care. However, all single-handed general practitioners cooperate in some kind of mutual deputising during weekends and holidays. The scope and type of work is similar to that in Denmark, New Zealand and the UK. Home visiting is still very much a part of the doctor's life and is expected by patients, particularly the elderly. In addition to the general practitioner, the district nurse and social workers all contribute to the care of patients in their homes, but with little cooperation between these groups. In turn they are helped by the following socio/medical workers: the district nursing aide, the home help, chiropodist and sometimes the physiotherapist. It is interesting that the pastor and 'the friendly visitor' (a volunteer who literally does what the word implies), who are non-medical, also play an important role, particularly in the care of the elderly (van Zonneveld, 1975).

Health centres and group practice

In 1977, it was estimated that there were 34 group practices and 40 health centres involving about 280 general practitioners (van Aalderen, 1977), but the majority of doctors still work as solo practitioners. In relation to health centres, the attitudes of the patients are rather positive and the few studies which have been carried out show that patients appreciate the better organisation and administration and the 24-hour service. However, patients fear that there may be a less satisfactory doctor/patient relationship (Van Es, 1976). In the future, group and partnership practice are likely to increase at a faster rate than health centres because they provide doctors with an opportunity to organise their professional and family life more reasonably without committing themselves to any integration with nurses or social workers.

Facilities

There is direct access to the radiology and pathology departments of the nearest hospitals, as well as reasonably easy referral to out-patient clinics for specialist opinions. In the Netherlands, patients are not able to attend out-patient clinics without first consulting their general practitioner.

Emergency care

The general practitioners have no set working hours, but it is customary for them to remain on duty until 18.00 hours. Informal rotas are arranged among themselves to cover off-duty, holidays and weekends, when they either transfer their telephone calls to a colleague, making use of an 'Ansaphone', or continue to receive telephone calls, agreeing to see some patients, e.g. maternity or private cases, but advising others to ring up the duty doctor. (Hall, 1975)

In the Hague, a deputising service is organised entirely by the general practitioners and involves no junior hospital staff. There appears to be good cooperation between the duty doctor and the patient's general practitioner – either by letter or by telephone.

Maternity service

The Netherlands is unique amongst the 'advanced' countries of the world in encouraging home confinements although this is changing (Table 9). Many doctors and health planners insist that improving maternal and neonatal mortality and morbidity rates can only be accomplished by increasing the percentage of hospital confinements (Finland, p. 137). The Dutch experiences explode this idea with, in 1972, a maternal mortality of 0.1 per 1000 live births (bettered marginally by Finland (0.08), and equalled by Denmark, Sweden and Australia) and a neonatal mortality of 8.8 per 1000 live births (bettered only by Sweden).

Ante-natal care is provided either by the midwife or by the general practitioner or at a district maternity centre (189 in 1970) organised by voluntary bodies known as the Cross Organisations (religious and lay organisations). '53 per cent of babies are still delivered at home – though the proportion drops to 35 per cent in Amsterdam, Rotterdam and the Hague. The smaller the town, the larger the percentage of home deliveries undertaken by the family doctor. All home confinements are attended either by a general practitioner or a midwife.' (de Bruïne, 1973) Midwives attend just over 37 per cent and are quite unsupervised by the general practitioner (Table 9). They are self-employed and totally independent of the medical profession, so inevitably there is rivalry and competition between the midwives and general practitioners for maternity cases in the community. From Table 9 it can be seen that it is the general practitioner who is losing out to the specialist while the midwives' share remains the same. The fees for the services of the midwife are paid by the insurance agencies, but those of a general practitioner will only be paid if there is no midwife available. One of the reasons why home deliveries are so popular and successful is due to the additional assistance received by the patient from maternity helpers or 'aides'. These girls are employed by the various Cross Organisations, and are present at the confinement. They carry out nursing and general household duties for two weeks following delivery. Although their general level of secondary education may be rather poor, they are given a two-year training for this work. This is considered to be rather important so that when they marry or retire, because of this further education, they remain as a sound and helpful influence in the community particularly in relation to general health matters.

TABLE 9 *Analysis of deliveries in the Netherlands*

| | Deliveries (%) | |
	1961	1973
Hospital	28.8	47
Home	71.2	53
General practitioner	46.4	32.5
Gynaecologist	16.9	30.3
Midwife	36.6	37.2

Source: Huygen, F. J. A., *Journal of Royal College of General Practioners*, **26** (1976), 244–8

Midwives are at liberty to call in a general practitioner or to seek the help of a specialist obstetrician in the case of complications: in such circumstances the fees will be honoured by the insurance agencies. Hospital confinements account for 47 per cent of the total, and the cost must be borne by the patient unless she has been admitted for medical reasons: clearly this is an additional reason in favour of home confinements!

Child care

General paediatrician first-contact care is entirely the responsibility of general practitioners, but preventive work is organised by a number of private Cross Organisations: White/Yellow Cross (Catholic), Orange/Green (Protestant) and Green (non-denominational).

They are all partially subsidised by the state. These societies are arranged in different provinces according to their religious background, and are spread throughout the whole country although in some large cities the local councils provide their own clinics.

There are 2700 'well-baby clinics' for babies under a year old, and nearly 70 per cent of all babies attend. Most clinics are staffed by general practitioners and special clinic nurses who have an additional training in social medicine and the problems of young families. The main emphasis is on developmental paediatrics, with eight examinations in this first year, as well as routine immunisation and general advice.

Child (toddler) health clinics, of which there are 2400, are also concerned with twice-yearly examinations up to the age of four years, with particular emphasis on sight and hearing tests. General advice on parenthood and time to discuss the normal difficulties of family life are appreciated by most young mothers.

Hospital service and primary care

At the end of 1972 there were 255 hospitals with a total of 75 575 beds for curative medicine and 27 197 for psychiatric use, 24 609 for the mentally retarded and 37 477 in nursing homes for the chronic sick. Private, non-profit-making organisations, usually Catholic, but sometimes Protestant, are responsible for 160 hospitals and 86 per cent of all hospital beds are privately owned, although the proportions according to specialty are not available. The remainder are public, usually operated by the local authority, or university hospitals which are heavily subsidised by the central government.

Hospital beds are divided into four classes of care: Class 1, 2a, 2b and 3. Compulsory health insurance (ZFw) only covers Class 3, but it is possible for private patients to be admitted to Class 3 beds. The chronic sick are cared for in nursing homes which are frequently staffed by general practitioners.

A report representing the views of patients, specialists, general practitioners and a university department of general practice concludes:

> 1. The family doctor can fulfil an important role for his patients in hospital. This role arises from his position as a doctor to the family, and is complementary to the technical specialist's work in hospital. The family doctor can, therefore, bridge the gap between hospital and home, and between the patient and his family.

2. A strict referral and hospital admission policy by the family doctor has important consequences and gives him a key position in health care. He can promote the shift from hospital-centred care to domiciliary-centred care which is now generally considered to be necessary. It seems likely that such a strict referral system means a better quality of medical care for patients.

This is a priority of the first order, greater than that of perfecting hospital medical care which will require an ever-increasing effort and cost for a decreasing group of patients. (de Melker, 1974)

But in reality what is the actual situation? General practitioners have no clinical responsibility for treatment, and very few wish to have this made available to them. Less than a third visit their patients in hospital with any regularity (i.e. 3 times per month). Communication between hospital and family doctor is poor, and specialists working in urban areas feel that general practitioners have little to offer in the way of help. This is an all too familiar picture which will be difficult to remedy without a great change in attitude within the medical profession itself.

Medical education and primary care

Medical training is the sole responsibility of the eight universities and the medical faculties attached to them (six state, one Protestant and one Catholic). The Netherlands College of General Practitioners was founded in 1956 as an association of physicians committed to raising the standards of general practice (soon after the foundation of a similar college in the UK (p. 50). It has played an important role in initiating a renaissance of and interest in general practice, and was instrumental in setting up the Netherlands Institute of General Practice in 1965, whose aim is to promote the development of general practice. The first Director of the Institute became the first professor of general practice in the Netherlands at Utrecht University in 1966. All eight universities now have their own departments of general practice with seven full-time professors. Their main task is seen as introducing students to general practice and increasing its academic status.

All undergraduates now receive some teaching and practical experience of general practice which depends to a large extent on the enthusiasm of the local general practitioners and the quality of care in the neighbourhood surrounding the respective universities. The department of general practice in Utrecht has led the way so that all students receive regular teaching with general practitioners through-out their undergraduate career. The other universities have gradually followed suit, although the degree of involvement is varied and teaching takes place at different stages in the curriculum. Vocational training has been obligatory since 1973 and at the moment is limited to one year: six months with a general practitioner trainer and six months in an appropriate hospital post, although in some departments the hospital period is eliminated and the whole twelve months is spent in general practice. This training involves one 'returnday' every week to a department of general practice where the trainees are helped to evaluate their experiences and discuss problems. It is well recognised, particularly by doctors in the College and attached to the Institute of General Practice, that this is insufficient and it is hoped to extend the training for a further year in the near future. After this period of vocational training the doctor can be registered as a general practitioner and be accepted by the various insurance organisation associated with the ZFw.

Personal assessment
The place of the general practitioner in the organisation of the health service is completely secure: furthermore, few countries can claim such a sound basis from which further developments and improvements can take place. Patients, politicians and the majority of the medical profession are convinced that one doctor – the general practitioner or 'house doctor' – is needed to provide first-contact care in order to take into account the personal and family background of the patient thus facilitating the diagnosis and initiating the most appropriate treatment. Home visits are still an integral part of the doctor's everyday life although they are not as frequent as in neighbouring Belgium (p. 67). According to recent estimates (van Aalderen, 1976), in 1961 the ratio of visits to consultations was 1 to 2 while in 1976 it had fallen to 1 to 5 or 6 (a similar rate to the UK). For 70 per cent of the population under the ZFw scheme all primary care treatment is free, including drugs: the only country in the world which can make such a boast.

But some aspects of the service act against and reduce the possibilities of expansion of primary care. First, the majority of general practitioners have too many patients, usually over 2500, often more than 3000 (and this does not include private patients). As the majority are working in solo practice, without close ties to district nurses, health visitors or social workers, the only reason for such a situation must be financial. Second, there is no incentive to provide good premises and improve the practice organisation: an identical situation to the UK prior to 1966 (p. 37). At the present time there are no clear plans to deal with these problems. Third, cooperation and the idea of integrating as a team is only just beginning although, in special practices, it has been in operation for almost a decade. There is still suspicion between nurse, social worker and doctor, and, probably not without some justification, the fear of medical domination is real. But the university departments of general practice, and particularly students, appreciate the need for cooperation and change. Fourth, a great deal could be done to improve the organisation of home nursing. At the present time White/Yellow, Orange/Green and Green Cross Organisations act in isolation so that in any area, particularly in the large towns, nurses from each organisation may be visiting patients of many doctors in different parts of the town. This is obviously wasteful of time and energy and an inefficient way to organise the service. The situation is well understood and Amsterdam has made a start by amalgamating the three Cross organisations so that each nurse is attached to a particular doctor. The next logical step, of course, would be to persuade doctors to restrict their practice area likewise! Fifth, when group practice really begins to develop, it would be an advantage to the patient if specialists held out-patient clinics in the health centres. It would act as a continuing education both for the specialist and general practitioner as well as being more convenient for the patient.

Note: In connection with the different methods of health insurance, I wish to acknowledge the very considerable help and information gathered from Maynard (1975).

5

SCANDINAVIA

The Scandinavian or Nordic countries consist of Denmark, Finland, Iceland, Norway, Sweden, the Faroe Islands and Greenland. Only Finland, Norway and Sweden will be considered in this chapter (for Denmark, see p. 67). These three countries have certain common characteristics: a high material standard of living, with relatively good housing conditions, freedom from serious environmental pollution and excellent recreational activities within easy reach of most of the people.

The population is divided into a number of differing ethnic groups, those of Norway and Sweden being very similar. The origins of the Finnish people remain obscure, and they exhibit a number of interesting and differing gene patterns which perhaps explains in part the abnormally high incidence of such conditions as coronary artery disease in certain parts of the country, the almost complete absence of phenylketonuria and the low incidence of the Rh negative blood group. The Lapps do not 'fit in' with any other European race, but the population in the northern parts of Norway, Sweden and Finland have certain genetic characteristics which have been influenced by the Lapps, who were originally nomadic.

Depopulation of rural areas and increasing urbanisation is a part of life in Scandinavia just as much as it is elsewhere in the world, although these effects are not as apparent in Scandinavia, which remains one of the least overcrowded regions of the developed world. Governments and health authorities have had an important role to play in ensuring that a balance is maintained between ecological and industrial pressures, as Scandinavia could well become the last bastion in Europe of developed countries which have not been ravaged by the problems of excessive urbanisation, overcrowding and industrial advances. In 1976, it was estimated that between 60 and 70 per cent of the population lived in Oslo, Bergen, Trondheim and the coastline of the Oslo Fjord; Stockholm, Uppsala, Malmö and along the Swedish coastline to the Norwegian border; Helsinki and its environs and the southern coastal belt of Finland.

The birth rates are low compared with other developed countries (Table 1) and with 'liberal' abortion laws this has produced an ageing population over the last twenty years (Table 2), which is relevant to the needs and demands of both the hospital and primary care services.

TABLE 1   *Birth rates per 1000 population, 1972*

Finland	Norway	Sweden	New Zealand	Canada	France	Republic of Ireland
12.74	10.30	13.82	21.90	15.90	16.90	22.40

Source: *Fifth Report on the World Health Situation, 1969–72*. Geneva, 1975

TABLE 2   *Population aged 65 years or more as percentage of whole population*

Country	1950	1970
Finland	6.3	10.1
Norway	9.7	11.4
Sweden	10.3	14.7

Source: Lääkintöhallitus Medicindstryrelsen (National Board of Health) Aupha Institute, Helsinki, 1975

The maternal and infant mortality rates are among the best in the world (Table 3), while in life expectancy, Norway and Sweden are again at the top of the 'health league'. The situation in Finland is less good, but the reasons for this are not clear.

Such excellent results are, of course, as much a reflection on an excellent standard of living as on the standard of health care, although for many years priority has been focused on maternal and child health services. As in other developed countries, the main causes of death are heart disease, malignant neoplasms, cerebrovascular diseases, accidents and respiratory diseases. The high incidence of heart disease in certain areas of Finland and in the Finnmark region of Norway is well known and is being studied.

TABLE 3 *Health indices*

	Infant mortality (per 1000 live births)	Maternal mortality (per 1000 live births)	Life expectancy M	F
Finland	11.27	0.08 (1971)	65.80	72.80
Norway	11.30	0.20 (1971)	71.40	77.60
Sweden	10.80	0.10	72.10	77.10

Source: *Fifth Report on the World Health Situation 1969–72*; these figures are for 1972

In Sweden, until the election of September 1976, there has been a long tradition of almost 50 years of Social Democratic government, while in Finland and Norway during the last 10 years the Social Democrats have always been a part of successive coalition cabinets. In all three countries, supported by the trade unions and Communists, the governments have had the overall support of the majority of the population for an egalitarian-type society with high rates of taxation and great expenditure on health and social services (Table 4).

It is accepted in all three countries that health care is the natural right of the whole population and that it is the duty of society (or the state) to provide and organise such health services. From Table 5 it can be appreciated that finance is produced from four different sources and the proportions in each country vary considerably.

The steeply rising cost of health care – particularly in Sweden – is a cause for great concern amongst the politicians, patients and doctors. Questions are being asked about the rationale of a health policy which has overemphasised the hospital services and technological medicine *vis-à-vis* medicine in the community. The folly of such action is most graphically seen in Sweden and will be considered later in the chapter.

TABLE 4 *Percentage of GNP spent on health and social services*

		1950	1960	1970
Finland	Health	1.5	2.4	5.0
	Social	7.4	8.3	13.0
	Total	8.9	10.7	18.0
Norway	Health	2.9	4.5	6.5
	Social	4.7	8.3	12.5
	Total	7.6	12.8	19.0
Sweden	Health	2.4	4.2	8.3
	Social	6.5	7.3	11.3
	Total	8.9	11.5	19.6

Source: Statistics about social expenditure in Northern countries. *Stat. Serv.*, 1950, 1960, 1970. Aupha Institute, Helsinki

TABLE 5 *Financing of health care in 1970: as percentage distribution*

	Central government	Local government	Employer	Insured[a]
Finland	41.2	31.7	13.3	13.8
Norway	22.1	31.5	17.2	29.2
Sweden	18.6	51.0	17.4	13.0

[a] Includes some direct payments from patients
Source: *Nordisk Medicin*, **89** (1974), 212–13

For the last twenty years Nordic countries have had a large number of hospital beds compared with other developed countries, and the situation in 1971 is shown in Table 6. Certainly there is now a realisation that the building of further acute hospitals must stop, as they are unnecessary and too expensive to build, staff and run. A consensus of opinion is also developing which feels that such hospital building that does take place should be directed almost exclusively towards the chronic long-term geriatric patient – certainly for the next decade or two.

Nordic countries state that they are short of doctors – but short in comparison with whom? It would seem that Norway and Sweden are slightly better off compared with Western Europe, and all three countries are worse off compared with Eastern Europe (Table 7).

TABLE 6 *Number of hospital beds (acute, general psychiatric and chronic) per thousand of the population*

Country	Hospital beds per 1000 population	Country	Hospital beds per 1000 population	Country	Hospital beds per 1000 population
Finland	16.2	Australia	12.4	Republic of Ireland	11.9
Norway	15.1	Canada	9.4	Italy	10.6
Sweden	16.9	France	10.5	N. Zealand	10.1

Source: *Fifth Report on the World Health Situation, 1969–72*. Geneva, 1975

TABLE 7 *Distribution of doctors*

Country	Habitants per doctor				(Projected)
	1960	1968	1971	1973	1980
Finland	1536	1080	849	876	490
Norway	900	740	690	670	570
Sweden	1060	800	700	625	415
France	964	807	730		
England and Wales	870	850	790		
Netherlands	842 (1959)	850 (1967)	760		
Czechoslovakia	571	510 (1967)	461 (1972)		
Bulgaria		570 (1967)	530		
Poland	1080	740 (1967)	640 (1972)		

Source: *World Health Situation*: 3rd, 4th and 5th reports. Geneva

It is impossible to assess the needs of primary care realistically without some reference to the nursing situation, and in this Scandinavia is well placed among developed countries (Table 8), only New Zealand having a greater proportion of nursing personnel.

So how valid is the belief that Finland, Norway and Sweden are short of doctors (and nurses)? Certainly on face value there is very little to support this view, but it will be seen later when dealing with the countries individually that *although there is no shortage of doctors, there is a shortage of man-hours worked by doctors*, either because each country is committed to a 37–40 hour week and there is an increasing reluctance on the part of doctors to work overtime, or because a large proportion of general practitioners only work part-time.

TABLE 8 *Distribution of nurses, 1971*

Country	Habitants per nurse	Country	Habitants per nurse	Country	Habitants per nurse
Finland	**170**	France	340	Australia	1030
Norway	**200**	England & Wales	300	N. Zealand	130
Sweden	**180**	Netherlands	400	Italy	420
		USA	620	Canada	670

Based on: *Fifth Report on the World Health Situation, 1969–72*. Geneva, 1975

FINLAND

For centuries Finland was part of Sweden, which gradually became weaker during the eighteenth century and was unable to protect Finland against her neighbour in the east. Finally, at the beginning of the nineteenth century, Sweden gave up Finland to Russia, and she remained part of the Russian Empire until the revolution of 1917. In 1919, by virtue of her newly proclaimed constitution, Finland became a sovereign republic. Although she is now a totally independent country, the influence of both her neighbours remains in many fields, and certainly in health care.

General introduction

Finland has a population of 4 634 000, and at the present time two languages are spoken: Finnish by 90 per cent and Swedish by 10 per cent of the population. The country is divided into 11 provinces and 470 communes. The people are represented in parliament by 200 deputies elected for four years. The head of state is the President of the Republic, who has the right to dissolve parliament. A particular and important feature of Finnish administration is that policy is decided centrally by the government, but the implementation of this policy is the direct responsibility of the local commune. This tradition applies to health, education and social policies in particular, and is a most highly cherished part of Finnish political life. Taxes are levied by the central government and at the commune level, while the provincial governments have no taxation rights. Thus the provincial government, which is not elected, is relatively weak and is mainly concerned with administration, acting as a full-time civil service. This principle of the decentralisation of the implementation of policies approved by parliament means that the representatives of the commune (elected every four years by proportional representation) have considerable responsibility in the field of health, social welfare and education.

Health policy is decided by the Cabinet and implemented at the Board of Health in Helsinki which is part of the Ministry of Social Affairs and Health. This policy, which is now produced on a regular five-year planning basis, must be approved by parliament, and it is then the responsibility of the commune to implement it to suit the needs of the local community. The commune is responsible for both hospital (excluding university, psychiatric and tuberculosis) and primary care services. Now obviously some communes are too small and poor to be a viable entity, so in such cases two or three may combine. Altogether there are about 210 health care areas. Equality of facilities and services throughout the country is another much valued ideal, and to fulfil this concept the poorer health care areas are subsidised by the central government on an agreed sliding scale, the current scale varying between 39 per cent in Helsinki and the surrounding areas to 70 per cent in Lapland. From Table 5 it can be seen that over 70 per cent of health care finance comes from a combination of central and local taxation.

Unlike most countries considered in this book, the importance attached to primary care is a reality and not an idle promise, as can be seen from the expenditure on medical care (Table 9) and the creation of new posts in the hospital and primary care service (Table 10).

The figures given in Table 9 only refer to central government financing, but there is no reason to suppose that the contribution from local government and other sources will differ from previous proportions.

It is important to note that by 1979 the capital investment in primary care will far outstrip that spent on hospitals. What other country can make such a claim?

As in the rest of Scandinavia, the district medical officer, incorporating the function of a general practitioner and public health officer, has been part of the medical scene in Finland for over two centuries. Medical training was started at the university of Turku around 1662, and by the beginning of the nineteenth century the regional development of hospitals was appearing. During the early part of the twentieth century, smaller 'cottage hospitals' were built to serve the needs of more isolated communities. But, in spite of this interest in matters of health, Finland was surprisingly slow in introducing any form of health insurance.

TABLE 9 *Expenditure on hospitals and primary care*

| | | Expenditure (Millions of F marks) | | | | | |
		1975	1976	1977	1978	1979	1980
Hospitals	Investment	160.5	130	100	75	85	110
	Running cost	1244	1440	1450	1500	1550	1600
	Total	1404.5	1570	1550	1575	1635	1710
Primary care	Investment	80	100	140	170	180	180
	Running cost	475	525	575	640	700	750
	Total	555	625	715	810	880	930

Source: Lääkintöhallitus Medicindstryrelsen (National Board of Health), Aupha Institute, Helsinki, 1975
Note. Costs are in 1975 money value: Exchange rate 1 US $ to 3.55 F marks.

TABLE 10 *Number of new posts in primary care (P) and hospital service (H) between 1975 and 1979*

| | 1975 | | 1976 | | 1977 | | 1978 | | 1979 | |
	P	H	P	H	P	H	P	H	P	H
Physicians	140	120	160	120	210	140	300	150	300	160
Community nurses	300	0	300	0	300	0	300	0	300	0
Hospital nurses	300	700	320	700	335	700	335	700	335	700
Laboratory nurses	70	50	70	50	70	100	70	100	70	100
X-ray nurses	60	40	70	40	70	60	80	60	40	60
Physiotherapists	60	40	80	40	80	40	80	40	80	40

Source: Lääkintöhallitus Medicindstryrelsen (National Board of Health), Aupha Institute, Helsinki, 1975

Health insurance

It was not until 1964 that the Sickness Insurance Act was passed. The whole population was covered, and contributions are paid equally by employee and employer on a graduated scale according to income. Sickness benefits during illness or accident are provided, and there is a percentage reimbursement of the cost of medical care. In 1976, patients were responsible for 40 per cent of doctors' fees, about 25 per cent of the charges for laboratory and radiological examinations and physiotherapy treatment and 50 per cent of the cost of drugs on a general list (but for those on a special list there is no charge). The sickness insurance agency fixes the fees in agreement with the Finnish Medical Association, and reimburses the doctors with the remainder of the fee. In recent years agreement has not always been easy to accomplish.

Doctors working in the hospital service are salaried, having been so for many years and, since 1972, doctors working in health stations are also salaried. All doctors work a 37-hour week. For the patient, there is a fixed charge of 10 F marks per day hospital care (the actual cost is around 200 F marks per day), 8 F marks per out-patient attendance, and 3 F marks per consultation in a health station, including all X-ray, laboratory and physiotherapy referrals.* Following an act of parliament in 1972, it is the intention that by 1979 all primary care facilities should be completely free, so that the only remaining cost to the patient will be a 'board and lodging' charge on admission to hospital.

It is important, therefore, to understand that health insurance, although a compulsory state requirement, is not involved in hospital or in out-patient services; in primary care (the physician consultation, laboratory, X-ray and rehabilitative services) the sickness insurance pays the reimbursement direct to the commune health station and not to the patient. The doctor is paid by salary. Only doctors working in private practice benefit from the compulsory state insurance: either a small and diminishing band of older general practitioners who have chosen not to work in health stations, or salaried hospital doctors who carry out private general practice on a part-time basis. Private general practice, including private laboratories, radiological centres and physiotherapists, is therefore heavily subsidised through the state: a

* In 1976 the exchange rate was 1 US $ to 3.20 F marks.

strange anomaly in a country like Finland, but the Board of Health appears to tolerate it because without this facility it would be physically impossible to satisfy the needs of primary care, particularly in the large towns. At the present time there are just not enough doctors working full-time from the local health stations, so the private sector not only serves a very necessary function, but prevents even more overloading of hospital out-patient departments. It also acts as a safety valve for doctors and patients, which is considered a necessary and inevitable requirement in any free society. But, as the number of doctors working full-time in the field of primary care increases, so the Board of Health hopes that the private sector will naturally decline. It appears that in reality this is slowly occurring. It is important to emphasise that there is no law or statute against private medicine, rather the National Board of Health intends to improve and develop the public sector so that the private sector will inevitably diminish.

Primary medical care

The Finnish Health Service, like that of the rest of Scandinavia, has had for many years a strong hospital emphasis, but it has been appreciated that this over-reliance on the hospital service is inappropriate to the medical needs of the country and is a very expensive and inefficient way to organise medical care. Since 1962, the re-allocation of both financial and manpower resources has been planned at the Board of Health and, as a result, in 1972 a new Public Health Act was passed. Up till this time, primary medical care was provided and organised separately by each commune, with the district medical officer of health being, in theory, the central figure and responsible for preventive and curative medicine. But such a situation was only a reality in a minority of communes and never in the larger cities, primarily due to a shortage of physicians prepared to work in this field.

The Public Health Act created administratively independent units, ideally of between 10 000 and 15 000 inhabitants, although in urban areas they can cover as many as 500 000 inhabitants (as in Helsinki). Such units are called health centres, and they are responsible for the administration and organisation of ambulatory care, preventive medicine, mother and child services, the local hospital, dental care, ambulance service and all medical aids for disabled people. The actual provision of medical care is made at community health stations, which cover populations varying between 10 000 and 30 000, depending on whether it be in an urban or rural situation. In other words, a health centre is an administrative area and may contain in the very large urban area up to sixteen health stations.

In principle, health stations are most comprehensive in concept. They contain consultation rooms for doctors and public health nurses, emergency treatment rooms, and usually X-ray, laboratory and physiotherapy departments. There are always dental departments included in the station – in fact, Finland has the highest ratio of dentists to population in the Western World. Since 1972, it has been planned that there should be 30 per cent acute beds for general medical observations (and a few maternity beds in outlying areas such as Lapland) and 70 per cent for chronic/geriatric patients. However, the proportions vary: in Lapland they were 50:50, while in some other communes perhaps 90 per cent of beds were solely for chronic/geriatric use. Wherever possible, the aim is to keep patients as close as possible to the community in which they live, and most communes plan to include homes for the elderly to be attached to the health station/hospital unit, as it is so often necessary and desirable to be able to transfer patients from one department to another. Such homes are the direct responsibility of the social services department, which also provides social workers, organisers for home care (i.e. meals, nursing help, wheel chairs and walking aids). All these facilities are centralised at the health station.

Depending on its geographical situation, a health station may have visiting specialists; this is a service which is desired by many doctors, and the Board of Health intends to increase the number and variety of specialists as and when it becomes possible. Operating theatres are also provided in the isolated stations for routine minor surgery (for example hernias, haemorrhoids and varicose veins). A small amount of acute surgery may be undertaken (for example appendicectomy and fracture work). Thus it will be seen that the health station is completely comprehensive in outlook, and in the future is likely to be used more and more in the training of medical students. It is difficult not to compare the Finnish health station, which is so close to the prophetic ideals of the Dawson Report (United Kingdom, p. 41), with the rather inadequate facilities of most health centres in the UK.

Staffing

On 1 January 1976, there were 1169 physicians, about 30 per cent working in primary health care, or 1 per 3963 inhabitants, which indeed represents a shortage, especially as doctors only work 37 hours per week. By 1 July 1976, the figure had risen to 1222, or one physician per 3792 inhabitants. It is the intention of the Board of Health to alter this ratio, and to encourage or direct newly qualified doctors away from the hospital service until the primary facilities are adequately staffed. This shortage is in fact compensated for by the greater number of public health nurses working in the health station who carry out much routine work, i.e. running hypertension and diabetic follow-up clinics or even providing first-contact care for the patient. The ratio of public health nurses to doctors may be as much as five or six to one, although the ratio for the whole country is three to one.

Health stations are open between 08.00 hours and 20.00 hours, and doctors spend the entire day in consultations and working in the attached acute hospital. Consultation time on average is four patients per hour, and for all practical purposes there is no home visiting by the doctor: any home visits that are considered necessary are done by the public health nurse. Inevitably, there is a waiting list to see doctors, and anything from one to even four weeks is commonplace, which is really quite unacceptable for an efficient primary care service. One doctor is always available for acute cases.

Emergency arrangements

Out-of-hours cover is provided at a health station, and one doctor in theory may be on call for as many as 80 000–90 000 patients – in other words, three or four health stations. Again this is totally inadequate, and many patients living in urban areas go directly to the local hospital's emergency department. As in many countries, hospital doctors feel that much of this type of work which they are forced to carry out is due to an inadequate or poorly organised service at primary care level.

Facilities

Particularly in the new health stations, facilities are superb, both in quality and quantity: some could even be described as lavish and unnecessarily extravagant. All health stations, since the 1972 law, are planned with X-ray, laboratory and physiotherapy departments. To give an idea of the orientation of investigative procedures away from the hospital towards the community, in 1973 the total number of X-ray examinations performed was 560 000, of which only 64 000 were done outside health stations. By 1975 the total had reached 700 000. The total number of laboratory tests in that year was 9 million – about 5.7 million in health station main laboratories, about 2.3 million in side laboratories (in other words, these were carried out mainly by public health nurses) and the rest (1 million) either in hospital, government or private laboratories outside the health stations (Kasari, 1975). By 1975, 17 200 investigations were performed. These increased figures give some indication of the relatively rapid growth of health station facilities which is a feature of the Finnish Health Service. Physiotherapy departments were large and planned with the latest equipment and facilities – but in a number of cases they seemed too large for the community they served and a waste of resources.

Other means of providing primary care

Primary care is also carried out by salaried hospital specialists working part-time as general practitioners after they have finished their hospital work. It is estimated that almost 30 per cent of patients use this opportunity (Aer, 1976) and, in addition, a number of patients are seen by a rapidly diminishing number of older general practitioners working 'solo' – perhaps only 3 per cent. All investigations and treatment – X-ray, pathology and physiotherapy – can be arranged by privately organised diagnostic centres, and directly subsidised by compulsory insurance, although the patient can decide to use the X-ray facilities of the local health station if he wishes.

Patients may also go directly to the out-patient (or polyclinic) department of their local hospital without any referral by a primary care physician. In 1976, there were 6.5 million visits to health stations (many of these include visits to the public health nurse), 1 million visits were made to hospital out-patient and emergency departments, and 3.3 million were seen by part-time specialists or general practitioners in the private sector. In other words, 60 per cent of all first-contact care took place in the health station, and about 30 per cent was treated in the private sector. Of the 1 million visits taking place in the hospital out-patient (polyclinic) and emergency departments, accurate figures are not known. Probably about 50 per cent take place in the out-patient departments and must be referred by a primary care physician. Only the remaining 50 per cent of visits to emergency departments are made without referral and of these only perhaps 60–70 per cent should be considered as primary visits.

Maternal and child health services

This aspect of primary care has been firmly established in Finland since the end of the Second World War, and it was already free of charge by the early 1950s. It has been a great success story, with the lowest maternal mortality rate and one of the best infant mortality rates in the world (Table 3).

In principle, maternity and child health centres are placed primarily in health stations and are staffed by public health nurses who by the middle of the 1970s combined the function of both midwife and health visitor. Depending on the catchment area of the health station, there may be also maternity and child health centres conveniently placed in the community. The public health nurse is mainly responsible for ante-natal care, working in close cooperation with the doctors in the health station. She usually makes the initial examination, seeing the patient regularly throughout pregnancy: the patient must be seen at least four times by a doctor. In order to make sure that all mothers attend regularly for ante-natal supervision, the maternity allowance is only payable if they have been signed up for a certain number of attendances.

Nearly all deliveries (99.9 per cent) take place either in specialist hospitals or the more remote health station maternity units in isolated areas. The public health nurse is responsible for care for twelve weeks after delivery. Babies and infants are also seen regularly at these centres with the general problems of baby management, vaccination, immunisation and simple developmental screening programmes (particularly sight, hearing and dental supervision), the under-one-year group being the most frequent attenders.

Since 1974, the work of these maternity and child care centres has been expanded considerably to include adult preventive medicine – particularly the follow-up of hypertension and diabetes – and they are now known as health education centres.

Hospital service and primary care

There are four levels of hospital developed on a regional basis:

(*a*) University hospitals serving a population of 500 000–1 000 000, with super-specialist and specialist facilities.

(*b*) Central hospitals, serving a population of 100 000–300 000 including all specialist requirements.

(c) Intermediate hospitals, serving a population of 50 000–100 000, with only departments of medicine, surgery, obstetrics and gynaecology and paediatrics.

(d) Hospitals attached physically to health stations serving populations up to 30 000. These may be acute or geriatric, and occasionally have beds for straightforward obstetrics and surgery.

All hospitals are financed by central government and the local communes. The state (central government) pays 10 per cent more subsidy to university than other hospitals to cover expenditure on teaching. For practical purposes, there are no private hospitals and no private beds in publicly owned hospitals.

> In 1975 about 7200 beds were in health station wards which are under the direct control of the primary physician working there. This represents about 20 per cent of all acute general hospital beds and 10 per cent of total hospital beds. The cost of a bed in a health station hospital at this time was 60 per cent cheaper than in a central hospital. (Kekki, 1976)

There is absolutely no doubt that such facilities close to the patient's home are appreciated by patients and enjoyed by doctors, and in fact both the doctor and patient benefit from the continuity of treatment which is possible under these circumstances.

Medical education and primary care

In 1976, about 600 medical students qualified from five medical schools attached to five different universities – Helsinki, Turku, Oulu, Kuopio and Tampere. Oulu (until recently the most northern university in the world) was only opened in 1960, whilst Tampere and Turku started to admit medical students in the late 1960s.

It was recognised during the late 1950s that Finland needed to increase her medical output very considerably – hence the opening of three new medical schools within ten years. It was also felt by the Board of Health that it should be possible to reduce the length of the basic medical education to $4\frac{1}{2}$ years without reducing standards, as it was intended that all doctors, including primary care physicians, should have a proper postgraduate training. In this way the number of doctors would be increased. This scheme never got off the ground, as it was bitterly opposed by the medical establishment at the universities because it was felt that it might reduce the status of the medical profession.

Exposure to general practice is variable, and to a large extent depends on the individual enthusiasm and interests of the departments of community medicine. In Kuopio, for instance, all medical students spend three months in every year (including premedical) at surrounding health stations: this has proved very popular with both students and the staff at the health stations. I also gained the impression that it not only boosted the morale of the doctors, but also improved their relationship with the university hospital staff.

After qualifying and completing a year's internship, a period of training is necessary before a physician can register as a specialist. General practice, or primary care, is now included in this programme, and consists of two years working in a chosen health station, followed by a further year in hospital – six months in a department of internal medicine and six months in a department of the doctor's personal choice.

Continuing education is haphazard and depends very largely on the inclinations of the individual doctor and the educational facilities available in his particular locality.

Personal assessment

Finland is the only non-Communist industrialised country which has placed an absolute priority on the development of primary care certainly until 1980, and almost certainly beyond that date.

> By the Community Health Act 1972, a systematic planning procedure was introduced into the health service whose aim was to bring about a uniform standard of care as to quantity, quality and availability of services throughout the country. It aimed to change from hospital orientated medicine towards preventive and outpatient care. It also introduced the concept of health centres as functional organisations in the community. (Kekki, 1975)

Health stations were to provide as far as possible a totally comprehensive system of health care so that as much patient care as possible should be kept away from the hospital. This, of course, as yet is far from a reality but, once the health stations have been built and staffed, the burden on the hospital out-patient departments will rapidly decrease, and the prospect of a really first-class primary care service should be possible. Very few countries can claim such definite plans to orientate staff away from the hospital service. Such positive and rational thinking is one of the most exciting prospects in the whole field of health care planning at the present time.

I was fortunate enough to see many health stations throughout the country, including Lapland, and was indeed able to vouch for the claim by the Board of Health that the underdeveloped and more remote areas of the country had been given priority in health spending. The standard of planning, decor, equipment, both for the medical and for the secretarial staff, was superb, while the radiological, laboratory and physiotherapy departments could not be improved. The dental department, as one would expect in a country with one of the highest dentist/patient ratios, was more than adequate, while the waiting areas for patients were ideal. But, have the authorities been too extravagant in design and equipment, and will there be enough money to complete future health stations? In the future the Board of Health will be trying to decrease the standard in design, size and decor in order to bring the communes back to a sense of reality (Aer, 1976). Laboratories are necessary in the more remote stations, but certainly in urban areas it seems wasteful not to centralise the facilities in the local hospital.

Involvement of the community in decision making, even though policy was decided centrally, appeared to work very well and produced an involvement of the local people in their health station/hospital.

There are a number of practical difficulties from the patient's point of view which are noticeable and unsatisfactory: basically, they are due to a relative shortage of doctors. A waiting time of one to four weeks to see a primary care physician and the virtual abolition of all home visits, even for the very young and elderly, is a feature of the primary care services which drives people into the private sector where the waiting time is perhaps one to two days and home visits are still carried out by diminishing numbers of old-fashioned general practitioners.

It is candidly acknowledged that the number of old people's hospitals is insufficient, and many of them are of a poor standard. I felt very strongly that many communes would have been more sensible to spend less money on the new health stations and then re-allocate the rest to upgrading the local hospital. Whether the Board of Health will bring pressure to bear for more realistic spending remains to be seen. Many old people's homes were inadequate, but here the problem is different. The responsibility for such accommodation is that of the

Department of Social Affairs and not the Board of Health, and while it is obvious that many of the old people should in fact be in hospital rather than in a home, it is not possible for the health authorities to provide staff or better facilities. A major preoccupation of many communes is trying to persuade the Board of Health to convert such places into geriatric hospitals. This, of course, is not a problem unique to Finland, but is something which must be solved quickly if a more adequate level of primary care is to be attained. The basic philosophy that all old people should be kept as close as possible to their own community is rational, humane and appreciated by both patients and their relatives.

To summarise – there can be few countries in the world where primary care services can be watched with more interest and hope.

NORWAY

In 1319, Norway and Sweden joined in a union, both countries later being joined to Denmark. Subsequently, Sweden freed herself from this triple alliance, but from 1380 Norway became even more closely bound up with Denmark, and did not establish her independence until the separation of the two countries in 1814. Norway's independence was brief, and in the same year she was again forced to accept union with Sweden. Finally, in 1905 her absolute independence was proclaimed, and she became a constitutional monarchy with political power being in the hands of an elected parliament (Stortinget).

General introduction

With an area equal to that of the UK and the Republic of Ireland, Norway had a population of only 3 922 000 in 1972: by 1975 it had passed the 4 million mark. About 35 per cent of the population live in rural areas in scattered settlements varying between 200 and 2000 inhabitants. Villages are almost unknown, and 60 per cent of the population live in and around cities and towns: the three main cities being Oslo (487 000), Bergen (213 000) and Trondheim (126 000). On the west coast and in the northern part of the country, the density of population is very low, and this presents particular problems, not only to the health authorities, but also for education, social services and transport. On the other hand, in the Oslo Fjord region, 35 per cent of the nation live in 4 per cent of their land. One in ten Norwegians live north of the Arctic Circle, and the problem of depopulation from this part of Norway has been a feature of life for the last twenty years. Ways and means of encouraging young people to stay have been thought about by successive governments, and the recent formation of a university in Tromsö (including a medical school) was a political act, carried out amidst considerable opposition, with this aim in view.

Agriculture, forestry (a quarter of the country is covered with forest) and fishing are no longer the main employments – in fact, only 12 per cent. The mining of iron ore and coal, manufacturing and building account for a further 36 per cent, and the rest is taken up by administrative and service industries. In addition, North Sea oil and the prospects of much increased prosperity is exercising the minds of politicians and people alike.

Norway is divided into nineteen provinces (or counties) with populations varying in size between 76 000 (Finnmark) and 487 000 (Oslo), with an average of 200 000. The provinces are further divided into 444 communes or municipalities, and it is the responsibility of each commune to provide and organise hospital and public health services. Local participation is the basis and foundation of the Norwegian Health Service, and has been so since 1860, when the first health law was passed. As in Finland and Sweden, taxes are levied both by central government and by the communes, the poorer communes being supported and subsidised by the national government.

Since 1945, the health and social services have been merged into the Ministry of Social Affairs, with a division for health care which is supervised by the Director-General of Health Services, who is a doctor. Each province has a full-time public health officer who is paid 50 per cent by the central government and 50 per cent by the province. He is responsible for carrying out the health policies as decided by parliament, for supervising all health personnel – except general practitioners – and for the overall administration of hospitals in his area.

At the health district level, there is a Board of Health composed of elected local politicians who organise and decide the implementation of health policies. The local district medical officer is the *ex-officio* chairman, and he is the only non-elected member of the Board. He is directly responsible to the provincial public health officer.

Medical insurance
Social insurance in Norway has developed in a haphazard

manner, evolving gradually; perhaps surprisingly, it was not until 1971 that a fully integrated, national social insurance system was launched. Accident insurance for industrial workers was initiated in 1894, and health insurance in 1909. In 1911, the very low income group was covered by a modified form of health coverage, but compulsory health insurance for the entire population did not become law until 1956. This involved many small insurance organisations and proved to be rather inefficient and cumbersome, so, in 1967, a start was made in joining all social insurance under one law, and this was fully accomplished in 1971, with the National Insurance Scheme, administered by the National Insurance Institution (Rikstrygdeverhet).

Social insurance covers sickness, injury, pregnancy, old-age pension, unemployment benefits and sickness benefits during illness: health insurance is carried out as an item-of-service payment mutually agreed and arranged between the Norwegian Medical Association and the Rikstrygdeverhet. Compared with most countries in the EEC (Chapter 4), there is excellent cooperation between doctors and the insurance agencies. Why this is so is not entirely clear, but the medical profession appears to be convinced by the philosophy of the welfare state and the absolute necessity, both for patients and doctors, to have total health coverage. In the past, older doctors experienced the depression of the 1930s, when often they remained unpaid even in kind, and this may well have been a contributory factor in the conspicuous lack of wrangling over fees. To give an idea of this cooperation, the Norwegian Medical Association is given the responsibility of investigating doctors who are thought to be abusing the system.

There is no charge to the patient for hospital care – in-patient and out-patient – or for laboratory and radiological investigations, either in hospital or on referral by primary care physicians.

There is partial coverage for general practitioners and district doctors, and specialists working on a part-time basis in the field of primary care. Specialists are paid at a higher rate than the general practitioner or the district doctor (Table 11).

The present arrangement is that the patient pays the difference between the actual fee and the amount the insurance will refund, and the doctor gets the refund direct from the local health insurance office. In this way it is made easier for the patient who does not have to find the full amount and then await a refund. There is a very wide range of drugs on a special list (all chronic and serious diseases) which are fully covered by insurance.

National insurance, including health coverage, is financed by premiums from the employee and employer, and by contributions from the communes and the state. The rates are decided by parliament.

TABLE 11 *Health insurance payments*

	GP/district doctor		Specialist
1st consultation	Health insurance pay	55%	60%
2nd consultation	Health insurance pay	70%	100%
3rd consultation	Health insurance pay	100%	100%

Source: Hümerfelt (1976)

Primary medical care

Historically, primary medical care in rural areas has been the responsibility of the district doctor, who combines the function of a general practitioner and public health officer. The District Doctor Law was passed by parliament on 26 July 1912. It divided the country into health districts composed of one or two communes, depending on the population density of the area. In 1976, there were 444 communes and 377 health districts with positions for 550 district doctors. By law, each health district must have at least one district doctor who is appointed by the provincial health department. He is chairman (*ex officio*) of the District and Commune Health Board, which is responsible for the supervision of environmental health, the control of communicable diseases, maternal and child health, school health service, health education, chronic sick and small 'cottage' or local hospitals often including a maternity department.

The district doctor is paid a relatively small fixed salary by the state for his administrative and public health duties, while for the curative, general practice side of his work he is paid by the usual item-of-service system. On average, he spends about eighteen to twenty hours per week on public health work, and many district doctors feel that this is probably in excess of what is necessary.

Consultation hours are usually 08.30–12.30 hours and 13.15–16.00 hours, when anything between 20 and 35 patients may be seen. Home visits are kept to a minimum, but the majority of district doctors, as opposed to their urban general practitioner colleagues who do none, would expect to make on average 12 home visits per week. They cover rural Norway. In the remote areas, especially on the west coast and northern parts of the country, they are the only doctors providing primary care, while in other areas general practitioners also work alongside the district doctor. Very often their areas cover many small islands, and much of their visiting is carried out by boat. It is estimated that about 100 work in single-handed practice, while the remainder work in pairs, or even in groups of three or four. They are assisted by their public health nurses, midwives and home nurses. An interesting scheme by which they are further supported is the use made of the internship period of study. After qualification, every doctor must work for a year in a hospital (but not a teaching hospital) and also as an assistant to a district doctor for a period of six months. Such help is particularly useful to single-handed doctors and helps to ease the burden of emergency cover. Off-duty arrangements at night and at weekends vary slightly, but generally are on a rota basis between district doctors, or, if a doctor is single-handed, then the intern assistant and public health nurse are included.

Until the early 1970s, one of the problems facing the new district doctor was the fact that the retiring doctor owned all his equipment (electrocardiograph, microscope, gynaecological examination couch, etc.) and often the furniture and accessories within the consulting room as well. The district doctor's home was owned by the commune and rented by the doctor. Obviously, this also posed difficulties for the health district in finding recruits prepared either to buy the old equipment or to provide their own. So, catalysed by this fact, as well as by rising costs and inflation, it is becoming the custom for the health district council to buy the premises and provide the equipment, allowing the incoming doctors to pay a reasonable rent. I found that all young doctors agreed with this idea and were pleased with such an arrangement.

The concept of the health centre, including accommodation for doctors, public health nurses and midwives, a small laboratory, sometimes physiotherapy and in more outlying districts often attached to a local hospital and old people's home, is becoming more popular. In 1976, there were 15 health centres owned by a number of communes in the skerries or small islands near Bergen, around Tromsö and also in Finnmark province.

Facilities

X-ray departments are not included in the health centre concept or in the accommodation usually provided for district doctors. Such services are centred on the nearest hospital. There are, of course, exceptions, usually where the health centre/district doctor accommodation and cottage hospital are combined. There is a waiting time of 3–6 weeks for such examinations as barium meals and enemas and intravenous pyelograms.

Pathology is centralised on the hospital service, and appears to be very efficient even though long distances may be involved. Most doctors would expect to have a small laboratory with a technician for simple blood and urine investigations.

Physiotherapy is largely organised on a private basis; departments are rarely found in a health centre, and never in a district doctor's office. As health centres continue to develop, it is hoped to include physiotherapy. Such services are covered by the usual insurance arrangements: the patient paying the difference between the actual fee and the amount the insurance refunds.

Urban primary care

The district medical officer has never played much part in urban primary care, so that before the Second World War it was the general practitioner who provided such services. This has changed, because during the sixties and up to the mid-seventies, the number of general practitioners steadily declined, and, to compensate for this loss of manpower, an increasing amount of first-contact care has been supplemented by salaried hospital doctors and a few specialists working as part-time general practitioners. In 1972, there were 932 general practitioners and 546 private specialists, some of whom worked partly as general practitioners. The majority of the general practitioners were over 50 years old, and an increasing proportion of them only worked part-time with the inevitable result that there was a declining and inadequate standard of primary care. This situation is most noticeable in Oslo, Bergen and Trondheim.

Between 1970 and 1972, manpower in primary care increased by 3 per cent, while in hospital it increased by 8 per cent. This trend has continued since the end of the Second World War. Although the total doctor/patient ratio between 1956 and 1972 steadily improved, this gives a false impression with regard to primary care where, in fact, the number of patients per doctor has increased (Table 12).

It can also be appreciated (Table 13) that, although between 1956 and 1972 the number of doctors increased by 2114, the number of general practitioners actually decreased by 44, and the combined total of general practitioners and district doctors by 3!

TABLE 12   *Distribution of primary care physicians*

	Population (million)	Population per doctor	Population per (GP+DD)	Population per (GP+DD+Int.)
1956	3.476	980	2601	2517
1966	3.770	843	3036	2797
1970	3.888	725	2956	2670
1972	3.922	689	2942	2613

Based on: Brunsgaard (1974)

TABLE 13   *Primary care physicians in comparison with total number of physicians*

	Total doctors	GP	DD	GP+DD	Int.	Total (GP+DD+Int.)
1956	3576	976	360	1336	45	1381
1966	4470	877	364	1241	107	1348
1970	5361	937	378	1315	141	1456
1972	5690	932	401	1333	168	1501

Source: Brunsgaard (1974)

A more encouraging feature of the medical manpower situation is that the distribution of doctors in primary care is fairly even (Table 14), although the distribution of specialists shows extreme differences (Table 15).

The traditional pattern of single-handed practice remains, and even though group practice and health centres are much talked about, there is little evidence that the general practitioner intends to change his style of work. There is no registration of patients, who are free to change doctors as frequently as they wish, leading to all the abuses, frustrations and inefficiencies of this style of practice.

TABLE 14 *Distribution of primary care physicians in absolute numbers and in relation to population, 1972*

	Population	Population per primary care physician
Norway	3 922 000	2613
3 northern provinces	456 000	2478
Oslo	477 000	2789

Source: Brunsgaard (1974)

TABLE 15 *Distribution of specialists in absolute numbers and in relation to population – 1972*

	Population	Total physicians	Specialists	Spec./ pop.	Private spec.	Private spec./ pop.
Norway	3 922 000	5690	2317	1:1693	546	1:7183
3 northern provinces	456 000	507	82	1:5561	8	1:57 000
Oslo	477 000	1691	953	1:501	242	1:1971

Source: Brunsgaard (1974)

Facilities are modest in comparison with other Scandinavian countries. The majority of laboratory investigations and all radiology are referred to the nearest hospital without difficulty, except the waiting time for patients.

The referral of patients to specialists presents some problems, particularly the long waiting time, and in some scattered areas there is also a real lack of certain specialists which adds to the patient's (and the general practitioner's) difficulties. In rural areas patients may go direct to the hospital out-patient department, but again problems may arise because of the long distances involved in travelling. In fact, what happens is that the busy specialist will usually insist on referral by a general practitioner before he sees the patient, in an endeavour to sift out the unnecessary cases. Others will see patients without referral: it is for the specialist to make the decision.

District nurses (public health nurses) have a varying degree of co-operation with urban general practitioners depending largely on the doctor's personal inclination. In rural areas there is a much better working relationship. Here district nurses are closely concerned with preventive work associated mostly with the maternity and child care service and the school health service.

Home nurses, who are responsible for patient care in the home, are employed by the local department of social affairs, and again the degree of cooperation varies: usually the home nurse contacts the general practitioner for information about patients. There are seldom daily routine meetings between nurse and doctor as increasingly take place in the UK.

Emergency arrangements

Few general practitioners in urban areas work beyond 16.00 hours on weekdays – many of the older ones working perhaps only in the mornings – while it is the rule not to work at the weekend or during public holidays. Who then does provide out-of-hours cover for the patients?

(*a*) First aid stations. These provide facilities similar to a hospital emergency department and are organised and staffed quite separately from general practice or the hospital service. A charge may or may not be made to the patient, depending on the town or city: in Bergen, a charge is made, while in Oslo it is free. One of the great disadvantages of the separation of the service from general practice is that there is no communication or information passed to the patient's general practitioner.

(*b*) In most provinces, the provincial or county medical officer of health, in cooperation with the local medical association, organises a deputising service which is staffed by younger general practitioners or hospital doctors and sometimes public health officers. In some cities the service is organised on a shift system – 16.00 to 21.00, 21.00 to 24.00 hours and 24.00 to 08.00 hours, and is used mainly by patients requesting a home visit. It is frequently said that the only way to get a home visit in urban areas is to wait until after 16.00 hours! Such an organisation is usually located in the main hospital of the district.

(c) In Bergen, there is a special out-of-hours service for children, between 17.00 and 23.00 hours. It is run on a rota basis by the paediatrician and the junior staff. Parents can take their children direct to the hospital. Between 20 and 60 children are treated each night (Hall, 1976).

Maternity and child health services

Health centres for mothers and children are organised on a flexible basis throughout the country. In rural areas, they are run in close cooperation with the district doctor, while in urban areas it is unusual for the general practitioner to be involved in the actual running of the centre. They are staffed by public health nurses who carry out routine ante-natal care, developmental screening of babies and infants and the usual advice concerning the management of babies and young children. The aim is for one centre per 3000 population. In both rural and urban areas ante-natal care is shared with the district doctor and the general practitioner, although 90 per cent of confinements take place in specialist maternity units, except in the far north and south of the country where confinements take place in 'cottage hospitals' or even at home. In the larger towns gynaecologists and paediatricians may visit these centres, giving support to the preventive nature of the work: curative medicine and treatment as a rule are not carried out.

Hospital service and primary care

Until 1970, the national government was responsible for building and running university, psychiatric and tuberculosis hospitals, while the province was responsible for acute and chronic hospitals. The day-to-day expenditure of all hospitals was financed mainly through the various insurance agencies and ultimately the National Insurance Institution (Rikstrygdeverhet). But with the ever rising costs, the difference between the Rikstrygdeverhet's support and the actual cost grew, so that increasingly the deficit was supplemented by local and central government taxes. Inevitably, provincial governments have been loath to commit an increasing percentage of their annual budget to the hospital service, so that the burden was borne by central government taxation. It is estimated that only 15 per cent is now financed by local taxes.

The Hospital Law of 1970 placed the responsibility for all hospital planning, construction and organisation firmly on the shoulders of the provincial government. There are four types of hospitals:

(*a*) Regional – including university – hospitals, with every specialist and super-specialist facility. They have between 500 and 1500 beds.

(*b*) Central or provincial hospitals, providing all specialist facilities with between 250 and 700 beds.

(*c*) Local hospitals with between 45 and 200 beds, according to population requirements, and with only medical, surgical, obstretric and gynaecological and radiological departments.

(*d*) Cottage hospitals with between 8 and 20 beds, situated in remote areas of western and northern Norway, staffed entirely by district doctors and supported by interns in training. Their function and level of care is almost identical to similar hospitals in Finland (pp. 134, 138) and the UK (p. 49). They are considered to be an absolute necessity by patients, doctors and health planners alike, and are extremely popular with the local population. Minor surgery and acute medical emergencies are cared for, and in the more remote areas there are maternity beds and delivery rooms. Wherever possible, old people's homes are being built in direct association with the hospital and, in the future, health centres will also be physically attached to the hospital (Kvamme, 1976). There is specialist support for these hospitals, with periodic visits by paediatricians, gynaecologists, ENT specialists, ophthalmologists and psychiatrists.

Medical education and primary care

Until 1972, there were only two medical schools: one attached to the state-owned university in Oslo and one in Bergen. But, in 1973, a new university was opened in Tromsö – the most northern in the world – followed in 1975 by one in Trondheim, both with medical schools. Even now, there are not enough graduates in medicine, and about one-third are educated abroad, most of whom return to Norway to practise.

Undergraduate education is under the financial and legislative administration of the Ministry of Education. The public health authorities, with the Ministry of Social Affairs, have practically no say in any phase of the decision-making process, except sometimes in the planning stage. The same holds true for the professional organisations. Decisions are made by medical faculties with representation by teachers and students, who have been represented on the faculty boards of both Bergen and Oslo medical schools since 1948. However, over the last few years students, under certain pressures, have periodically withdrawn from faculty meetings as a means of political protest. Nonetheless the needs of general practice have been recognised. In 1969, a Chair in General Practice was set up in Oslo, followed in 1972 by Bergen, while in the two new universities, at Tromsö and Trondheim, departments of general practice have existed from the beginning.

Each medical school has experienced difficulty in finding space in the curriculum for general practice as many recognised disciplines were reluctant to give up time. In Bergen, for instance, general practice teaching is still optional, does not begin until the final year and involves teaching both by the small full-time staff in the department and by a number of selected district doctors. It is planned in the future to attach a student for a week with district doctors in the surrounding area. In 1977, general practice teaching was incorporated into the first clinical year (Hümerfelt, 1976). In Tromsö, an entirely different scheme is afoot, and there has been a definite attempt to get away from the traditional curriculumn. From the first year, students see district doctors at work, and throughout the course they are involved with the problems and aims of primary care. In fact, at the beginning of his clinical studies, a student spends six months away from the university – two months with a district doctor and four months in a local and/or cottage hospital. The curriculum is experimental, with integration being the aim of all those involved in the teaching of general practice (Forsdahl & Telje, 1976). The success or failure of the scheme is being watched closely, not only in Norway but throughout the rest of Scandinavia.

In order to qualify as a specialist in general practice, it is necessary for doctors after their 18 months internship period to spend:

(a) 2 years in primary care, usually attached to a district doctor;

(b) 1 year hospital training in relevant disciplines (internal medicine, paediatrics or psychiatry) usually for three-month periods. The intention is for this year to be flexible;

(c) a further continuous period of study over the next 5 years, including 3 months in hospital and 200 hours' additional training. This is easily accomplished in Bergen, where special weekend and various 3–5-day courses have been organised by the department of general practice. In Oslo, and to a lesser extent in Tromsö and Trondheim, regular day courses are arranged so that there are sufficient post-graduate sessions for any general practitioner or district doctor who wishes to attend.

District doctors and general practitioners who have already been in practice five years are not required to undergo this training in order to become specialists in general practice, but in future, for all new entrants, it is planned to make this obligatory, although the final decision has not yet been taken. The physician is then officially called a general practitioner member of the 'Norske Laegeforenung'. He is then entitled to charge more for consultations and it may give him a higher status amongst his colleagues, and perhaps the patients.

Personal assessment

General practice in Norway is in a critical situation, mainly because the recruiting of young doctors to this field of medicine has decreased drastically over the past years. From 1955 to 1966, the total number of general practitioners decreased by 100, while the number of hospital jobs increased by 1000. The age distribution of the GP's has changed in an unfortunate way. In 1956, about 30 per cent of GP's were more than 50 years old; ten years later, almost 60 per cent were over 50 years and close on 10 per cent were over 70 years. In a nutshell, one may describe the situation as follows: in a period when people seek doctors more frequently than ever before, the actual number of GP's has decreased, the average age has increased and the working capacity consequently decreased. We have been drawn into a vicious circle which must be broken if General Practice is to be regarded as a necessary part of the Norwegian Health System, and very few, if any, would question that. (Borchgrevink, 1970)

But between 1970 and 1975 (since these words were written) there was a growing interest in general practice from the new generation of young doctors, so that although there is still an overall shortage of primary care physicians, the future looks more hopeful (Hümerfelt, 1976). It is anticipated that by 1984 there will be one general practitioner/district doctor per 2000 population, which will require approximately 30 per cent of all new graduates to enter general practice (Brunsgaard, 1974). Whether or not this can be accomplished remains to be seen. At the present time there is still a shortage of new entrants to general practice in cities and towns, while nearly all district doctor posts are filled in rural areas. In the spring and summer of 1976, a number of vacancies suddenly and unexpectedly appeared in the northern Arctic regions: it is hoped this will be only a temporary phenomenon (Hümerfelt, 1976).

Why is there usually no problem with recruiting district doctors? Mainly, it seems to me, because they are held in high esteem by the local community and enjoy a much more professionally satisfying life than their urban general practitioner colleagues. They must be prepared to accept responsibility for most of the medical and social problems of the community, and they are able to practise medicine in a less restrictive way and withstand pressures in such matters as prescribing antibiotics and tranquillisers. It is largely up to them how they 'train' their patients, while in a city the patient can pressurise his doctor by changing if he does not get the treatment he wants. The district doctor still feels that he can influence the life of his community and really get to know his patients. From an economic point of view, as he is in part paid by salary by the state, he receives a good pension at the age of 70 years. The problems of urban practice are most noticeable in Oslo, Bergen and Trondheim, both for the patient and the doctor. In smaller towns the care is much better. From the patient's point of view, the main complaints are the long waiting time to see the general practitioner, the poor out-of-hours service provided by the general practitioner, the inadequate care of patients with chronic illness and social problems, and the almost total lack of home visiting. For the young doctor, the difficulties of setting up practice are largely financial, with high rents and even higher prices for buying premises, plus the additional burden of buying all the necessary equipment. In order to pay off his debt, he must work what are considered excessively long hours, and the newer generation of doctor is not prepared to do this, particularly as partnership, group practice and health centres have not become established in Norway. It is an interesting fact that patients are suspicious of health centres, even though the alternative may be poor. In a survey in Tromsö it was found that only 5 per cent of patients had a good, continuing doctor/patient relationship before a health centre was opened, and yet 40 per cent of the population still did not use the centre even though there was no waiting time (Telje, 1976). The reasons are obscure.

Most doctors and health planners feel that the only hope for the future of urban general practice lies with the idea of the Oslo Department of Health – the Mellbye plan – and its extension throughout all towns in Norway. It is advocated that Oslo should be divided into 150 districts and each district be provided with a district doctor, having similar responsibility, commitments and contracts to his rural colleagues, and working in close cooperation with a public health nurse and social worker. Whether or not this dream becomes a reality depends largely on money and deciding on priorities of spending. A bad mistake was made in 1970, when the New Hospital Law was introduced, in that no provision or mention was made of primary care. How different from the situation in Finland!

An interesting feature of the 18 months pre-registration period for newly qualified doctors is the fact that they must carry out their period of training only in non-teaching hospitals. Furthermore, the mandatory six months' attachment period to a district doctor during this training period is unique in Europe. It means that all doctors, whatever their eventual specialty, must spend some time in primary care. Such far-sightedness on the part of the Norwegian authorities could be followed with benefit by every country in Western Europe.

SWEDEN

Sweden is a constitutional monarchy with the government appointed by the king, taking into account the state of the different parties in parliament (Riksdag). The present Social Democratic party has been in almost continuous power since 1932, and the country has a very long tradition of stability and peace: in fact, she was last at war in 1814.*

General introduction

Sweden had a population of 8 129 000 at the end of 1972, and covers an area almost twice that of Norway. The population is homogeneous, although there are a considerable number of immigrant workers – mostly from Finland and Eastern Europe – estimated to be 20 per cent of the work force. The rate of population growth over the last century has been low: from 3.5 million in 1850 to 5 million in 1900 and 7.5 million in 1960. The birth rate is low, so the increase in population over the last 70 years has been as much due to a fall in the death rate as to anything else. This means that for the foreseeable future the under 15 years age group will continue to decrease, while the over 65s will

* In the general election of 1976, the Social Democratic party lost power.

increase (Table 2). Such trends, of course, have an important bearing on the future planning of the health service.

The population of Sweden is unevenly distributed: in Lapland there are 3 inhabitants per square mile; in Scania there are about 200 per square mile. According to the latest figures, almost 5 700 000 people lived in urban areas in 1970, compared with 3 285 000 in 1950. The three largest cities are Stockholm (population 1 352 000), Göteborg (685 000) and Malmö (449 000). The shift of population from the countryside to a few expanding areas around the main cities has been taking place in fact since the middle of the nineteenth century, and, in 1976, 86 per cent lived in the southern third of the country. But this movement is not solely an urban drift, and people move in both directions. Young people move more than older, the talented and well educated more than others, and blue-collar workers more than white-collar workers. Mobility also appears to be higher in eastern rather than western Sweden (Lindmark, 1976).

The distribution of population between the different sectors of the economy is industry 42.7 per cent, agriculture 9.5 per cent, distribution and services 47.8 per cent. Forests (60 per cent of the land is forest and lakes), iron ore and water power are at the heart of Sweden's economic prosperity, which provides her with one of the highest material standards of living in the world. Industrialisation did not overtake agriculture until 1930, and one of the characteristics of Swedish industry is that most firms are of small to medium size – over 90 per cent only employing between 5 and 100 workers – so that there are few industrial cities and the extremes of urbanisation which have taken place in other industrialised countries have not occurred in Sweden.

The country is divided into 24 districts (or counties), together with Stockholm, which has a special status. As in Finland and Norway, public health and medical care are decentralised, so that the medical care board of each county is responsible for providing and organising all health services.

Although health policy, priorities of spending and manpower distribution are decided at the National Board of Health and Welfare in Stockholm, the implementation of these policies is at county level. The governing body of the county council (or *landsting*) is elected every three years and meets at most five times a year. Therefore, the executive committee takes the day-to-day decisions and reports back to the *landsting*; the medical executive committee or medical board is perhaps the most important and powerful, as it spends nearly 80 per cent of the county's annual budget. It should be remembered that in Sweden 51 per cent of the total health service budget comes from local or county taxes (Table 5).

Health insurance

For such an egalitarian society, it is surprising that comprehensive health insurance was so long in coming. It was not until 1955 that a national health insurance scheme was passed through parliament and it was further extended in 1967. In 1968, patients were for the first time able to receive a refund on drugs prescribed by doctors, while in 1970, a uniform tariff for doctors' fees was agreed and introduced. From 1 January 1974, a national dental insurance scheme was added, covering all citizens from the age of 17 for 50 per cent of the fees: under that age, all dental treatment is free.

As in Finland and Norway, all doctors working in hospital are salaried, and since 1970 all district doctors working in health centres or employed by the county councils are paid by salary, the scale being the same for both hospital and primary care work. Since 1975, all doctors work a 40-hour week (passed by law). This is not enforceable or attainable in all areas, and many work at least a 50-hour week, for which they are given additional overtime remuneration. Because the rates of taxation are so high, very few doctors are inclined to work more than this and if it is necessary for them to do so, they take extra holidays rather than further payment (compare Finland where this practice is forbidden by law). In 1976, patients paid 15 S. Kr. (1 US $ to 4.45 S. Kr.) for each visit to a health centre. This was paid direct to the county council, the social insurance system in turn paid the county council a further 60 S. Kr. This includes both consultation and any radiological or laboratory investigations that might be necessary. In hospital the patient makes a token payment. Physiotherapy is reimbursed at 75 per cent of the actual cost. Compensation is made for travel in connection with all medical and dental consultations and treatments, and is calculated according to the cheapest means of travel that can be used in view of the patient's health. Refunds on prescriptions for drugs are made directly by the pharmacy. Such refunds are calculated on one or more prescriptions presented to the pharmacy simultaneously and made out to the patient by one doctor. The maximum sum payable by the insured person on each occasion is 20 S. Kr. Certain drugs are entirely free of charge: this list is comprehensive.

Visits to private practitoners working in the field of primary care – who may be general practitioners, salaried hospital specialists or industrial medical officers working on a part-time basis – come under a separate and higher reimbursement list. As in Finland, there is the odd situation whereby the state insurance scheme supports and subsidises private practice.

Insured persons pay a fixed amount per year plus a variable amount depending on income. In 1974, the average combined charge worked out at 650 S. Kr per year. The employer's contribution for health insurance was 3.8 per cent of the employee's pay, and in addition the state contributes an increasing amount each year.

Primary medical care

The county councils are responsible for the planning and provision of both hospital and primary care services. Until 1963, primary care was under the direct control of the National Board of Health, who were in the midst of pursuing a policy of widespread hospital expansion with a parallel emphasis on specialisation and the training of increasing numbers of specialists. The reasons for this obsession with the hospital service, almost to the exclusion of all other aspects of the health service are familiar. It was thought that, with a shortage of doctors, it was rational, economic and more effective to centralise their expertise in one place. The Swedish Medical Association was able to persuade both politicians and general public alike that specialisation, and therefore the building of more hospitals, was an absolute prerequisite of modern health care. Once such a policy had been set in motion, it was extremely difficult to stop or even slow down, particularly if there was no incentive on the part of the medical profession to do so. 'Hospital specialists, isolated from the real medical needs of the people, train students to become their mirror image, and the students eventually follow their teachers' example and become specialists themselves. A career in primary care is thought to indicate failure, and those who seek it are branded as "non successes".' (Haglund, 1974) Such comments are common to many countries, but apply particularly to Sweden. In about 1963, when the new law concerning primary care gave the responsibility to the county councils, it was beginning to be realised by a few physicians and administrators that a fundamental mistake had been made, but the vast majority of the general public and politicians, although they sensed that something was wrong, still remained convinced by the image of scientific, hospital-orientated medicine. In fact, as recently as 1970, Sweden's answer to the organisation of modern health care was started – the building of a 1400-bedded hospital in Stockholm. It is of course now realised that this ultimate folly of health care planning – a form of medical madness – can never solve the real health needs of the people, nor can any nation, even one as prosperous as Sweden, afford to build and staff such a hospital. Nor indeed can any country afford the dubious luxury of organising primary care through the hospital service.

In 1972, the National Health Board planning committee stated that, partly due to the rapidly escalating costs of the hospital service, it was necessary to redress the balance between the hospital primary care services and also to increase the provision of chronic sick homes instead of acute hospitals. But the National Health Board only acts in an advisory capacity, and the responsibility lies with the county councils who, as yet, and perhaps not surprisingly, have been slow to make fundamental changes in policy, for, at the local level, the medical profession is still able to exert tremendous influence in order to maintain a hospital-dominated health service.

How then is primary care delivered in Sweden? First, through hospital out-patient departments, where it is estimated that just over 60 per cent of all doctor/patient contacts in primary care take place. Patients need no referral, and there are long waiting lists – often up to six weeks. Doctors in the hospital service much resent this constant overburdening of the out-patient system, especially as it is felt that 80 per cent of these patients should have been seen in the setting of general practice. The basic facts need no elaboration.

Second, first-contact care is carried out by a variety of doctors. It is exceedingly difficult to obtain accurate figures on manpower deployment, even from the National Board of Health. In 1975 there were about 13 000 physicians in Sweden, of whom 1800 were district doctors or general practitioners. There were 9000 salaried doctors working in hospital, of whom nearly 550 worked in addition as part-time private specialists after they had finished their hospital duties (40 hours per week). In addition there were 1300 private specialists and general practitioners and 500 full-time industrial medical officers, who practiced privately or on a part-time basis. There were, therefore, 4150 doctors (district doctors, general practitioners, hospital specialists and industrial medical officers) who provide primary care (Gunnarson, 1976).

Each county is divided into health districts, which are served by one or more district medical officers (district *läkare*) who combine both the work of a general practitioner and a public health officer. In 1976, there were about 1800 full-time salaried district doctors employed by the county councils. The number of patients they were responsible for varied enormously: 1:3600 population in Dalby, 1:4170 in the Tynered district of Göteborg, 1:4600 in the Ornsköldsvik area, while in some rural areas and in Stockholm the ratio was only 1:2500.

In the future it is planned to organise the services of district doctors from health centres covering a population of between 15 000 and 50 000. The aim is to provide one district doctor per 3000 population, with public health nurses (1:3000 population), social workers and psychiatric nurses working as a team. In addition, visiting specialists (paediatricians, gynaecologists, psychiatrists, orthopaedic surgeons) will be included on the staff – depending on the needs of the particular locality. In many ways, such health centres are similar to the poly-clinics of the USSR and Eastern Europe (Chapters 6 and 7), with radiological, laboratory and physiotherapy departments. In 1976, there were 750 health centres, but a considerable increase is needed if there is to be any chance of fulfilling the objective of organising primary care along these lines, for example in Stockholm there were 10 health centres and the aim is to build a further 40 by 1980 (Stockholm City Council, 1976).

There is a great variety in the size of health centres, many in rural areas have only one district doctor supported by two or three public health nurses, depending on population size. Such health centres would usually have a laboratory capable of doing most routine blood tests; physiotherapy would also be easily available, but radiological examination would be carried out at the nearest hospital or larger health centre. The future policy favours increasing the size of centres, thus reducing the number of doctors working in isolation.

Consultations take place throughout the day: it is the usual practice to allocate 15 minutes per patient. Waiting time to see district doctors varies between one and four weeks. It is usual for one doctor on the staff of the centre to be on emergency call each day for acute cases. It is fair to say that virtually no home visits are now made by doctors.

The public health nurse plays a most important role in the organisation of first-contact care, and her time is divided in the following way. In the early morning there is a set time for answering the telephone, either giving advice to patients, suggesting they come into the health centre or go to the local hospital. She also deals with some initial consultation, seeking help from the doctor when necessary, and she is increasingly used in all aspects of preventive medicine, for example paediatric counselling, routine paediatric development assessment and inoculations. In some places, there may be a special nurse allocated to adult hypertensive and diabetic screening programmes. If home visits are required by the elderly, it is the public health nurse who carries these out.

The extent to which primary care is dependent on the nurse can be seen from the following figures: in 1972, there were 5 400 000 patient consultations with district medical officers and 5 300 000 with public health nurses.

The large new health centres which I saw were without exception of the very highest quality in equipment, facilities and decor. By any standards they were superb, with beautiful interior furnishings, but the planning was in some respects disappointing, often with great waste of space and sometimes a very strange sense of priorities, for example in Lidingo Sjukhus in Stockholm there is an enormous waiting area for the large and prestigious X-ray department and a small waiting area for patients attending the district doctor. Even more astonishing was the fact that there was no emergency room for the treatment of even minor casualties. Mention should also be made of the excellent receptionist and secretarial staff available to help the doctor.

General practitioners – about 850 – work independently of the county councils. They are paid on an item-of-service basis through the health insurance scheme. They are a declining and ageing group of doctors often working long and irregular hours. Recent reports indicate that this is the medical service most appreciated by patients (Freedman, 1975). Mostly centred in large cities, they work in solo practice, usually with a small laboratory, but with very little in the way of ancillary staff, and more often helped by their wives who act as secretary/nurse. Any payments for referrals for radiology and laboratory investigations or physiotherapy treatment are refunded to the patient in the usual way. Referral of patients to specialists in hospital cannot be done privately.

Specialists, including industrial medical officers, make up the largest number of doctors working in primary care – about 56 per cent as opposed to 44 per cent district doctor and general practitioner combined. They are usually internists, paediatricians or gynaecologists, and they work very much on a part-time basis, as can be seen by the number of consultations in primary care in 1974 (outside the hospital out-patient departments) – 87 per cent with the district doctors, general practitioners and public health nurses, and 13 per cent with specialists.

Industrial medical officers also provide primary care.

> All major industries in Sweden employ whole time medical officers. They perform the public health requirements of the various factory acts as well as giving medical care. Many smaller industries tend to form groups and share a common medical centre, perhaps with more than one doctor. They work a 40 hour week, with similar salaries to health service staff, but have freedom from obligatory or on-call duty. (Freedman, 1975)

Emergency arrangements

Out-of-hours cover – usually from 17.00 or 18.00 hours to 08.00 hours on weekdays, all Saturday and Sunday, also public holidays – is arranged in the following ways. First, many patients go direct to the emergency department of the nearest hospital. Second, increasing numbers of health centres organise their own emergency service. One doctor is 'on call' at the centre and all patients are brought to him by car or ambulance. There is no home visiting, which is hardly surprising, as one doctor may be covering a population of up to 70 000. Most doctors do not accept extra pay for this work, but for every hour on-duty, an extra time off-duty is allowed, for example for one Saturday, the entitlement is three extra days' holiday. Lastly, in large towns, for example Stockholm or Göteborg, a special deputising service is organised. This is quite separate from the hospital and health centre part of the service, and has its own staff of doctors and nurses. Twenty-four hour cover is provided, and the staff work on a six-hour shift system. Home visits are carried out, and it would seem that this is the only time a patient is able to receive this service. There are no reliable figures available which show the proportion of patients using the different available facilities. The impression is that the majority of patients use the emergency department of the hospital to the greatest extent.

Maternal and child health service

The care of mother and child has always been at the forefront of health services in Sweden, which in part explains the excellent maternal and infant mortality rates over many years, so that since 1966 they have always been at the top of the 'health league'. In fact, as early as 1901 the first infant welfare centre was established. This was followed by others until, by the time of the Second World War, most towns had one. By the mid-1950s, both maternity and child health services were free, and in 1969 new regulations were authorised by the National Board of Health.

Maternal health care is provided by:

(*a*) Maternal health centre Type I, which is incorporated within a hospital department of obstetrics and gynaecology.

(*b*) Maternal health centre Type II, which is usually situated within a health centre or the office used by a district medical officer. Wherever possible, it is combined with a child health centre. In 1971, there were 667 maternal health centres Type II.

All mothers receive complete ante-natal and post-natal care provided mainly by midwives or specially trained public health nurses. It is obligatory for them to attend a doctor on at least three occasions during pregnancy. Nearly all confinements (99.9 per cent) take place in hospital.

Child care service is provided by:

(*a*) Child health centre Type I, associated with a department of paediatrics, wherever possible at a children's hospital.

(*b*) Child health centre Type II, often combined with maternal health centre Type II at a health centre or on purpose-built premises. In 1971, there were 1273 such centres catering for children up to the age of five years.

Centres of this type provide immunisation and general advice about feeding, the development of babies and the upbringing of young children. Such activities are carried out by the public health nurse. Developmental screening is organised and performed by a doctor (usually the district medical officer) who makes four to seven examinations in the first year, two in the second, and one yearly thereafter.

Office hours and telephone arrangements at maternal and child health centres are decided by the county council or City Board of Health in consultation with the chief physician. It is emphasised that coordination and the exchange of information between these centres and the appropriate maternity and paediatric out- and in-patient departments is absolutely essential if a good service is to be provided. Everything is done to encourage women to attend, and in the more remote areas with poor communications, special free transport is arranged.

Hospital service and primary care

For the purpose of hospital organisation, Sweden is divided into seven regions, each with an average of slightly over one million inhabitants. Each region has a regional hospital of 1200–2300 beds, with all super-specialist facilities. At the next level comes the central general hospital with all specialist departments, and in the rural areas there are general hospitals with departments of medicine, surgery, anaesthetics and radiology.

There is virtually no direct relationship between the primary care physician and the hospital service, although the hospital plays a very significant part in the actual provision of primary care services. Only in rural areas are patients under the care of district medical officers: in chronic/geriatric hospitals. There are no acute hospital beds attached to health centres.

Medical education and primary care

The idea that there is a shortage of doctors in Sweden has become an accepted fact of life. In fact, compared with other developed countries (except Eastern Europe and the USSR), this is simply not true: the shortage is relative, and directly linked to the 40-hour week. At any rate, it is now accepted by the Swedish Medical Association and the National Board of Health that during the period 1970 –90, the number of physicians must increase from 11 100 to 29 900. Sweden is a rich country, but whether she will be able to afford such expansion, or whether such expansion is necessary or desirable, is a matter for debate.

At the present time, there are six medical schools attached to universities at Stockholm, Göteborg, Uppsala, Lund, Umea and Linköping. Whether the increase in student intake over the next 25 years can be accommodated by the present medical facilities is still undecided.

Undergraduate training lasts $5\frac{1}{2}$ years, and is almost exclusively specialist and hospital orientated. There is no primary care teaching or involvement of district doctors, with the exception of the University of Lund, which has appointed a professor of primary medical care based on an experimental research health centre at Dalby, near Lund.

Postgraduate training, after a year's internship, consists of 21 months in a variety of posts – 6 months' internal medicine, 6 months' psychiatry, 3 months' paediatrics and 6 months working in a health centre. Following this, there is a further 5 years' specialist training. Since 1973, vocational training has been started for primary care. It is a 3½-year course, involving 18 months in an internal medicine department in hospital, 6 months in the psychiatric unit of a hospital and 3 months in paediatrics, 6 months with a chosen district doctor and a 9 month elective – either in hospital or primary care. This was initiated at the University of Lund but has not spread throughout Sweden.

Personal assessment

It may seem churlish to criticise a country whose population is so obviously healthy, and whose maternal and infant mortality rates and life expectation are so good. But, unfortunately, it is difficult not to come to the conclusion that primary care is in a poor state and in urgent need of evaluation.

The most serious problem facing Sweden is the re-education of both the general public and the medical profession away from the principle that only the hospital can deal with the majority of illness. Since the war, two generations have been persuaded that only a hospital or a specialist can really give the best advice and correct treatment, even for comparatively minor illness. In a new experimental health centre at Tynnered in a suburb of Göteborg, the main problem experienced by the primary care physician was changing the attitude of patients away from hospital care and from considering district doctors as second-class physicians (Berg, 1975). It will be an extremely difficult and painful process, as initially those doctors who are striving to produce a renaissance in primary care will be opposed by the majority of their colleagues. Politicians can help at this point, particularly when they visit other countries and see that 80 per cent of all illness can be treated successfully outside the hospital. But probably the rapidly rising cost of the hospital service will bring back some sanity more quickly than anything else.

Even amongst those who are in favour of strengthening primary care, there is a difference of opinion as to whether the doctor of first contact should be a generalist or a specialist. The National Board of Health favours a small but definite increase in the number of specialists working in primary care, and it is planned that the visits to general practitioners and district doctors should decrease from 87 per cent to 83 per cent, while specialist consultations should increase from 13 per cent to 17 per cent. Some doctors would go even further and say that all district doctors, if they are working in a team, should specialise in paediatrics, gynaecology, internal medicine or psychiatry (compare with some group practices in the USA, Chapter 8). But there are also many doctors who feel that what is needed is a generalist who can look after the whole family (Gunnarson, 1976). This view would seem to be supported by the patients' opinions expressed in newspapers and magazines, and was the impression I gained after discussing the subject with nurses and social workers. There appears to be confusion about the role of a specialist. The majority of patients want a 'family doctor', and would like to see the same doctor as often as possible. There is no evidence that they wish to see different doctors for different diseases and different members of their family. In addition, they would like home visits, particularly for the very young and the elderly. In health centres which had developed this specialist outlook and were concentrating on the follow up of such diseases as hypertension and diabetes, there was excellent continuity of supervision for a number of diseases, but virtually no continuity of care of people and their families.

But a really excellent feature of primary care was the concept of having research health centres, without which it is felt that it is impossible to make any realistic plans for the future. A wide variety of subjects are under scrutiny at the moment: clinics for diabetes, hypertension and psychiatric disorders, all primarily organised and run by nurses; the need for cooperation between social workers and doctors and the best way to achieve this; emergency and out-of-hours care, and how best it should be organised; the value of laboratory investigations; the care of the dying, and the management of cancer patients; the problem of waiting time to see a doctor (is the delay due more to the patient or the actual difficulty in making an appointment?); organising the flow of patients in a health centre and analysing the different habits of doctors in such matters as follow-up consultations, specialist referrals and prescribing of drugs.

That the Swedish Health Service has overemphasised the hospital and specialist services for too long is not disputed by independent observers. A minority of the general public and politicians are also beginning to realise that fundamental mistakes have been made. The National Board of Health appears to be ambivalent, and there is not much evidence that the priorities of spending are going to change radically in the future. But there is a small but increasing band of dedicated and enthusiastic physicians, nurses and social workers who see the need for primary care and are aware of its true potential. It is amongst these people that the hopes for the future lie.

6

UNION OF SOVIET SOCIALIST REPUBLICS

The Union of Soviet Socialist Republics covers an area of 8 603 852 square miles, and in 1972 had a population of 247 500 000. It occupies about one-sixth of the inhabited surface of the world, and straddles half Europe and most of Asia, having boundaries with many countries in both continents. It experiences extremes of climatic conditions, from the permafrost of the Arctic belt to the stifling heat of the Central Asian Desert.

The USSR is divided into fifteen republics, and is composed of over a hundred nationalities. A wide variety of languages are spoken – Russian, Ukrainian, Georgian, Armenian, Uzbek and Kazakhs – and many of the hundred separate nationalities have their own particular dialects. In spite of this diversity, three-quarters of the population is made up of Caucasian Slavs, who are found not only in western Russia, but in every republic. The most recent census, in 1970, showed that 46.1 per cent of the population were male, and 53.9 per cent female, and less than 10.0 per cent were over the age of sixty years, although it was recognised that this percentage would steadily rise over the next twenty-five years. It was estimated that 58 per cent lived in cities and towns, and 42 per cent in rural areas, many of which were very sparsely populated.

No country in the world has a better doctor to population ratio (with the exception of Israel). In 1972 there were 698 000 doctors, giving a ratio of 28.2 doctors per 10 000 population. In fact, the figure is somewhat misleading, because two grades of dentist are included as physicians and, in addition, there are wide variations between the different republics – Georgia 34.6 and Kirgizia 18.8 – and between urban and rural areas. By 1975, the figure was 32.6 per 10 000 population. As far as can be judged from official sources, it is the intention of the Soviet authorities to continue producing 43 000–44 000 physicians yearly, with the expected ratio of 34–5 per 10 000 population (Venedikkov, 1973). About 70 per cent of physicians are female, but whether this ratio will be maintained is uncertain. This appears to take no account of the enormous numbers (2.1 million) of middle grade health workers – *feldschers*, midwives, nurses, pharmacists – already working in the health service, and poses a number of questions and doubts about Soviet planning.

The main causes of death are similar to those in all developed countries – cardiovascular disease 45 per cent, malignancies 15.8 per cent, and respiratory problems 12.7 per cent – and infant mortality has fallen from an estimated 279 per 1000 live births in 1916, to 23 per 1000 in 1971. During the same period of time, the life expectancy has risen from thirty to seventy years (male and female). Such are the bare facts. The vastness of the country and the variety of such different regions as Siberia, Armenia, Ukraine, Uzbekistan and Georgia, each with its own language, customs, traditions and architecture, are to most visitors quite staggering. But, equally amazing is the uniformity and the standardisation which has occurred in many spheres of human activity, and particularly in the medical services.

The health service in the USSR has developed over the last fifty years, immediately following the revolution in 1917. Prior to this, it was disorganised and fragmentary, and the only pre-revolutionary figure remaining to the present day is the ubiquitous, time-honoured *feldscher*. In accordance with the aspirations of the revolution, and because the organisation could be started literally from nothing, the health service has developed in a logical and sustained manner, to produce an integrated, comprehensive state service, which is universally available and free to the patient at the time of use, both in hospital and in the field of primary care. One of its salient features is the great emphasis placed on preventive as well as curative medicine. The service is financed through the state budget (Union and republic budgets), although small charges are made for dentures and there is a percentage payment for prescriptions (with exceptions for children, expectant women, old people, certain chronic diseases) as well as a token charge for therapeutic abortions. Private practice is not forbidden, although it is officially discouraged. It is carried out in two ways:

first, in large cities there are a few polyclinics which patients attend on a fee-paying basis. The staffing of these polyclinics is arranged by the state, and is obviously a great financial advantage to the doctors concerned although direct payment between patient and doctor does not take place. Second, some private practice is carried out from the doctor's private flat or house. All doctors are salaried.

Each of the fifteen republics has its own Ministry of Health under the overall control and direction of the Ministry of Health in Moscow. Although they accept the policy as outlined and decided in Moscow without demur, they do appear to have some control over local spending. Administratively, each republic is divided into *oblasti*, or regions, covering a population of one to five million. Some cities, such as Moscow, Leningrad, Kiev and Novosibirsk, with populations of well over a million, also function as *oblasti*. Each *oblast* is divided into *rayoni* or districts, with populations ranging from 40 000 to 150 000. The *rayoni* are further sub-divided into *uchastocks* or neighbourhood medical districts, which vary in size according to different functions, i.e. the *uchastocks* for paediatric, adult and women's care vary in size. Basically, primary care takes place at the *uchastock* level, secondary care in the *rayon* hospital and tertiary care in the *oblast* or republic hospital or institute. The regionalisation of health care, both administratively and operationally, is one of the most noticeable features and remarkable achievements of the Soviet system, and is a direct result of being able to plan without hindrance from the past. The same pattern exists in principle in rural areas, although there are differences in detail. (See rural health service.)

Primary medical care

The USSR is committed to the principle that the doctor of first contact should restrict his work to a particular age group or sex of patient, i.e. there is no family doctor or general practitioner, all being considered specialists in either paediatrics, adult medicine or gynaecology. There is no free choice of primary care physician for the patient.

The key to the provision of primary care in urban areas is the polyclinic, which combines both primary and secondary out-patient care. There are separate polyclinics for children, adults, industry, and consultation clinics for women.

In addition, there are 'dispensaries' which in fact are highly specialised polyclinics, concerned with such conditions as tuberculosis, heart disease, mental illness, venereal disease and cancer. Of course, they can only be justified, and therefore are only found, in very large cities, such as Moscow, Leningrad and Kiev. Although patients are free to seek help directly from a 'dispensary', in other words to use them as access points to primary care, more usually they are referred from a polyclinic by another doctor. These 'dispensaries' include both in- and out-patient departments, and are an essential part of the 'dispenserisation scheme'.

This scheme, which was originally given this name because the work was originally based on 'dispensaries', is now a major part of the work carried out in paediatric, adult and industrial polyclinics. It is considered to be the most important method of preventive work in the USSR. Essentially it amounts to establishing regular medical surveillance of certain groups of the population. Many sectors of the population are now covered by the 'dispensarisation scheme', including pregnant women, children of pre-school age and school children, particular groups of workers, athletes, scientists and politicians.

The scheme also follows up patients with known medical conditions, irrespective of their job; for example tuberculosis, diabetes mellitus and neoplasms. Patients are initially chosen for 'dispenserisation' when they attend the polyclinic for any reason. It is eventually hoped that every citizen in the USSR will be covered by the scheme and examined on a yearly basis.

Each polyclinic covers differing catchment areas according to its function, for example paediatric or adult, and is not usually attached physically to a hospital. A 'women's consultative clinic' can be considered as a polyclinic, but may often be described as a 'dispensary', although in reality such distinctions are merely an exercise in semantics. The staffing consists of primary care physicians with the addition of all categories of specialist, but it is important to realise that such a specialist has a different function from one in a country such as the UK. It is estimated that there are proportionately ten times as many specialists in the USSR as in the UK or, to put it in another way, the clinical experience of a specialist in the UK is likely to be ten times greater than in the USSR, as this experience is gained from a population ten times the size. In addition, the staff of a polyclinic do not work in hospital, which considerably limits the extent of their experience. It is only the specialists working in the *oblast* or *rayon* hospitals who have the same degree of clinical experience and expertise as their British, Danish or Dutch counterparts.

There are always full X-ray and pathological services in a polyclinic, as well as the services of a large physiotherapy department.

Paediatric service

It is planned that one *uchastock* paediatrician should care for between 700 and 1200 children under 15 years of age. Although this aim has been realised in many republics, there are still exceptions, for example urban Kazakhstan has 1 paediatrician per 2030 children (Popov, 1969). To quote Popov (1971): 'The number of paediatric *uchastocks* more than doubled between 1955 and 1968, the figures being 15 397 and 33 153 respectively. In 1955, on an average, the number of children covered by an urban paediatric *uchastock* was 1350, while in 1968 the figure had fallen to 1008.' Each paediatrician works seven hours per day for five days a week, with an occasional weekend duty depending on the size of the polyclinic. There is no night work between 20.00 hours and 08.00 hours, this being covered by the emergency service. Work is divided between consultations in the polyclinic, home visits and health education. Each paediatrician has an attached paediatric nurse, who works in the polyclinic both as a nurse and as a secretary. She accompanies the doctor on all home visits, which are carried out by means of an ambulance car provided at the polyclinic.

The service is uniform throughout the country: Paediatric Polyclinic No. 14, Tashkent, capital of Uzbekistan, is described in some detail as an example of the facilities and services provided. It is in no way unusual. It was built in 1970 on the outskirts of the new city, and covers a population of 16 000 children. The catchment area is divided into eighteen *uchastocks* with roughly 900 children per *uchastock*. In addition, the polyclinic is responsible for the medical supervision of twenty-one *crèches* and kindergartens and eight secondary schools. As in all Soviet medical establishments, the staffing appears luxurious to most outside observers. There are two senior paediatricians in charge of organisation, and eighteen *uchastock* paediatricians, with the attached nurses, providing primary care: i.e. one paediatrician and nurse per 900 children. All necessary specialised services are available, as well as four dentists and their appropriate staff. As in all polyclinics, there are X-ray, laboratory and physiotherapy departments. There is no appointment system, nor is there any intention of starting one, as both patients and doctors seem content with the usual queuing. Patients are all registered by secretarial staff, and a folder is provided for each patient's clinical notes, which are used both by primary care physicians and specialists with the obvious advantage of continuity.

Function of 'uchastock' paediatrician

1. Treatment of minor illness in the polyclinic or the child's home, and, if necessary, arrangement for admission to hospital. Domiciliary visits are encouraged to the extent that parents are positively advised by health education posters not to bring a feverish child to the polyclinic. Requests for visits are for the usual childhood diseases (for example measles, mumps, scarlet fever and chickenpox), upper respiratory tract infections and undiagnosed fevers (Barisova, 1971).

The *uchastock* paediatrician is not trained or encouraged to accept much clinical responsibility, and it appears to be routine policy that many children under two years of age who are seen with a fever are admitted to hospital, and any clinical problem not immediately resolving itself is also admitted. Inevitably, this means that there is a much higher paediatric bed ratio per population than in any other country. It is interesting to note that all mothers are expected to stay in hospital with children under the age of three years. Paediatricians and nurses were astonished to hear that this is not the usual practice in many countries, and could not understand how children of this age group could be satisfactorily looked after without the help of their mother.

2. Examination of normal babies and children, and referral to specialist paediatricians in the polyclinics when necessary occupies a great deal of time. After discharge, following confinement in hospital (nearly 100 per cent in urban areas, 85 per cent in rural areas), the *uchastock* paediatrician makes the initial examination when she visits the mother and baby at home on three successive days (this is a minimum period and is obligatory), and thereafter as necessary. After this, the following examinations are carried out.

Every month for the first year – this includes inoculations against tuberculosis, poliomyelitis, measles, smallpox, tetanus and diphtheria, which are all completed within the first year of life.

At three months, there is a special orthopaedic assessment. Between one and two years, the minimum number of examinations is two.

Between two and seven years, examinations are yearly. Between six and seven years there is an examination by a team of specialists at the polyclinic: ENT specialist, ophthalmologist, cardiologist and neurologist.

At school, further examinations are carried out by the specialist team at eight, nine, ten and fifteen years. The day-to-day care is under the supervision of the *uchastock* paediatrician.

3. Health education and the 'dispenserisation scheme', which involves the systematic follow up of all children with known abnormalities and repeated screening to detect abnormalities.

Adult service

Adult care is provided by three separate organisations – the district polyclinic, the industrial polyclinic and the women's consultative clinic.

Uchastock adult service

The adult polyclinic is concerned mainly with the care of retired people, non-working mothers and the chronic sick and disabled. The adult working population is encouraged to attend the industrial polyclinic at their place of work.

The primary care physician is known as the *uchastock* therapist or *terapevt*. She works from a polyclinic, in rotation with a colleague, usually on a seven-hour shift; in theory she covers a population of about 2000 people. Whether this 'norm' has been reached is open to debate, as it is difficult to find accurate information for the entire country. The average for the USSR was 3020 persons, and may even have been more than this (Ryan, 1972). This would seem to be confirmed by the following quotations:

> Nevertheless, the rate of growth of the urban system of polyclinics is still not high enough: it is markedly less than that of the hospital system and is failing to keep pace with the rapid growth of the urban population. In a number of places, in addition, the *uchastocks* are lagging behind even more and are not fully staffed with medical personnel . . .
>
> The lack of proportion between the development of outpatient care and that of hospital care, and the comparative backwardness of the former, is shown by the following figures from the Ministry of Health of the USSR:

Number of physicians (thousands)

Year	Total	Outpatient care	Hospital
1947	140.4	99.6	40.8
1960	334.1	221.2	112.9
1968	495.8	330.4	165.4

These figures show that, over the period 1947 to 1968, the total number of physicians providing medical care increased by a factor of 3.5; the corresponding figure for physicians in outpatient care was only 3.3, as compared with 4.1 for physicians in hospital. (Popov, 1971)

As in the paediatric services, the *uchastock* therapist works a five-day week, occasional weekends and no night duty. Between 20.00 and 08.00 hours, when use is made of the emergency service, there is in fact an emergency call room in most polyclinics, which deals with minor illness and enquiries, and is staffed by a *feldscher* or a nursing sister. The usual X-ray, pathology and physiotherapy departments are found, along with the usual surgical and medical specialists.

Polyclinic No. 22 is situated on the western side of Kiev, capital of the republic of the Ukraine. It covers a population of 50 000, which is divided into eighteen *uchastocks*. From a staffing point of view and in connection with the availability of diagnostic facilities, it is unremarkable, although it has one unusual feature, in that it is attached to a 200-bed hospital containing medical and surgical beds. The staff consists of two physicians concerned with organisation, twenty-five *uchastock* therapists, i.e. three therapists per two *uchastocks*, or one therapist per 2000 population, and about ninety specialists in every branch of medicine and surgery. Even in this situation, with a physically attached hospital, the specialists stick rigidly to working either in the polyclinic or in the hospital. The limitations imposed by such restrictive organisation need no further elaboration.

The type of work encountered by the therapist is predominantly respiratory, cardiovascular, alimentary and rheumatic/arthritic (Vasilperna, 1971), and is similar to my own experience of general practice in the UK. The difficulty in correlating morbidity statistics can be seen in a survey carried out in the town of Stupino (Bobakhoddzaev, 1971), in which there is no mention of rheumatism/arthritis (which is such a dominant feature of most countries throughout the world) and in which angina pectoris is included under the heading of the respiratory rather than the circulatory system. One enormous difference found throughout the entire length and breadth of the USSR is the unusually small attendance rates at the polyclinic for psychoneurotic/anxiety-type illness, which is such a time-consuming factor in primary care in the Western World. It is far from certain whether this is because in a socialist environment the anxieties and tensions which are thought to precipitate or cause such illness do not exist (as the Soviet authorities claim) or because, as the critics would say, such illnesses are not encouraged or even allowed.

Uchastock therapists divide their time between 3½ hours' consultation in the polyclinic, and 2½ hours' domiciliary visiting, averaging perhaps six to eight calls per day (Vasilperna *et al.*, 1971), and similar figures are quoted for different parts of the USSR: between 1967 and 1968 in Rostov-on-Don, Bendery, Orel and Kishinev in the Ukraine, observations were carried out on twelve *uchastock* therapists, showing that they divided their time in the following proportions: 52 per cent in the polyclinic and 48 per cent in domiciliary consultation (Ryan, 1972).

Paramedical support is provided in the polyclinic by the attached nursing sister, who works in a similar fashion to the paediatric nurse. Domiciliary nurses are provided by the Red Cross Organisation. These nurses are trained for one year only, and are mainly used to help old people and the chronic sick. There are usually two Red Cross nurses per *uchastock*, and they provide general care for the patient, washing and housework, help with cooking, collecting medicines and routine 'popping in' on the old or chronically sick.

Industrial health service
This is an essential part of primary care. Most large industrial concerns have their own polyclinic and even a small hospital. Small industrial 'enterprises' cooperate, sharing the use of a polyclinic and its staff. The organisation is similar to the average district polyclinic. The number of medical and paramedical personnel employed is much greater than is usually found in other countries. According to a WHO Fellowship Group: 'a factory employing 10 000 workers has 62 doctors and 161 nurses and nurse-aides, and a factory employing 20 000 work-

ers (with 25 000 dependants) has 135 doctors and 853 paramedical personnel' (WHO, 1960).

The following basic range of prophylactic and therapeutic measures is provided for workers in industry and other special categories.

(a) Study of morbidity among workers (for example coal miners, chemical workers, sportsmen and university and technical teaching staff) and the prevention of various diseases in specific industries.

(b) Checks to ensure that medical and psychological requirements are satisfied in certain dull repetitive work: exercise breaks are now very popular to reduce nervous and muscular stress.

(c) Environmental checks: minimum dust concentration and maximum limits for noise and vibration.

(d) Supervision of selection of workers.

(e) Primary medical care for acute illness or accidents, with treatment and investigation at the factory polyclinic.

(f) Assessment of unfitness for work.

The following are examples of two industrial polyclinics in Irkutsk, capital of East Siberia.

Polyclinic No. 3 (reserved for scientists and staff of institutions and colleges of higher education and research) covered a population of only 8500 and had a high staff ratio: six *uchastock* therapists and twenty specialists, with the usual diagnostic and therapeutic facilities. This was explained by the fact that the patients did not live in one area of Irkutsk, but were spread throughout the city. This gave rise to more home visits because of the greater distance of the polyclinic from the patients' homes: it was estimated that there were twenty domiciliary visits by *uchastock* therapists per day, plus nearly thirty by a nursing sister or *feldscher* under supervision. Perhaps another explanation, not quoted by the authorities, is that scientists, along with other groups such as coal miners, politicians and sportsmen, are given special or privileged care.

Polyclinic No. 1 (in the Kirov district) covered a population of 40 000, working in heavy machinery, plastics, tea-packing and light engineering. The district was divided into fourteen *uchastocks* with a similar number of therapists. Most of the industrial concerns have additional medical posts near the site of work staffed by *feldschers* and nurses. Doctors attend these medical posts for the convenience of patients and the supervision of the *feldschers*; it is obligatory to attend three times a week.

Women's consultative service

This provides comprehensive therapeutic and preventive care for the female population. Each consultative clinic covers a population of up to 200 000, which is considerably larger than either the paediatric, adult or industrial polyclinic. The policy in the future is to try to build such clinics and women's hospitals as one unit. This will help patients and allow a much freer exchange of staff between the hospital and clinic. As a general policy at present, obstetricians and gynaecologists working in the consultative clinic alternate their work on a six-month rota basis, but never work in the hospital and polyclinic at the same time. Basically, the following services are provided:

(*a*) Investigation and treatment of any gynaecological disturbance.

(*b*) Routine ante-natal care during pregnancy, with great emphasis placed on psychoprophylaxis. There is almost a 100 per cent hospital confinement rate in the main urban areas with normal deliveries undertaken by midwives under the supervision of obstetricians. The average length of stay in hospital is between six and ten days. Breast feeding appears to be the rule rather than the exception.

(*c*) The abortion service is not free, and is not encouraged, but is on demand by the patient. The law was re-introduced in 1955 and is interpreted in different ways, in spite of official propaganda. Although few doctors are perturbed about the moral implications of abortion, worries are expressed about the medical complications and problems that can and do arise. There are also wide variations in the different republics, in some of which women are actually discouraged from having abortions. The reason for this is to try to increase the population of the smaller republics. Families with five, six or seven children are common in Uzbekistan, Turkestan, Armenia and Georgia.

(*d*) Contraceptive advice is available, although it is not dispensed with the same evangelical fervour as is currently found in many Western societies. Condoms, caps and spermicides are in common use, while the intra-uterine contraceptive device is becoming more popular. As yet, the contraceptive pill is still regarded with some suspicion, and many doctors remain unconvinced about its long-term safety. Probably, as lower-dose pills become available, they will be used more frequently and eventually pressure will be exerted by the patient.

(*e*) Routine screening for cervical cancer (plus breast examination) is carried out twice every year from the age of twenty years until sixty years. These examinations are carried out in the consultative clinic or in the industrial polyclinic. Are such frequent cervical smears and examinations necessary? Certainly argument continues but, unfortunately, in the USSR, where so many examinations have been performed, it is difficult to discover if any real evaluation of their policy has been carried out.

Rural health services

Quite obviously, it is not possible to provide the same comprehensive organisation of primary care in rural areas. There are two main stages in the provision of medical care for the rural population.

First, this is provided by personnel not qualified as doctors, i.e. a *feldscher*/midwife or a *feldscher* working in a *feldscher*/midwife post. Most villages, communities or collective farms have such posts, depending on the distance from the nearest rural hospital.

The *feldscher*/midwife post is normally staffed by a *feldscher* and a midwife, although often one person combines the two roles. Sited in remote areas, they provide personal and continuing care for a population of up to 2000. There may be maternity beds available (up to five) and a labour room, but this very much depends on the distance of the post from the nearest rural hospital. The work is mainly concerned with minor ailments, preventive inoculations, 'dispenserisation' and the supervision of hygiene and sanitation. Serious illness or anything with which the *feldscher* feels she cannot cope is transferred to the nearest hospital. It is usual for visiting primary care physicians to attend regularly to supervise the *feldscher* and sort out any problems. On some collective farms, a physician may also be found working in conjunction with the *feldscher*.

The second level of care is the responsibility of doctors working in a rural hospital (combined hospital and polyclinic facilities). Such hospitals usually have 20–40 beds, and serve surrounding villages and collective farms within a radius of about ten miles (population 5000–7000). They have a resident staff of primary care physicians and the basic team is composed of paediatrician, therapist, gynaecologist and dentist. Depending on the individual situation, there may be, in addition, a surgeon and a radiologist. There is close cooperation between such hospitals and the nearest district or *rayon* hospital, where specialists are available in emergencies. Road or air transport facilities are usually good and the patient can, of course, be evacuated to the *rayon* hospital when necessary.

Every rural hospital is responsible for a number of *feldscher*/midwife posts which are attached to the hospital: for instance, in Urik in East Siberia, the hospital covers a population of 5000 people and is staffed by a therapist, paediatrician, gynaecologist, surgeon and radiologist, with eighteen nurses and midwives. Eight *feldscher*/midwife posts are attached to the hospital. In this situation, patients are admitted to hospital much more readily than in urban areas (Poblinkov & Litvinova, 1972). To quote from a report on a sample survey taken in 1967/8 on hospitalisation and the higher rate found in rural areas: 'the much broader indications for hospitalisation of rural inhabitants arises from their reduced opportunities to receive qualified extra-hospital care, and the greater return rate of rural inhabitants with one and the same disease' (Romenskii, 1970).

Whatever the reasons, there can be no disputing the facts, and it would seem to me that the bed and staffing ratios were grossly over-inflated.

Emergency medical service

This is a completely separate service from the hospital and polyclinic, staffed by a separate group of doctors who are specially trained for this work. It is universal in urban areas and extremely well organised in all the major cities. Emergency Medical Centre No. 1 in Kiev will be described in detail as a general example of urban emergency care. This is the centre through which all emergency calls pass, and there are eight other satellite centres in different parts of the city, i.e. Kiev, with a population of 1 250 000, has nine emergency centres (Moscow, with a population of 6 500 000, has thirty-three centres). It is accepted that one ambulance car per 10 000 population is necessary, therefore the total in Kiev is 125. The service provides cover for:

(*a*) Emergency calls in general on request from doctors, the general public, police and fire service.

(*b*) A specialised emergency service which is only used after a request by the *uchastock* therapist or paediatrician or from one of their own ambulance cars. It provides specialised ambulances with appropriate equipment for the following categories of emergency: accident and resuscitation, myocardial infarction, maternity (with incubator for neonates), acute psychoses and poisoning.

(c) Transportation of non-urgent cases to hospital.

Staffing and equipment

There is a special training for three months before entering the service, and physicians are not usually accepted until they have done at least three years' postgraduate work following the initial year's internship after qualification. Once in the service, they spend two months every year in hospitals as a continuing training and education. The only exceptions to this rule are the cardiologist and anaesthetists working in the coronary care ambulance, who also work regularly in hospital.

Each ambulance car contains simple equipment, for example nitrous oxide with oxygen mixture, oxygen, splints, emergency drugs; it has one doctor, one *feldscher*, one nursing orderly and one driver. The specialist ambulances are similarly staffed, but obviously contain additional equipment according to the type of service, for example electrocardiograph, defibrillator, anaesthetic equipment, plasma and incubator.

Initially, all incoming calls come through to Centre No. 1, a system that is usual throughout the USSR. Similarly, dialling '03' is universal. Calls are received by a team of eight receptionists who take the messages; they are simultaneously recorded on tape in case of mistakes and are then passed to a doctor. He decides what action to take and which of the peripheral emergency centres to contact. He is also available for advice should it be thought unnecessary to send out an ambulance. Working alongside the doctors are a further four receptionists: one has direct contact with all city hospitals so that emergency warning can be given about impending admissions; another has a direct line with the police, gas and electricity departments, and the remaining two help the doctor and recheck calls. In another room, and quite separate, a further receptionist deals solely with arranging non-urgent admissions to hospital. Unnecessary use of the service is estimated at 15 per cent.

In a rural area, the emergency service is based on the rural hospital, with one ambulance covering roughly the same population as in urban areas. Sometimes very large distances are involved, and in these cases the flying doctor service is used, particularly in West and East Siberia and in the Soviet Far East. Ambulance aircraft are subordinate to the *oblast* hospital, but the patients may be taken to either the *oblast* or *rayon* hospital, whichever is appropriate in the circumstances. Doctors, who always accompany these aircraft, are supplied from the hospital and not the emergency care service.

Medical education and primary care

The Soviet system of medical education presents some specific features, and to understand these fully it is necessary to understand the objectives of the whole health service in its organisation. The emphasis on the integration of curative and preventive measures, on the special needs of certain groups of the population, such as mothers, children and industrial workers, and the need for large numbers of specialists in all branches of curative and preventive medicine, has resulted in a system of training which differs from the usually accepted practice in other parts of the world. (WHO, 1960)

Since 1930, medical education has been the responsibility of the Ministry of Health, and it is not the concern of universities but of separate, independent medical institutes. On admission the student must choose between three different faculties – general medicine, paediatrics or hygiene. The curriculum, which is uniform throughout the country, lasts six years and is followed by one intern year. Students showing exceptional talent in their undergraduate studies, or absolute reliability and conformity in their political views, are rewarded by admission to a research or teaching institute; otherwise, they serve a compulsory three years in the rural health service.

Postgraduate training for primary care physicians is entirely hospital-orientated, which seems strange in a country so conscious of the importance of first-contact care. It is equally inappropriate when it is recognised how little clinical responsibility is expected from the *uchastock* therapist or paediatrician. Many physicians have expressed their dissatisfaction with their postgraduate training, which is entirely organised by hospital specialists, while others have intimated that within the present framework of primary care organisation, only by combining hospital and polyclinic duties could their interest be maintained and job satisfaction regained.

The Union Ministry of Health, moreover, has stipulated that district physicians shall spend prescribed periods working in hospital; for a district paediatrician, the fixed period is (or was in 1965) three to four months of every 1½ to 2 years. But this norm seems to be honoured more in theory than in fact; one district paediatrician writing to *Meditsinskaya Gazeta* asserted that she had an opportunity to work in the adjacent hospital for only three months every three to five years. She recommends a return to an earlier system whereby the district doctor worked in hospital for two hours every day, after which she went to the polyclinic and then out in the district. Without such an involvement in stimulating clinical work, the correspondent concluded today's district physician is 'threatened with transformation into a qualified dispatcher'. (Ryan, 1972)

Finally, mention can be made of the view that the pendulum should swing back from the narrow specialist towards a broadly trained physician of first contact. This school of thought was represented in a letter to *Meditsinskaya Gazeta* which included the following assessment:

It is no secret that unwise use of the specialisation principle frequently results in the patient trapesing from one specialist to another, each giving this or that prescription, which are at times contradictory. Here then is the question: Who should summarise and generalise the findings received from different specialists? In my opinion, the district *terapevt*. In addition, it seems to me that the district doctor can be not only a *terapevt* but a doctor of any specialty, possessing high organisational qualities, along with a wide knowledge in the area of internal medicine

Personal assessment

Whatever criticisms are levelled at the Soviet Health Services, no-one can dispute that primary medical care is available and accessible to the entire population. This is a phenomenal achievement, particularly when considered in relation to the ruin and chaos immediately following the 1917 Revolution, as well as the purely logistic difficulties in such a vast country. It must be recognised that the USSR has gone a long way to solving the organisational problems of primary care in large urban areas which, after all, remains a major problem in most industrialised countries. But, with regard to continuity (the third essential component of primary care) the situation is less promising. The inevitable fragmentation of care, which is a direct consequence of the present organisation, may be too high a price to pay for total preventive and therapeutic care. With the pattern of disease changing from the acute to the chronic, incurable, degenerative problems of middle age, it would appear to be more essential than ever to have a primary care physician who can assess the needs and requirements of the whole family. As has already been seen, there is a dissatisfaction amongst some doctors, who are unhappy with the present role of the district doctor. But what is the likelihood of change? Almost none, as this questioning appears only to involve the *uchastock* therapists themselves and as yet has not permeated the establishment of Soviet medicine. My opinion, after talking to a considerable number of primary care physicians in many parts of the USSR, is confirmed by a report which states

> The need to enhance the status of the *uchastock* doctors is increasingly recognised. For example the Ukrainian Minister of Health recently stated, 'it is necessary to make the work of the *uchastock* doctor more interesting and feasible'. The mainstream of current thinking appears to be that he shall develop his responsibilities *vis-à-vis* other specialists becoming in some sense a counter balance to them. One example of this school of thought is provided in the following quotation, 'The *uchastock* doctor must bring together and evaluate the specialist's combined findings. He alone can have comprehensive information knowing better than others the anamnesis of the illness and the patients' life history, his occupational path, style of living, psychogenetic factors and so on.' And what does the patient feel? This is very difficult to find out, but there are occasional murmurings in the Soviet press, particularly concerned with the problems patients experience when they are needlessly pushed from one doctor to another. (Bradshaw, Ryan & Thomas, 1975)

What lessons can be learnt? As in all things it is a matter of assessing priorities and discovering what is needed within the context of a particular society. Although Soviet health planners may not recognise that the comprehensive nature of their primary care service produces problems, there is now evidence that some patients and some primary care physicians are more aware of the situation than the Ministry of Health in Moscow. It is perfectly possible for one family to be attending four separate primary care institutions at the same time: grandmother at the *uchastock* polyclinic, mother at the women's consultative clinic, father at the industrial polyclinic and one of the children at the paediatric polyclinic! Furthermore, it is possible for a worker to attend both the *uchastock* and industrial therapist at the same time, without informing either, although the authorities say this rarely happens.

There is no doubt, however, that the personnel from the three separate divisions of adult primary care never meet and, for that matter, rarely communicate with each other about a patient. Perhaps the authorities would benefit by giving consideration to the role of a 'generalist' family physician instead of the present tripartite structure. Certainly there is an opportunity and need for some experiment.

Within the polyclinic system, both adult and paediatric, the registration of patients, the use of the same folder for a patient's notes by both specialist and primary care physician, the ease of access to X-ray, laboratory and physiotherapy departments, the ease of referral to specialists, and the continuation of home visits are all excellent features from which many countries can draw lessons.

It is also of interest to study the Soviet attitude to old age.

> In planning the volume of work in a polyclinic concerned with people aged 60 and over, one shall consider from 69 to 70 visits per person per year as necessary. Because of general weakness and limited mobility an essential part of medical care should be rendered at home. For people aged 60 and over 24–35 per cent of visits are home visits and for those aged 80 years and over 50 per cent of all are home visits. 45 per cent of home visits by therapists are to people aged 60 and over. Expansion of medical care at home will be achieved by increasing the number of visits by paramedical personnel. (Revutskaya, 1975)

It would be difficult to name one country in the world whose old people would not benefit from such a realistic approach.

It is axiomatic that good primary care cannot exist without an adequate secondary level of care, and in this respect the USSR is fortunate in the organisation of the hospital service, with its rational approach to the differing levels of specialist care so that there are few gaps in the service.

My main criticism lies in the apparent lack of assessment throughout the entire service, with its almost blind faith in the directions and planning of the Ministry of Health in Moscow. Is it necessary to go on producing doctors at the rate of 43 000 to 44 000 per year? Is it necessary or desirable to examine obviously fit children so frequently? Is the 'dispenserisation scheme' worth the time and manpower involved? Is the aim of extending this scheme even further to cover the whole population desirable or even useful? If the answers to these questions are yes, then is it a profitable way (in a non-economic sense) for doctors to spend their time? Are twice-yearly cervical smears necessary?

Surely it is an unnecessary luxury for a nurse always to accompany the *uchastock* therapist or paediatrician on home visits? If a nurse or *feldscher* can do initial home visits in rural areas, why not, under supervision, in urban areas? Could not a more useful role be found for nursing staff in urban polyclinics? Is the disturbingly high hospital admission rate (particularly in paediatrics and rural areas) really necessary?

The Soviet authorities are unwilling or unable to answer these questions. It is, therefore, extremely difficult to decide whether, in fact, any evaluation of the service is taking place and this, in turn, makes it almost impossible to make any reasoned judgements about the future.

7

EASTERN EUROPE

The boundaries between Eastern and Western Europe have been in a state of continuous flux throughout the last hundred years. But, following the end of the Second World War, eight countries came under the influence of the USSR, both politically and economically, and instituted a form of government known as a People's Democracy. For this reason they are now considered as a definite political entity. The countries are Albania, Bulgaria, Czechoslovakia, the German Democratic Republic, Hungary, Poland, Romania and Yugoslavia. Since the immediate post-war period, Albania has turned exclusively to the Republic of China for help and support, while Yugoslavia has adopted a totally independent policy towards the USSR.

There is considerable ignorance about the lives of over a hundred million of our fellow Europeans (9 per cent of the world's population). Understandably, much to their irritation and sometimes despair, these intensely individualistic and talented peoples, each with their own language, culture and tradition, are merely grouped together as part of the 'Communist bloc', without any consideration of their separate identities. In relation to medical services, however, there is some excuse for taking this view because to a visitor it is extremely difficult to appreciate the more subtle differences and nuances in organisation and delivery of medical care which occur in these countries.

Before the Second World War, the influence of German medicine was strong, particularly in Czechoslovakia, Hungary and northern Yugoslavia, with its rather remote attitude to patients and its autocratic, hierarchical organisation in the universities and hospitals. Everything changed with the chaos which followed the Second World War,

187

accompanied as it was by the rapid expansion of Soviet influence. In the field of health care, there has been debate, both within and without Eastern Europe, as to whether the Soviet system is appropriate for countries so different and diverse in their historical perspectives as well as in their previous levels and organisation of medical care. Such argument is totally academic, for the situation is unlikely to change radically in the foreseeable future. The USSR was in a good position to advise on the organisation and building up of a medical service from nothing, following their experience of the post-revolutionary period 1917–23. They were able to identify essential priorities – maternal and child care, the control of infectious and communicable disease, preventive medicine in its widest context and, later, a strong industrial health service. The governments of Eastern Europe were able to carry out such policies which were to the great benefit of the mass of the population, even if there was inevitable opposition from some pre-war physicians.

Theoretically, the attitudes of people and society in general should have changed over the last twenty-five years with the advent of a socialist society, but people cannot be separated from their past and, consequently, some traditions die slowly. Although the relationship between doctor and society, doctor and patient, and doctor and other health workers is entirely different from pre-war days, it is difficult to decide how fundamental these changes have been. Certainly patients accept free access to medical care as normal, and no longer is the physician placed on a pedestal, yet, in spite of doctors being salaried, the doctor/patient relationship remains intact and does not appear to depend on the exchange of money as so many people maintain; this is my opinion, after attending numerous primary care physicians both in consultation sessions and in home visits. And, contrary to popular belief, private practice is permitted to a varying extent. In Hungary and Poland, full-time state-employed doctors are permitted to practise privately out of hours provided permission is granted from the health authority. In the German Democratic Republic private practice is also legal and widespread, while in Czechoslovakia it is restricted to retired physicians. Only Bulgaria and Romania have forbidden private practice by law.

> In general, these countries (Czechoslovakia, Hungary and Poland) are experiencing the same trends, patterns of morbidity and causes of death that are evident in all so-called 'developed' countries. If birth

rates in the range of 13–18 and death rates of 10 and under (per 1000 population) are indicative of social progress, if a rising prevalence of chronic degenerative disorders and falling incidence of acute infectious diseases reflect improved standards of living, if lengthening life-spans for women (but not as decisively for men) are hallmarks of the 'have' nations, then these three countries must be so characterized. Such status is all the more remarkable in view of the severe economic handicaps with which the new regimes got under way in 1945.

While annual statistics on causes of death indicate there is still something of a time lag between these Eastern European countries and the more affluent Western countries, the emergence of cardiovascular and neoplastic diseases as the prime killers and cripplers of the population defines the major current tasks facing the new medical care systems.

Behind such disease statistics lie the hard facts of modern industrial, urban, 'civilised' life, which have been identified as major health problems by authorities in Budapest, Prague and Warsaw as sharply as by those in Washington, London and Stockholm. A special word should be added to this discussion on health standards concerning the problem of housing. In each of the countries visited, the shortage of housing for urban families was designated as a major – perhaps the major – domestic issue. This involves not only the unavailability of apartment units and the inadequacy of space within such units, but also a lack of privacy, tranquility and aesthetic surroundings. The relationship of poor living standards to emotional disorders, antisocial behaviour, the transmission of infectious disease, and the difficulty of home care for the acute or chronically ill is all too obvious. (Weinerman, 1968)

Such remarks apply equally well to Bulgaria, the German Democratic Republic, Romania and Yugoslavia (there is no information concerning Albania), and illustrate the problems facing their primary care services.

Financing of health care

The financing of health care differs considerably and these differences are directly related to the extent of compulsory health and social insurance which existed in these countries before the accession of their Communist party governments. Bulgaria and Romania, before the Second World War, were very poor agrarian countries, with virtually no health insurance and appalling health statistics; infant mortality varying between 179 deaths per 1000 live births in Romania and 147 in Bulgaria. Not surprisingly the financing of health services since the end of the Second World War has been largely a government responsibility, amounting to 96 per cent in Bulgaria (1973) and 81 per cent in Romania (1968), while insurance payments in both countries were less than 1 per cent. On the other hand, the German Democratic Republic and Hungary had extensive compulsory sickness insurance for the majority of manual and white-collar workers and their families, which were as comprehensive and developed as in most countries of Western Europe. Consequently, social insurance provides a considerable proportion of health finance – 48 per cent in the German Democratic Republic (1968) and 46 per cent in Hungary (1968), with Poland and Czechoslovakia occupying an intermediate position – 13 per cent and 23 per cent respectively (1973) (Kaser, 1976).

Organisation of health service

All Eastern European countries, with the exception of Yugoslavia, have faithfully followed the organisational pattern of the Soviet Health Service, at national, regional or provincial, district and community levels. This applies both to the political participation in health matters as well as the structural organisation. All policies are decided centrally by the Ministry of Health in conjunction with the overall planning laid down by the national governments. In addition, they have adopted, within the possibilities of their own countries, the principle of primary, secondary and tertiary levels of care in a logical attempt to rationalise the use of manpower and resources.

Principles and objectives of socialist public health services.

(a) Health care and treatment of the sick are not merely a personal concern for the individual member of society. They are equally the responsibility of the state.

(b) All health services should be free and accessible to the whole population.*

* This objective was not reached for many years; the rural populations and self-employed farmers being largely excluded. In 1966, a fully comprehensive and available service was introduced by law into Czechoslovakia; in 1968 in the German Democratic Republic and Romania; in 1971 in Bulgaria; in 1974 in Poland; and, finally, in 1975 in Hungary (Kaser, 1976).

(c) The health service is unified. All health institutions come under the Ministry of Health regarding organisation and methods of work. Health planning is decided at national level, but the operative management of such policies is delegated and entrusted to the district and community levels.

(d) A distinctive feature is the stress laid on preventive medicine (particularly certain priority groups, for example mother and child, industrial workers) and health education.

(e) Involvement of the public in the active participation of local health measures is essential, for it is realised that the health service could not function adequately without the interested support of the general public through the Red Cross and trade unions.

Such basic principles apply to all Eastern Europe. The primary care services of three of these countries will now be described in rather more detail.

BULGARIA

Amongst the countries of Eastern Europe, Bulgaria is perhaps the most orthodox in its association with the USSR, and this applies to its health service. It has a population of 8 100 000, over a million living in the capital, Sofia, and at the present time about 42 per cent of the population are urban dwellers. In 1939, it was a backward peasant country with only a rudimentary health care system, and in the space of almost forty years great strides have been made in matters of health. Poliomyelitis, malaria and diphtheria are diseases of the past. The death rate has fallen from 13.4 (per 1000 population) in 1939 – probably more than this, but the returns were incomplete in those days – to 9.4 in 1973. Life expectancy was only 51.7 years in the period 1935–9, while between 1969 and 1971, it had reached 71.1 years. Infant mortality rates have dropped from 138.9 per 1000 live births in 1939 to 25.9 in 1973. The number of physicians increased from 3516 to 17 601 between 1944 and 1973, and the number of qualified nurses from 372 to 29 681. Such are some of the bare statistical facts.

The service has been free for the entire population, except for a small tax on prescriptions, since 1971. Private practice is forbidden, but it should be noted by rigid devotees of a 'free' health service that in country districts a small token payment is levied from the patient if the doctor considers the call to be unnecessary, or should routine treatment be demanded out of hours. The money is paid to the doctor and patients can appeal against the decision, although most seem to consider these payments to be perfectly reasonable. A small payment is also required for a termination of pregnancy on non-medical grounds.

Primary care

Since 1968, there has been a real attempt to provide similar care in both rural and urban areas, even if the organisation is inevitably different. The basic health team, which is responsible for 4000–5000 people, consists of:

(*a*) internist and one nurse who look after the adult population;

(*b*) paediatrician and two nurses caring for children up to 15 years;

(*c*) gynaecologist providing care for two or three health teams (i.e. population varying from 8000–15 000 people), who is assisted by a number of midwives;

(*d*) dentist and assistant.

In each urban health team, doctors work on a shift system of seven hours, and therefore there are two internists and two paediatricians working in rotation: one working at the centre in the morning while the other does home visits, and vice versa in the afternoon. The emergency out-of-hours work is carried out largely by another special team of internists and paediatricians working from the nearest polyclinic. Depending on the local situation, the health team works whenever possible from a neighbourhood polyclinic.

The next level of care in the urban community is the polyclinic, which covers a population of 30 000–50 000: in other words, serving between six and twelve health teams. They provide primary care for the urban population as well as specialist referral facilities. Rural patients requiring specialist treatment may use either the nearest district hospital or polyclinic, whichever is more convenient. Polyclinics contain all the basic specialties and diagnostic departments. Some are attached to hospitals but, for the most part, they are physically separate. Specialists do not combine work in the polyclinic and the hospital: they work in a rota, nine months in the polyclinic and three in hospital. There is, therefore, no continuity of care by specialists between the out- and in-patient care. Polyclinic 15 in Sofia covers a population of 32 000 with six health teams. There are eleven specialists, also X-ray, pathology and physiotherapy departments. Patients are referred to specialists by members of the health team, or they may go directly.

In rural areas it is impossible to have such a team, and in these situations there is one doctor (similar to a general practitoner as in Denmark, the Republic of Ireland, Norway and the UK), one dentist, a midwife, nurse and/or *feldscher*. They work from a health centre. The doctor is on call all the time and off-duty is arranged mutually with the nurse or *feldscher*.

Rural health centres

Visits were made to a number of these centres and the following are given as examples.

The first centre was at Lopian, a village on the northern foothills of the Balkan mountain range about 100 miles from Sofia. The nearest hospital at Botevgrad was a journey of fifty minutes by ambulance. The population was about 2700 including two smaller outlying villages. The actual centre was in a modern building which had been built since the war. It was clean and had all the basic equipment including two maternity beds for normal confinements and a dispensary with the necessary day-to-day drugs. In addition to the basic medical staff already mentioned, there was an ambulance driver to take the doctor on home visits and patients to hospital. All surgical emergencies were dealt with in the district hospital at Botevgrad, and such an arrangement was usual in all rural areas.

The other centre was at Polikraistle, a rather larger village of about 3000 inhabitants with a surrounding population of 1500, situated 16 miles from the nearest hospital at Turnovo, the old capital and a town of fantastic natural beauty in the centre of Bulgaria. Here the staffing was slightly increased, the additions being three *feldschers* and a nurse. The working day in such rural centres was as follows: 08.00–12.00 hours and 16.00–17.00 hours, consultations at the centre; 13.00–15.00 hours, home visits. Average attendance figures at Polikraistle were given as twenty-five consultations and four to five home visits daily.

Industrial health service

This service is now very comprehensive, with separate polyclinics supplementing the basic health service to a considerable extent. Particular interest is taken in women and adolescent workers. Arrangements are made for all ante-natal care and cervical smear examinations to be carried out at the industrial polyclinic and, more recently, 'dispenserisation schemes' (similar to the USSR) have been introduced. These polyclinics are sited at large industrial concerns or may be shared by a number of smaller factories.

Type of work at primary care level

As in the rest of Eastern Europe and the USSR, the care of the population is divided between therapist, paediatrician and gynaecologist. There is exactly the same emphasis on preventive medicine, with the routine examination of babies and children, immunisation programmes, cervical cytology, ante-natal care and the introduction and spread of the 'dispenserisation scheme', initially within the industrial health service but in the hope of eventually extending it to cover as much of the population as possible.

> Since 1972, the Ministry of Health has embarked on a pilot project in the Gabrovo District, with the object of identifying new approaches to health care delivery and of evolving an even more efficient system of organisation of the health services. Gabrovo is a major textile producing centre, and considerable emphasis in the project has, therefore, been placed on the control of occupational diseases, especially those caused by noise and vibration. The entire population, about 200 000 in number, is subjected to health check-ups aimed at differentiating between persons who, although apparently in good health, are probably suffering from a particular disease, and persons who are free from disease. All those found to be suffering from a disease and 'at risk' groups, including all women, receive care under the 'dispenserisation scheme'. Children under fifteen years of age and women are required to undergo these compulsory examinations once every year, while men are examined every two years. Workers are examined two or three times every year, or at even more frequent intervals if necessary.
>
> Another objective of the Gabrovo project is to introduce working methods which will relieve qualified medical personnel of certain tasks that can be entrusted to auxiliaries. (Ezban, 1975)

The spectrum of disease presented to the internist and paediatrician of the health team are similar to other developed countries in Europe. They have easy access to X-ray, electrocardiography, pathology and physiotherapy facilities; specialist advice is readily attainable. There is no discouragement of home visits. There are problems though in relation to the status of the primary care physician, his relationship with the specialist working in the polyclinic, the use of specialists as first-contact doctors, and the dangers of fragmentation and duplication of care because of the separation of medical services at the primary level. But these difficulties are not confined to Bulgaria; they exist in the other countries under consideration, and will therefore be discussed in general terms at the end of the chapter.

Health education is regarded as a social and professional obligation for all doctors – clinicians as well as public health workers – and particularly primary care physicians (Gargov, 1970). Every doctor is obliged to carry out health education in his daily work and contact with people, consisting of advice regarding smoking, exercise and overeating. District paediatricians are responsible for carrying out this work in schools, while industrial therapists spend a great deal of time lecturing and advising workers. The volume and content of health propaganda obviously depends on local needs, and the director of every health establishment – hospital, polyclinic, health centre – is responsible for health education in the region served and has a special programme for this purpose. How successful such policies have been is difficult to say, but there is no evidence to suggest that they are any more effective than in the rest of the world.

Medical education and primary care

There is no specific training for primary care in the undergraduate curriculum over and above the courses on social and preventive medicine taught in the fifth and sixth years, even though primary care is recognised as a specialty – in theory at least.

> Front line care puts complicated and responsible tasks to the doctor in connection with the health of the individual, the family and society. The district physician must have a broad medical culture, and be trained in prevention, early diagnosis, rapid and efficient therapy. He has to deal with medical and social problems. 'Dispenserisation', sanitation of the environment, health education and psychological methods are exceptionally important in his work. The requirements for the constant improvement of his qualifications are increasing. (Bratanov & Vulchev, 1966).

It is believed that the therapist and the paediatrician in urban areas, the general practitioner in the village, and the therapist in the industrial health service all have different tasks to perform, and therefore all require different postgraduate training programmes. How far this has been achieved is open to question. It is relatively easy to pinpoint the problem, but much more difficult to produce a satisfactory answer and, at least on the evidence available, this has not occurred. It would seem that the postgraduate courses for primary care physicians are, in fact, stereotyped and too hospital- and specialist-orientated. Again, not a problem unique to Bulgaria!

CZECHOSLOVAKIA

Lying at the heart and centre of Europe, with Prague a living architectural reminder of the past eight hundred years of European civilisation, Czechoslovakia has had a chequered history, involving loss of independence in 1620 after the Thirty Years War, followed in the nineteenth century by a gradual revival of autonomy against the Austro-Hungarian Empire. In 1918, Czechoslovakia was re-established as an independent state, but for all too short a time. There followed the disgrace of Munich, the terror of the Nazi occupation, the eventual withdrawal from the influence of Western Europe at the end of the Second World War and the formation of the Socialist Republic of Czechoslovakia in 1949.

The Charles University in Prague was founded in 1348, the first to be established in Central Europe, and from the very beginning it had a medical faculty. In 1135, the first hospital was built in Prague, so there has been a long tradition of medical care – in fact, more than in most of the other countries of Eastern Europe. In addition, the concept of social and health insurance goes back to 1888 when assistance was organised for workers and their families during illness, maternity and old age with an attempt at expansion in the years between the two World Wars. Since 1951, the health services have been organised along the lines of the People's Democracies of Eastern Europe, and in 1966 a new health care law was passed which further expanded the public health service, particularly stressing the relationship between living and working conditions and health, and the importance of the individual in accepting responsibilities over health matters in his local community (MOH, Prague, 1966).

The health services are planned. Long term plans for fifteen years, five year plans and plans for the next year are worked out. Being part of the state economic plan, the health plan has the force of law. Thus it is possible to train and place medical personnel according to the needs of the population and the national economy, to modify the health institutes and to provide the funds and equipment necessary for the work of the health services. It was possible substantially to improve in a planned fashion, within a short time, the health care for certain groups of the population, especially children, and to eliminate the main shortcomings of the health services in formerly neglected areas of the country. For example, in Slovakia since 1949 the rate of increase in the number of hospital beds has been three times that in Bohemia and Moravia, and the increase in the number of doctors twice as rapid. Forty per cent of all funds is spent on building health institutions in Slovakia. Since the beginning of 1949 the number of doctors in the industrial area of Ostrava has tripled, although on a national scale, the number of doctors has only doubled. (Stich, 1962)

How successful in fact has the Czechoslovak Health Service been? Certainly there have been enormous advances in the standard of health care as shown by the usual criteria. An increase in life expectancy from 54.9 (male) and 58.7 (female) in 1938 to 67.8 (male) and 73.6 (female) in 1965, a decline in infant mortality from 33.5 in 1957 to 21.4 in 1972 and maternal mortality from 0.63 to 0.17, these are the cardinal signs of an 'advanced' country, coupled with the increasing problem of the degenerative diseases of middle age.

The population of 13 750 000 has remained almost static over the last fifteen years: this would seem to have been possible because of the general policy and widespread acceptance of 'abortion on demand'. The country is made up of the Czech Socialist Republic (Bohemia and Moravia with a population of approximately ten million) and the Slovak Socialist Republic (with just under four million population). At the present time there are six cities with populations of more than 100 000, the largest of which are Prague, Bratislava and Brno. Administratively, both politically and medically, there is a similar pattern to the rest of Eastern Europe. The country is divided into eleven provinces (or regions): seven in the Czech Republic, three in Slovakia, with Prague counted separately – each composed of a little over one million people. From a health service point of view, Bratislava is considered as a separate region, so there is a total of twelve. At this level, the main medical institution is a Type III hospital, usually with more than a thousand beds and including all specialist and super-specialist services. Patients are either referred directly from polyclinics in different parts of the region, or from other less specialised hospitals. Tertiary care takes place at regional level which is divided into districts (*okre*) with populations varying between 50 000 and 200 000, providing secondary care through district hospitals (Type

II, containing 500–1000 beds, including all major specialties and Type I, with 100–500 beds, providing only facilities for internal medicine, paediatrics, obstetrics, gynaecology and surgery). The districts are finally subdivided into 20–40 health communities which are the base line of the health service, and in fact are the level at which primary care facilities are provided.

All services are free, although there are small charges for prescriptions for children, pregnant women and the elderly, and the patient must pay for emergency treatment given as a result of drunkenness. Private practice is definitely 'frowned on' and is virtually restricted to specialists in hospital, a few polyclinics and retired physicians.

Primary medical care

It is a densely populated country with good transport facilities to connect towns with rural areas. The population is distributed fairly evenly throughout the country and, as a result, there is little difference in the organisation of primary care in town or country.

The urban and rural population is organised on the basis of the health community system, in which each community has on average 3750 people and is under the supervision and care of the health community doctor (internist) who looks after the adult population. Working with him and under his administrative control are a community paediatrician, a gynaecologist and a dentist. The paediatrician usually provides care for two health communities, while the gynaecologist covers five or six. The heads of the appropriate departments in the local hospital or polyclinic are responsible medically for giving advice and help to the health community internist, paediatrician and gynaecologist. Specialists from the polyclinic can be called in by the health community team to help with any difficult diagnostic problem.

The community doctor works, as do the paediatrician and gynaecologist, from the community health centre, which is a building with only the basic requirements for clinical examination, and no X-ray, pathology or physiotherapy facilities.

There are separate consulting rooms for the internist, paediatrician and gynaecologist. Each doctor has his own nurse who does the secretarial work, dressings, injections and also accompanies him on domiciliary visits. If the health centre in a scattered rural area is not easily available, then medical posts are established in the outlying villages. These are visited on a regular basis by the community doctor, and similar centres are set up in the paediatric and women's services. In some urban situations, the health community team works from the neighbouring polyclinic, and is in direct liaison with the appropriate specialist departments. When primary care doctors are based on the polyclinic, this has for them the added advantage of easy access to X-ray, pathology and physiotherapy departments. The community doctor is responsible for the curative and preventive care of the adult population in his area. The pattern of disease does not appear to differ very much from other developed countries, and the curative work is carried out either at the health centre or the patient's home. There is no discouragement of home visits. The 'dispenserisation scheme' is limited to the follow-up of certain chronic diseases (hypertension, diabetes and ischaemic heart disease).

As in other socialist countries, there is a well-developed industrial health service which caters for the working population. Patients are free to consult either the factory doctor or the health community doctor according to convenience or preference. The factory health centre has much the same facilities as the community health centre, but the doctor concentrates his attention more on preventive and 'dispenserisation' work, health education and the general supervision of the factory. He deals only with very minor accidents or illness. Industry is divided into three categories: the first includes coal mining, heavy metal and chemical plant, the second engineering, and the third all remaining industry. The number of doctors varies according to the category. 'Current goals aim at ratios of one industrial physician for every 1000 workers in mining, for every 1400 in heavy industry and for every 2000 in other activities.' (Weinerman, 1969) To most Western observers, such staffing ratios are exceptionally high and the problem of boredom must surely be present as a health hazard to the doctors themselves! Surely this is an extravagant and wasteful way to employ such skilled personnel.

Czechoslovakia has a well-organised paediatric health service, encompassing both curative and preventive medicine. The community paediatrician and the paediatric nurse look after the children in two or three health communities (varying between 1000 and as many as 3000 children). The average figure is 1650 which is still considered too high, and will presumably be reduced in the coming years to 1100 (Lingeman, 1973).

The work of the paediatrician involves the care of sick children, both in the health centre and in the home, routine examinations, particularly in the first year of life, inoculation programmes, 'dispenserisation', recall of children with chronic disease (rheumatic fever, asthma and congenital defects) and the running of the school health service, except in some areas of Prague and Bratislava where separate school doctors are employed. Kindergartens and *crèches* are also the responsibility of the community paediatrician. It is interesting to note how the attitude of the government towards *crèches* is changing. For years great emphasis has been placed on the importance of *crèches* where children between the ages of six months and three years can attend whilst their mothers are at work. Every district in a town and most villages have at least one *crèche*. The government and the health authorities have encouraged mothers to use these facilities, not that they needed much encouragement, as most mothers are compelled to work for economic reasons. The demand for *crèches* is now as strong in Western countries as in Eastern Europe and the USSR – particularly from the more militant women's organisations. But in Czechoslovakia in recent years young mothers were being actively encouraged to stay at home to look after their children. A new law was passed in September 1971 granting a mother, who temporarily gives up work to look after her child, a weekly payment equivalent to a third of her expected wage had she continued to work, plus the safeguard that she cannot be dismissed from her former job for at least one year. If the family has another child who attends school, then the payments will also continue for a second year. Paediatricians say that this is not enough, but at least it is a start. The Czech experience with *crèches* shows that morbidity is higher in children attending regularly in the first year of life. In addition, there is retardation of emotional development and often speech as well, while physical development (sitting, walking, etc.) is sometimes advanced. Paediatricians had quickly come to the conclusion – certainly by the early 1960s – that *crèches* were a poor substitute for the home, but social pressures, resulting from the economic difficulties of the family, prevented any change until recently (Ošanec, 1973). Such facts may, of course, seem almost too obvious to those who are concerned with the sound upbringing of children.

As in the paediatric field, gynaecology has been established at the primary care level within the health community system. At the present time, one gynaecologist is responsible for five or six health communities averaging about 9000 women. It must be remembered that a considerable amount of ante-natal care and examinations, such as cervical smears and breast examinations, are carried out within the industrial health service, depending on which is most convenient for the patient. A midwife assists with routine nursing and secretarial work, although in some rural areas she carries out most of the clinical work under the supervision of the gynaecologist. The general scope and content of the work is similar to Western countries, involving ante-natal care, general gynaecology and cervical smears. There is almost 100 per cent hospital delivery rate, and any particular problem, such as pre-eclamptic toxaemia, diabetes or suspected placental insufficiency, are referred to the nearest polyclinic or hospital. Contraception still presents a medical problem, as the 'pill' is not in widespread use and 'abortion on demand' is the commonest form of birth control.

> About 30 per cent of pregnancies are surgically interrupted. Of the total number of abortions, some 80 per cent are performed on married women and about 80 per cent are for non-therapeutic reasons. Although the induced abortion rate in Czechoslovakia is considerably below that in Hungary, there is currently much concern at its extent and hope that newer oral and intra-uterine devices can be substituted. (Weinerman, 1969)

The polyclinic follows the same essential pattern as is found in the rest of Eastern Europe. Most of the older polyclinics were built in isolation, but there has been an attempt in recent years to build polyclinics as near as possible to hospitals or, if it is possible, physically attached to them, in order to rationalise the use of specialist staff and integrate out-patient and in-patient care. Patients can go directly to the polyclinic, thus bypassing the primary care physicians in the community health centre. This is one of the unsatisfactory aspects of the polyclinic and will be discussed later in the chapter. Emergency care is organised through the polyclinic, which may be responsible for between 40 000 and 100 000 people. In some rural areas, out-of-hours and weekend work is the responsibility of the health community doctor, who thus finds himself 'on call' much more than his urban counterpart. On the other hand, working in country areas has its rewards and there is a much warmer relationship with patients; the doctor is held in high regard within the community.

Medical education and primary care
Czechoslovakia, unlike the USSR and some of her East Euro-

pean neighbours, follows the usual Western pattern of medical schools being integrated within a university. At the present time, there are nine medical schools, five of which are affiliated with the Charles University in Prague. There are no specific departments concerned with primary care in any of the medical schools, so at the undergraduate level it is the social medicine part of the curriculum which introduces the student to the influence of the family, the environment and various social factors which affect the aetiology and progress of organic disease.

After qualification, every doctor must do one year in hospital as a 'houseman' or 'intern', followed by a further three years in hospital in one of the primary specialties. This leads to first degree certification. A further four years in a subspecialty – cardiology, neurosurgery, ophthalmology, nephrology – followed by appropriate examinations leads to second degree certification. All district doctors must now be trained to second degree level, and there are only a small number of pre-war or early post-war doctors who have not reached this standard. Although this may seem a very satisfactory situation compared with the paucity of training in many Western countries, a large number of district doctors and a few enlightened people in academic circles are far from satisfied with the training (Ošanec, 1973). They believe that it is too hospital-orientated and fails to recognise that primary care is a separate specialty which cannot be considered as merely internal medicine in the community! Whether there will be a radical change in the vocational training of the district doctor remains to be seen. Throughout their whole professional life, all doctors working in the community must spend six weeks working in hospital every three to four years and, whenever possible, must spend half a day every month working in the appropriate hospital department: the only difficulty being that many doctors find it impossible to get away as no locum is provided.

HUNGARY

Although for many hundreds of years Hungary was essentially an 'Eastern' country because of its occupation by the Mongols and later the Turks, its more recent history has been characteristically European, with its incorporation into the Austro-Hungarian Empire in the nineteenth century, and its entanglement in the tragic events of the last forty years. Certainly there was a close association in medicine between Vienna and Budapest, involving such famous names as Semmelweiss and Billroth. Later, Budapest was integrated into the 'German School' at the end of the nineteenth and early part of the twentieth century. The tradition of Hungarian medicine is, therefore, inescapably rooted in the West, and this can be seen in one or two variations on the Eastern European theme of medical care. First, the tradition of the specialty hospital (tuberculosis, children's, cancer, eye and 'spa centres' for all manner of Central European cures) remains and this has inevitably caused an unevenness in the hospital service with gaps and less uniformity in the organisation of secondary and tertiary care than is found in the rest of Eastern Europe, except perhaps in Poland. This is entirely in keeping with the individualistic nature of the people. Second, private practice exists in two forms, even though since 1975 there has been totally free health care for the entire population: there is a prescription charge of 15 per cent per item, with the exception of expensive drugs such as steroids and some antibiotics, while certain groups of patients (old people, children, expectant mothers) can claim a refund. The government allows one hour per day private practice at the end of the day's work, regulates the fees and lays down the required standards for consulting rooms (usually in the physician's own home). Private practice exists mainly among specialists working in the larger towns, although it is also carried out by primary care physicians, almost exclusively in Budapest. As in Poland, where it is also fairly widespread, it is extremely difficult to estimate its extent. The second form that it takes is the giving of 'gifts' and small amounts of money, particularly to nurses and doctors in hospital, and also frequently to those working in the primary care field, where elderly patients seem to feel that doctors are underpaid and in this way hope to show their gratitude. I gained the impression that this practice was not a means of bribing doctors as 'it is alleged to be a remnant of the pre-war system when little decent service was obtainable except with direct payment' (Weinerman, 1969). Rather, it seemed a simple way of giving thanks. Third, the almost equal financing of health care between central government (48 per cent) and social insurance (46 per cent is a reminder that some of its economic policies are firmly rooted in the ideas of Western Europe.

Hungary has a population of just over ten million, two thirds of whom live in rural areas, and two million are concentrated in Budapest. In 1970, the doctor/patient ratio was 1:520 but still there is a shortage of doctors in rural areas, as most would prefer to practise in the capital, or at least in one of the few larger towns such as Debrecen and Szeged. In fact, Budapest with 20 per cent of the population uses 40 per cent of the medical resources and, although this may in part be explained by the fact that patients are referred to various specialist centres from all over Hungary, nevertheless it also means that there is still some maldistribution of manpower and resources.

Primary care
The country is divided into about 3300 health communities or medical districts, each containing about 3000 patients under the care of the district doctor working from a district health centre or, in some situations, from a neighbouring polyclinic. There is no choice of doctor although, in exceptional circumstances, a change can be made. Also working at the district level are the district paediatrician and gynaecologist carrying out the usual curative and preventive work for two (2300 children) and eight (24 000 population) health districts respectively.

District doctors work a seven-hour day, usually in pairs so that consultation hours and home visiting alternate. They may see between thirty and sixty patients in a consultation session, and have perhaps six to ten home visits. Groups of district doctors, usually eight, have been formed for educational purposes, under the supervision of a 'leader' who is generally a specialist internist from the local polyclinic. The success of such groups depends on the enthusiasm of individual members, so that supervision may mean nothing more than a very occasional visit to the district health centre or may involve regular clinical meetings and discussions. The 'dispenserisation' scheme is not so widely followed as in the USSR or in the rest of Eastern Europe.

The district gynaecologist works alongside the district doctor with the assistance of one or two maternity nurses. The work is unremark-able, with a tendency to refer everything but the simplest problem to the hospital or polyclinic. One of the most controversial questions is the very high abortion rate which produces all the well-known difficul-ties, both for the patient and the gynaecological services, as well as a serious demographic problem for the government. Almost all con-finements take place in hospital. In many rural areas it is not possible to divide the responsibility of care between therapist, gynaecologist and paediatrician, and one doctor looks after the whole population. He is a true general practitioner, and these country doctors definitely enjoy the diversity of their work as compared with their city counterparts. The 'status' of doctors in the community is high, as has always been the case in Hungary, even though today the pay is relatively poor, and in country areas they are held in particularly high regard. To offset these professional benefits, it must be remembered that the general social amenities are very poor indeed, and for the doctor's family the pull of Budapest or Debrecen is very strong.

Following the Eastern European system, there is the usual additional general medical service for industrial workers in factories and other large industrial enterprises. The organisational pattern and concern for preventive as well as curative medicine is the same as already described in Bulgaria and Czechoslovakia. An additional feature of the industrial health service is the great number of hospitals or sanatoria which are reserved for special categories of workers, although the number of doctors involved in this work is not quite as high as in Czechoslovakia. 'Dispenserisation' is emphasised rather more than ordinary care, which is normally provided by the district doctor. 'Spas' play an important role in maintaining the health of workers. The therapeutic properties of these springs (particularly surrounding Lake Balaton) are taken for granted, although there is no scientific evidence to support the claims that are made. Nevertheless, they are widely used for such diseases as hypertension, ischaemic heart disease, rheumatism and arthritis – the type of illness so often dealt with under the 'dispenserisation' recall system.

Primary health care – in fact all levels of health care – for children is organised and delivered through a separate system with its own health centres, polyclinics and hospitals: this exactly mirrors the situation found in the USSR, and is different from the rest of Eastern Europe. Whether it has made any difference to the quality of the service or improved the general health of Hungarian children *vis-à-vis* their Polish, Czechoslovak or Romanian neighbours is extremely doubtful. Infant and neonatal mortality remain comparatively high at 33.2 and 27.1 per 1000 live births respectively in 1972. While some blame can be laid at the feet of the obstetric service and the policy of widespread abortion, with a definite relationship between the high incidence of prematurity (about 13 per cent of births) and perinatal and neonatal mortality, the paediatric service has reason to be concerned.

Each district paediatrician is allocated to two health communities (about 2300 children) and he works from a special paediatric health centre covering up to ten communities. In other words, in urban areas up to five community paediatricians may work from the same premises. In the rural areas this is impossible and, in fact, the paediatric work may be done by a 'general practitioner'. The care of children in kindergartens and schools is the responsibility of a separate school health service, but *crèches* and nurseries caring for children up to three years of age continue to come under the orbit of the community paediatrician.

Polyclinics follow the same pattern as in the rest of Eastern Europe, with the exception of paediatrics. They have the same staffing problems owing to their separation from the hospital service, and are often large, containing between 100 and 120 specialists. All emergency services in urban areas are organised by the polyclinic, which may cover a catchment area of 50 000 people or roughly sixteen health communities.

Medical education and primary care

There are four medical schools attached to universities in Budapest, Pécs, Szeged and Debrecen. The undergraduate curriculum is common to all, and consists of two years' pre-clinical, followed by three years' clinical study, with the final sixth year devoted to special vocational training in the major specialties (internal medicine, surgery, gynaecology). Primary care or general practice is not represented as a separate discipline within the curriculum. Nevertheless, each university takes advantage of the experience of local district doctors who contribute either by formal lectures or, occasionally, by involving the students in some 'teaching units'.

Each university has a slightly different approach, and, at the present time, the undergraduate curriculum is under urgent reform. For instance, at the Semmelweis University, Budapest, a recent report stated:

> it is rather a decisive part of the task of the university to educate physicians answering the expectations of society. Teaching and training must reflect two principles: firstly social demand, and secondly change in the progress of medicine. General practice should be built into the curriculum and we estimate the teaching of General Practice as essential. In our experience, the choice of General Practice takes shape only very late by our students. For this reason we are organis-

ing a vocational guidance system in order to help students understand the problems of our health service. We wish to increase a training system in the curriculum which is more orientated towards the public health demands of our country. (Szatmari, 1976)

It will be interesting to watch the progress that is made in Hungary.

General practice has been recognised as a specialty only since 1973, and at present postgraduate vocational training is only optional for those entering general practice. Thus it is perfectly possible for a newly qualified physician to go into general practice without any special training. Again, change is 'in the air', stimulated to a large extent by the Societas Medicinae Generalis Hungaricae established in 1967.

Postgraduate education is formal, and very often without much relevance to the work of the district doctor. It is organised through the National Institute of Postgraduate and Continuous Medical Education, Budapest, and involves four weeks in every five years, the lectures and clinical work usually taking place within the hospital environment.

Personal assessment

Primary care and the specialist services provided in the polyclinic are closely integrated, in the belief that this produces a better service for the patient. The concept of a polyclinic is sound, with ease of referral to specialist colleagues, as well as direct access to X-ray, pathology and physiotherapy facilities. This should enable a larger proportion of illness to be investigated, diagnosed and treated within the community. But what happens in reality would appear to be a long way from this ideal, for not only is there excessive referral to the polyclinic by the district doctor or paediatrician, but also in turn a large number of patients find themselves in hospital who could or should have been dealt with in the polyclinic. This problem arises not because there is anything wrong with the polyclinic principle, but because there is confusion of the role and function of the polyclinic specialist. He does not work in hospital at the same time as providing out-patient care, neither does he have access to hospital beds or responsibility for the patient in hospital. Admittedly, he may work on rotation in the hospital, but this is not the same as looking after the patients that he has seen in the polyclinic. Such limitations are particularly frustrating and obviously have a demoralising effect on him and his attitude to medicine, restricting the type of case with which he can deal. For example, an ophthalmologist can spend most of the day carrying out simple eye tests or treating minor eye conditions, while an experienced surgeon deals with simple casualty work and the occasional inspection of haemorrhoids to brighten his day! Such specialists in fact carry out a great deal of unnecessary work which in most Western countries would be seen and treated by a competent general practitioner. Their function is still further distorted by the fact that patients can consult them directly. This means, in effect, that they are performing tasks which should be carried out by the district doctor, paediatrician or gynaecologist. Lastly, the catchment area of the polyclinic is too small to give the specialists enough experience with the clinical problems that they might expect to encounter. Until the role of the polyclinic specialist is redefined, and the integration of hospital and polyclinic staff is solved, ambulatory out-patient services will be unsatisfactory.

How beneficial is it for the patient to have three separate services at the primary level, with the inevitable fragmentation of care? Certainly it can be argued that the service is accessible and available to everyone, but at the cost of continuity. It is possible for one family to be under the care of three separate doctors – in fact four if the industrial service is included (USSR, p. 184). Does this matter? Apparently many specialists and health planners think it does not. This might well be so if in fact primary care consists merely of a certain basic minimum knowledge of these three specialties, but this view completely misunderstands the nature and scope of primary care (Chapter 2). Of course, it is essential for the primary care physician to have a sound clinical training, but equally primary care physicians should have a much wider concept and understanding of illness than is possible from a specialist point of view. That social, economic, cultural and, most of all, family conditions play an important part in any illness is now universally acknowledged, and so what is needed is a physician who understands and knows the whole family and is thus able to interpret more readily the interplay of these factors on the patient's illness. To divide the care of a family into three is to place almost insurmountable obstacles in the path of the physician.

And what do patients want? In a study of the relationship between the patient and the primary health care team, it was found that

> patients laid great stress on the first-line doctor's role of 'adviser and confidante', and also accorded great significance to how they were

spoken to. The majority of them expected that the doctor would interest himself not only in the complaints they themselves were stating, but also in other personal, family and working problems related to their state of health. We found a close agreement between these views and the expectations of the public and the attitude of the first-line doctors. (Inst. Soc. Med., 1972)

If this is what patients want in Czechoslovakia, and there is nothing to suggest a different response in the rest of Eastern Europe, then this surely is a *cri de coeur* for the return of a general physician who will take responsibility for the whole family and supervise their general medical care.

Within a medical system which repeatedly states that primary care is so important, and one which has also been able to throw off many of the shackles of previous medical orthodoxy, it is disappointing to find that so much reliance and trust is still given to specialisation, to the extent that two thirds of all physicians are 'specialists' working in the polyclinic or hospital service. In addition, poor facilities in the community health centres inevitably lead to a poor level of diagnosis with an enormous amount of unnecessary referrals to the polyclinic and a consequent overloading of this service. Such referrals also give 'ammunition to the specialists' in their criticism of the standard of primary care. And so, regrettably, the status of first-contact doctors is low, particularly amongst students: this is a familiar story throughout the world, and is not confined to these countries. What is so disappointing, though perhaps not surprising, is that these attitudes should continue in these countries and until the myth of specialisation is exploded, there will be no fundamental change.

But it would be quite wrong to give the impression that nothing has been achieved, for the reverse is true. 'Free' medical treatment has eventually been provided for everyone and it is easily available and accessible. This is no mean achievement and there are few countries in the world who can make such claims. Critics of the 'socialist' system of medicine frequently make great play about the lack of choice of doctor, but refuse to admit that there is a similar problem under the 'free market' system, but for very different reasons! If the type of work and level of care at the health centre and polyclinic could be delineated more accurately, thus reducing the number of unnecessary referrals, it would considerably improve the service. Furthermore, if the confusion of function and role between the first-contact physicians and the specialists could also be solved, coupled with the upgrading of the district or community doctor so that he had much more comprehensive care of the family, then Eastern Europe would have a sound comprehensive system of primary care.

8

UNITED STATES OF AMERICA

The United States of America extends 3000 miles from the Atlantic to the Pacific Oceans and 1500 miles from the Canadian border to the Gulf of Mexico, encompassing great geographical and climatic differences: the prairies of the mid-west, the deserts of Arizona and Nevada, the fertile valleys of California, the Arctic wastes of Alaska, the subtropical regions of Florida and the vast urban sprawl extending from Boston through New York to Washington, from Los Angeles to San Francisco, and around the Great Lakes from Milwaukee to Chicago and Detroit. It is estimated that two-thirds of the population live in these spreading conurbations. A highly industrialised country with immense manufacturing expertise and potential, it also has enormous natural resources: coal, oil, natural gas and a wide variety of minerals which, until quite recently, were all thought to be infinite. In addition, highly productive and efficient agriculture – wheat, maize, cotton, rice, tobacco and citrus fruits – has made the USA the richest country in the world.

Inevitably it is a land of contrasts: of affluence, energy, hard work and great technological achievement alongside poverty, social indifference and apathy. The population also reveals differences in tradition, religion and social and cultural values which are a direct result of differing historical backgrounds. Apart from the American Indians, the forebears of this mighty continent were either buccaneers from Spain, explorers and traders from France or Puritans from England. Following them came the slave trade from the west coast of Africa, resulting in the present population of nearly 23 million Negroes, and during the last 150 years the country has become a haven for refugees from every type of tyranny, persecution and natural disaster in Europe. Furthermore, large ethnic groups, including 5 million Mexican-Americans, 2 million Chinese, numerous Puerto-Ricans and Japanese have settled in various parts of the land. Although the pioneering adventure spirit of the early settlers, with their tough, independent individualism which drove men to discover the west coast, appears to have disappeared in the morass of the consumer-orientated, luxury-style, almost mindless extravagance of the twentieth century, nonetheless such ancestors may in part explain the philosophy of American society and, in turn, its attitude to health care: every man should be able to fend for himself and those that are unable to do so have only themselves to blame. This may seem too categorical a statement, but this kind of thinking is reflected in a number of government health programmes.

The USA has a written constitution, a two-chamber legislature – the Senate and the House of Representatives, which together are known as Congress – and an elected Presidential Head of State. It is a federal system of government with three basic levels – federal, state and county (local): each having powers to levy taxes of which the largest is the federal tax. Historically both the federal and local governments are the creation of the states and in a number of respects – legal, social, educational, health and environmental – the states have considerable independence and autonomy. The federal government is thus in a position of relative weakness. This is reinforced by the fact that some laws which are drafted, approved and passed by Congress, are often 'watered down' by powerful pressure groups to such an extent that they can be interpreted by different states in different ways: this has certainly been the case with some welfare and medical legislation (see Medicaid, p. 233).

Demographic and health statistics

The population has grown from 180 million in 1900 to 207 million in 1971 and 213 million in 1976. Like other developed countries there has been a steadily increasing population of the over-65 years: 4.1 per cent in 1900, 6.8 per cent, in 1940, 10.0 per cent in 1968 and nearly 11.0 per cent in 1976. In other words, between 23 and 24 million Americans are over 65 years old and it is estimated that by 1985 the figure will rise to 25 million. During the last five or six years, population growth has been virtually zero with a decreasing population of under-5 years, so the implications of these findings at each end of the age range should be important factors in future health planning.

Of the total population, 75 per cent live in urban and 25 per cent in rural areas. The mobility of people can be gauged from the fact that 37 per cent move their place of residence every five years (Goldsmith, 1977); also refer to Table 1. This pattern of mobility, which has been steadily increasing over the last twenty years, also applies to doctors, and under such circumstances it is more difficult to provide continuity of primary care.

TABLE 1 *Percentage of population who change place of residence by type of change (USA March 1969–70)*

Type of change	Percentage of population
Same county	11.7
Different county	6.7
Within same state	3.1
Between states	3.6
Abroad	0.8

Source: US Department of Commerce. Bureau of Census Population Characteristics. *Census Population Report Series* P-20, No. 210, Table 1, p. 7

In addition, the drift from the rural to urban areas has affected the USA perhaps more than any other developed country and has been further complicated by other factors. After the end of the Second World War, with the increase in the mechanisation of agriculture, a great number of negroes working in the southern half of the country, left the land and migrated to the north in the belief and hope of finding work, and also with the knowledge that more generous welfare programmes existed in that part of the country. They tended to congregate in the poorer 'down-town' areas of large cities and at the same time there was a mass exodus of the middle classes from the decay, pollution, poverty and violence of the inner cities for a 'clean life' in suburbia. Subsequently other minority groups – Mexicans and Puerto-Ricans – have also gravitated to these inner-city ghetto areas. Such changes in population distribution have directly affected the accessibility and availability of primary care as the great majority of doctors now live and work in suburbia.

The USA has one of the highest GNP *per capita* incomes and the second highest unemployment figures amongst the major industrialised countries in the world. The most recent figures of levels of income and the differences between the black and white populations are shown in Tables 2 and 3.

TABLE 2   *Percentage distribution of families and unrelated individuals by income level and colour (1969) Dollars (USA 1950 and 1969)*

Income ($)		Distribution of families (%)	
		1950	1969
Under 3000	White	21	9
	Black	51	20
3000–4999	White	25	10
	Black	30	22
5000–9999	White	42	33
	Black	17	36
10 000 and over	White	12	48
	Black	2	22

Source: US Department of Commerce. Bureau of Census Population Characteristics. *Statistical Abstract of the United States 1971* (Washington DC, 1971), No. 500, p. 318

TABLE 3   *Median main income of families by colour of head of family in constant (1969) Dollars (USA 1950 and 1969)*

		Income ($)	
		1950	1969
	White	5290	9774
	Black	2848	6191

Source: US Department of Commerce. Bureau of Census Population Characteristics. *Statistical Abstract of the United States 1971* (Washington DC, 1971), No. 500, p. 316

On Inauguration Day, 20 January 1977, a leader in the *New York Times* commenting on a report from the National Urban League stated that 'while 10 per cent of whites are in poverty, 31 per cent of blacks live below the poverty line. While blacks comprise 11 per cent of the labour force, they accounted for 20 per cent of unemployment. Mr Carter faces deeply rooted social and economic deprivation, hard-core unemployment, inner-city deterioration and competition between blacks and whites at the lower end of the economic spectrum.'

In all health statistics there are considerable minority/white differences (Table 4). These simple figures show beyond all doubt where one emphasis in medical care should be directed: towards the black and other under-privileged groups.

TABLE 4 *Health statistics*

			1950	1960	1970	1975
Life expectancy	Other	M	59.1	61.1	61.3	62.9
		F	62.9	66.3	69.4	71.1
	White	M	66.5	67.4	68.0	68.9
		F	72.2	74.1	75.6	76.6
Infant mortality	Other		44.5	43.2	30.9	22.9
	White		26.8	22.9	17.8	14.4
Maternal mortality	Other		2.21	0.97		
	White		0.61	0.26	0.22	0.11

Source: Vital Statistics Rates in USA 1940–60. *Monthly Vital Statistics Report: Annual Summary for USA 1975.* Nationa Centre for Health Statistics, Department of HEW

The commonest causes of death are the same as in most other developed countries: heart disease heads the list, followed by malignancy, cerebro-vascular disease and accidents. This merely emphasises the universal problems of 'advanced societies'.

Cost of medical care

It is difficult to dispute the often-heard claim that the cost of medical care is out of control. The facts speak for themselves. In 1950, total health spending amounted to $12 billion (4.6 per cent GNP) or $78 *per capita* per year, and by 1975 it had risen to $118.5 billion (8.3 per cent GNP) or $550 *per capita* per year. Even taking into account the effects of inflation this represents an enormous increase in 'real' money terms. The health service industry now employs nearly 5 million people and it is estimated that by the mid-1980s, it will consume between 10 and 12 per cent GNP if spending is allowed to continue at the present rate.* The increasing involvement of the federal government can be seen from Table 5 and the manner in which personal health care is financed from Table 6.

TABLE 5 *Distribution of national health expenditure: by source of funds (in billion $)*

Source of funds	1966		1974	
	Expenditure (billion $)	% %	Expenditure (billion $)	% %
Private	31.1	74	62.5	60
Federal	5.5	13	28.1	27
State and local	5.5	13	13.6	13
Total	42.1		104.2	

Source: Worthington, N.L., National health expenditures, 1929–1974. *Social Security Bulletin*, Feb. 1975

During the fiscal year 1974, hospitals accounted for 40.9 per cent of national health expenditure, with physicians' services using 19.0 per cent, pharmaceuticals 9.7 per cent and long-stay nursing-home care 7.1 per cent. The remaining 23.3 per cent was shared between dental services, research and medical education.

Between 1950 and 1970 the consumer price index rose by 61 per cent (food 54 per cent, housing 63 per cent, transport 65 per cent) and medical care by 125 per cent. The difference between the general price increases and medical fees has been most marked in the last fifteen years (Table 7).

Clearly expenditure on health cannot continue to increase at the same rate as it has done over the last 15 years and, therefore, a number

* It is impossible to compare directly the GNP between different countries: for instance, in the USA and the UK the former includes nursing, home care (equivalent to Part III accommodation in the UK), medical education, research and private spending, which are all excluded from UK calculations.

TABLE 6   Financing of health care: 1974

	Total (in billion $)	Govern- ment (%)	Private health insurance (%)	Direct payment (%)	Philan- thropy (%)
Hospitals	40.9	53	35	11	1
Physicians'services	19.0	24	37	39	0
Pharmaceuticals	9.7	8	6	86	0
Dental services	6.2	5	9	86	0
Other services Nursing home, Research medical Education	14.5	46	3	46	5

Source: *Current Federal Health Policy Issue*, September 1975, for fiscal year 1974, Department of HEW

TABLE 7   Increase in consumer price index and medical fees

	1960–65	1965–71	1971–74ª	1975
Consumer price index	1.2	4.1	5.5	9.3
Physicians' fees	2.7	6.4	4.2	12.3
Hospital costs	5.9	13.1	6.8	18.0

Source: *Budget Options for Fiscal Year 1977*. A report to the Senate and House Committees on the Budget. Congressional Budget Office. 15 March 1976.
ª During this period the Economic Stabilisation Programme was in operation, which kept hospital costs under some control and actually reduced physicians' fees compared with the price index for the only time in 15 years.

of questions must be asked. Is the USA getting value for money and if not why not? Should society through the federal and state governments say 'enough is enough' and impose a limit on the percentage of the GNP being allocated to health care? Should there even be a cutback on spending? Such questions have never been seriously asked before because in many ways they are alien to the whole philosophy of American society. Until recently, both government and people appeared to believe that every medical problem was solvable provided enough money was spent on research, that better health inevitably meant more money and that in a predominantly free market system an appropriate level of need would be demanded and met. These assumptions have proved to be false, and increasingly it is felt that spending without planning can only lead to out-of-control costs. Similarly, if the physician controls the cost of what he provides for the patient by creating his own demand for investigation, treatment and operation, then two undesirable consequences follow. First, by the simple expedient of over-investigation and over-treatment, combined with a favourable fee-scale, the physician may practise in an over-doctored area without any serious financial disadvantage. Second, in a free market economy the consumer normally has some control over what he buys. Yet with medical care, which in the USA still remains a consumer product, there is no way of knowing whether the patient or society is being sold an essential or non-essential product. There is no protection against professional advice which may be influenced too much by financial considerations. Serious doubts have been voiced for a number of years, and in 1974 the Office of Technology Assessment was set up by Congress 'to help legislative policy-makers anticipate and plan for the consequences of technological changes and to examine the many ways, expected and unexpected, in which technology affects peoples' lives'. Amongst many differing problems, medical technology has been scrutinised, including cardiac transplants and renal dialysis, as well as the more prosaic question of automated laboratory analysis. Unfortunately, the reasons for ordering laboratory investigations, how many are necessary and how far the procedure-orientated method of insurance may have contributed to their enormous growth, has been barely touched upon. Such an omission is strange, particularly when it is recognised that laboratory investigations are increasing by 15 per cent per year and in 1975 amounted to 10 per cent of the total health service budget. Perhaps the reason may be found in the composition of the advisory committee – predominantly technological and procedure-orientated doctors and scientists.

Inevitably

> the United States is allocating resources in such a way that its standards of care are very uneven. While tackling, often in an extravagant way, some problems that are enormously expensive, it neglects to provide some needed and relatively inexpensive services such as

ante-natal care in poorer communities. In the health care field the law of diminishing returns seems to apply: the higher the level of care already prevailing the more expensive becomes the next improvement. The United States is using vast resources at certain points where incremental improvements can be achieved only at great expense while ignoring other points where the ratio of benefit to cost would be more favourable. (Maxwell, 1975)

Health costs are now too large a proportion of the nation's budget to be left solely in the hands of the medical profession and, if it does not cooperate and provide some leadership and objectivity in considering this complex problem of needs and resources, then planning may well be taken out of its hands and its worst fears of government control may be realised. Few people can now disagree with the medical director of Blue Shield California when he stated; 'If we doctors don't demonstrate a genuine concern for the public interests, if we don't determine what it is they really want and try to meet their needs, we don't stand a chance of escaping an imposed monolithic bureaucracy.' (O'Donnell, 1975)

No country illustrates more vividly the dilemmas and paradoxes facing medicine today: that the richest and most powerful country in the world has not provided adequate primary care for all of the poor, the elderly, the chronic sick and the unemployed, and that for a variety of reasons the care which the rest of the population receives is often needlessly expensive, both in investigation and treatment. Numerous estimates have been made as to what percentage of the nation falls into the former group – varying from 20 per cent to 40 per cent according to the statistics and criteria used. To quibble over the accuracy of these figures would appear to be merely an academic luxury and a means by which some sections of society can voice the feelings and fears of many: that health care for everyone would bankrupt the country. Surely what matters is that society recognises that such people exist, that they are clearly identifiable and that their needs should be met. To quote from a Congressional Report in 1972, 'in simplest terms there are men, women and children in the United States for whom doctors, nurses, clinics and hospitals simply do not exist' (DHEW, 1972). Little has changed since that time except that inflation has increased, so if anything the position is more serious.

Particularly in the USA the dramatic advances in medical technology and in scientific research have not been matched by similar advances in the organisation and provision of health services and there has been only a slow awakening to the associated socio/economic problems. The glamour of scientific medicine has encouraged doctors and lured patients into believing that progress in this direction alone would inevitably bring an overall improvement in the nation's health (compare Sweden, p. 165). The fallacy of the belief that if only more money could be spent on further research and hospital medicine then a solution to the health needs of the majority of people would be found, has been finally laid bare. And yet, in spite of the serious and dramatic rise in medical costs, and in spite of the evidence of epidemiologists concerning poverty, nutrition, housing and employment, as well as the benefits of an alteration in personal patterns of living, the general public refuse to accept the facts.

Background to present position of health care

A brief survey of the influence of the last 75 years may help to identify some of the reasons for the inadequacies of the present-day medical scene. At the end of the nineteenth and during the first decade of the twentieth century, general practitioners, often poorly trained, provided care for those patients who could afford it. In 1910, in response to a feeling of disquiet about the quality of medical training, Abraham Flexner, under the auspices of the Carnegie Foundation, produced his report on medical education in the USA and Canada. There was felt to be a need to integrate all medical schools into the universities with the intention of improving standards of teaching. It was also decided that medical education in the future was to be based on science and research, and until the late 1960s medical schools slavishly adhered to these principles with the inevitable and predictable consequences that while many of the outstanding advances of American medicine can fairly be claimed to be the direct result of the Flexner Report, so equally it has in part led to the present chaos in medical manpower. Specialist teachers have produced too many specialists and super-specialists for the needs of the country and this has been accompanied by the steady decline in the number of general practitioners.

Following the First World War came the successful treatment of diabetic mellitus and pernicious anaemia, and the discovery of sulphonamides, and with the Second World War there were great improvements in surgical techniques followed by advances in anaesthesia and subsequently the widespread introduction of antibiotics. Medical scientists then became mesmerised with biochemistry and investigative procedures, while the pharmaceutical industry produced many new drugs so that it was rightly assumed that specialists were needed to carry out and understand all these advances and wrongly assumed that the majority of patients and their illnesses, therefore, required specialists to look after them.

The federal government, until comparatively recently, has remained conspicuous by its lack of leadership in health policy. In 1912, the Public Health Service was formed and incorporated into the Department of the Treasury and in 1934 transferred to the Federal Security Agency. In 1954, the Public Health Service was finally assimilated into the newly formed Department of Health Education and Welfare. At no time have health matters had a strong place in government. While many European countries – Denmark, the Federal Republic of Germany, Hungary, the Netherlands, the UK and New Zealand were introducing various forms of health insurance for certain groups of workers, the USA remained committed to the view that individuals should be responsible for the payment of medical fees and those that cannot pay must rely on charity. At least this policy was consistent with their general philosophy that the government that governed best was the one that governed the least! It is interesting to note that the first big initiative in health by federal government was in the early 1930s when financial support was given for research at the National Institutes of Health. Even at the beginning of the severe depression which affected the whole country for almost a decade, research was thought to be more important than organising mother and child care.

The initial impetus for some form of health insurance came just before the First World War and, in 1916, the Association of Labour Legislation suggested compulsory medical insurance cover with sickness benefits which were to be voluntarily introduced at the state level. It was intended to cover some employed people and their families and was to be paid for by federal and state taxation with contributions from the employers. Initially, this plan appeared to have universal support, but by 1919 the American Medical Association (AMA) had galvanised public opinion and successfully quashed the idea. The next big impetus came in the middle of the depression and followed the Report of the Committee on the Cost of Medical Care, which had highlighted the enormous financial problems for an increasingly large section of the population. So in 1935/7 the federal government tried to introduce some form of national health insurance which was again thwarted by the self-interest of the AMA. In 1939 and 1943 two further pieces of legislation, both introduced by Senator Wagner of New York, which were concerned with the state obligation to care for the poor combined with a federally supported health insurance scheme, were yet again to be demolished by the lobbying of the AMA. In 1948, the Murray–Wagner–Dungell bill, which was intended to provide a comprehensive national health insurance plan for the entire population, funded by payroll taxes and administered by the federal government was narrowly defeated in the House of Representatives: again largely due to the AMA. With hindsight, if the bill had only encompassed the poor and medically indigent, it would probably have been passed and preceded Medicaid legislation by nearly 20 years. Further attempts, during the Republican administration of the 1950s, to introduce some form of federally controlled or sponsored health insurance continued to be opposed by 'organised medicine' but gradually the pressures of society for reform became greater than the narrow, but powerful, vested interests of the AMA. It became accepted that society should be responsible at least for those patients who could not afford private medical insurance and that this should be the collective concern of the state. This change of emphasis was in part brought about by the rising cost of medical care, which made an increasing proportion of the population aware of their own inability to pay. Eventually, even the AMA could no longer successfully oppose this essential piece of social legislation and finally, in 1965, Medicare and Medicaid were introduced for the care of the elderly and the very poor.

Medical insurance

Health insurance in the USA is the despair of the tidy mind, a nightmare for those who do not have it or cannot afford it and often a frustration and disillusion for those who do. The main defects are: too limited coverage for primary care services, inadequate coverage for long-term and chronic illness, too great an emphasis on in-patient hospital investigation and treatment and a reimbursement scheme which is concerned more with 'procedures' than service. Lastly, Medicaid has provided less than satisfactory coverage for the medically indigent, for low-income families, for those who find themselves temporarily unemployed, and for those who are high medical risks. At the present time the USA remains the only developed industrialised country in the Western World without compulsory health insurance.

To a section of the general public, personal medical care has become an expensive luxury to be had only when absolutely necessary. Although an increasing amount of personal health insurance now covers the needs of many, much is left uncovered. 'In 1968, of 180 million Americans under 65 years (not eligible for Medicaid) 36 million had no hospital insurance, 39 million had no surgical insurance, 61 million had no in-patient medical insurance, 89 million had no laboratory or X-ray insurance, 102 million had no insurance to pay for family doctor office or home visits, 108 million had no insurance for prescription drugs and 173 million had no dental insurance.' (Smith, 1972) By 1975, according to the Department of Health Education and Welfare (HEW), of 191 million Americans under 65 years, 141.34 million (74 per cent) have some form of private insurance, 21.01 million (11 per cent) are covered by public programmes (Medicaid, veteran associations, armed forces), 9.55 million (5 per cent) supplement their public coverage with private insurance and 19.10 million (10 per cent) have no coverage at all (Fox, 1977). This last group are too 'rich' for Medicaid, too young for Medicare and too poor to afford the premium of private insurance.

The deficiences and inadequacies of coverage for those that do have hospital insurance are as varied as the number of agencies or intermediaries available for patients to choose from, and it is impossible to do more than outline the principal drawbacks. Sometimes there is a dollar limit (between $10 000 and $30 000 in 1976) and often a restrictive clause on the number of days of hospitalisation for each illness, or the patient is responsible for the first four weeks, or all payments stop after six months. Catastrophic illness until recently has been a problem, but protection against this is now one of the fastest growing components of private insurance. There is also too great an emphasis on in-patient care – both for treatment and diagnostic investigations.

Regarding primary care, the gaps are enormous.

> In 1974, leaving aside 'courtesy' visits (usually office but occasionally home), for which no charge is made, approximately 50 per cent of all clinic and physician office visits made by persons of all ages are paid for entirely by the patient or his family. About 11 per cent are paid for entirely by private insurance and just over 12 per cent by Medicare

and/or Medicaid. Some 14 per cent are paid in part by the individual patient, in part by public or private insurance. The remaining 13 per cent of total visits are covered by accident insurance, Workman's Compensation, local, private and public welfare programmes other than Medicaid and federal programmes for such special beneficiaries as civilian dependents of servicemen, merchant seamen, American Indians and veterans. (Piore, 1975)

As with hospital coverage, there is an overemphasis on procedures and investigations while preventive medicine and health education are virtually ignored: a familiar situation in many countries. Similarly, the cost of drugs is only partially covered and, in 1976, 67 million Americans were without any coverage at all for prescribable drugs.

It would be misleading and wrong to assume that improvements have not been made both in the reduction of direct out-of-pocket expenses and the associated increase in third-party insurance (Table 8)

TABLE 8   *Direct out-of-pocket and third-party payments for health services 1950–75*

| | Personal health care expenditure (million $) | Direct out-of- pocket (%) | Total third party (%) | Third party Private Public | | | |
				Health insur- ance (%)	Philan- thropy (%)	Federal (%)	State (%)
1950	10 400	68.3	30.9	8.5	3.0	9.4	10.0
1960	22 729	55.3	44.6	20.7	2.3	9.2	12.4
1970	60 113	40.4	59.7	24.0	1.5	22.3	11.9
1972	74 688	37.6	62.4	24.9	1.4	24.3	11.8
1974	90 281	35.4	64.6	25.6	1.4	25.5	12.1
1975	103 200	32.6	67.4	26.5	1.2	27.7	12.0

Source: Worthington, N.L., National health expenditures 1929–74. *Social Security Bulletin*, February 1975

as well as some increase in the access to care amongst the poorer sections of the population (Tables 9, 10, 11 and 12). From Table 9 it can be seen that there has been a radical shift in the number of physicians visits by low- compared with high-income families between 1959 and

TABLE 9 *Number of physician visits (doctor/patient contacts) per person per year by family income*

| Year | Physician visits per person | |
	Low income[a]	High income[a]
1957–9	4.6	5.7
1963–4	4.3	5.1
1966–7	4.6	4.6
1969	4.8	4.5
1974	5.9	4.9

[a] 'Low' and 'high' are $2000 v. $7000 + for 1957–9
$3000 v. $10 000 + for 1963–4
1966–7
$3000 v. $15 000 + for 1969–74.
Source: Fox, P. & Bice, T. Socioeconomic status and use of physician services revisited. *Medical Care* (1976) **14,** Aug.

TABLE 10 *Number of visits (office) per person by family income and age*

| Year | Age | Office visits per person | | |
		Income $5000	Income $5000–$9999	Income $10 000+
1969	0–16	2.8	3.4	4.2
	17–44	4.5	4.1	4.2
	47–64	5.5	4.6	4.3
	65+	6.1	5.8	7.5
1974	0–16	3.7	3.7	4.5
	17–44	5.9	5.2	4.5
	47–64	6.5	5.8	5.2
	65+	6.3	6.8	7.7

Source: Fox, P. & Bice, T. Socioeconomic status and use of physician services revisited. *Medical Care* (1976) **14,** Aug.

TABLE 11   *Number of physician visits per person per year by race*

Year	White	Non-white
1957–9	5.2	3.5
1966–7	4.5	3.1
1974	5.0	4.4

Source: Fox, P. & Bice, T. Socioeconomic status and use of physician services revisited. *Medical Care* (1976) **14**, Aug.

TABLE 12   *Percentage of population with one or more physician visits within a year of interview*

	July 1963 June 1964	July 1966 June 1967	1969	1971	1973
Colour					
White	67.4	69.3	70.3	73.3	75.1
All other	56.2	59.0	62.9	65.6	70.7
Education of head of family					
Less than 5 years	55.1	58.0	61.2	64.1 ⎱ 68.3
5–8 years	59.4	62.1	63.4	66.0 ⎰
9–12 years	67.4	68.8	69.7	72.2	74.0
13 years or more	75.8	76.2	76.2	79.1	80.5

Source: Physicians visits. Volume and interval since last visit United States – 1971. *Vital and Health Statistics*, Series 10, No. 97, p. 2, National Centre for Health Statistics, Department of HEW, March 1975

1974: in fact an overall difference of 40 per cent. But these figures must be viewed with caution as they take no account of the 19.11 million who cannot afford medical aid and whose need is probably greatest of all, nor do they indicate where the visit took place. It would certainly seem likely that the increase in access for the poorer section of the population has not taken place within the organisation of main-stream medicine (i.e. the consulting room), but in the unsatisfactory atmosphere of the 'Medicaid mills' (p. 234) or emergency rooms of hospitals. But such statistics cannot be ignored and certainly they show a trend towards easier access for the poor, although it could also indicate that the middle income people are finding it far more difficult to cope with medical costs.

Methods of insurance

In 1975 third-party insurance accounted for 66.2 per cent of payment for health services of which 39.7 per cent was from public funds (Medicare/Medicaid) and 26.5 per cent from various forms of private insurance.

Private insurance

This is provided by the Blue Cross/Blue Shield Organisations and commercial insurance companies in almost equal proportions. The premiums of the majority of all privately insured people are now paid on a group basis by employers so that health coverage has become a major element in all wage negotiations between the large labour unions and industry. Inevitably, many decisions on health matters are in danger of being made on an employment basis rather than in relation to health needs and requirements. In 1976, the biggest expense for General Motors Car Company was not the cost of buying steel to build cars but the cost of insurance premiums paid to Blue Cross/Blue Shield for health insurance for their employees! The premiums of the remaining minority are paid either partly by employers and partly by employees, or completely by employees.

1. Blue Cross and Blue Shield are non-profit-making voluntary organisations which now operate throughout the country. They also act as intermediaries by contracting with the federal and state governments in the administration of Medicare and Medicaid.

Blue Cross was started in California and Texas in the late 1920s to enable the wealthier section of the population to insure against hospital costs which, even in those days, were a major problem. It is still largely concerned with hospital costs and contracts with individual hospitals which have previously agreed to an accepted schedule of charges. The apparent direct relationship between Blue Cross and the American Hospital Association caused considerable concern and criticism for many years as it was felt that this could be one of the main factors in the uncontrolled and escalating costs of hospital care. In 1972, this liaison was officially ended.

Blue Shield was founded in California in the mid-1930s as a direct response by private medical practitioners to the attempt by the Governor of California to introduce a state medical insurance programme which was seen as a threat to private medicine. Basically Blue Shield is concerned with professional fees and contracts with individual doctors while the patient is the subscriber. A physician under contract agrees to abide by a recognised fee schedule and the patient is fully reimbursed. But the patient is quite free to consult an independent physician (non-member of Blue Shield) who does not have an agreed fee schedule and can, therefore, charge a higher fee – the patient being responsible for the difference. Fees, which were originally decided through the California Physician Service, came to be known as the 'usual, customary or reasonable fee'. In 1950, the California Relative Value Fees Guide for medical services was accepted, first in California and then nationally. It has remained the main arbiter in determining the relative values of fee schedules although not the actual level of payment. It is also responsible for the insistence on procedures rather than services. This is not surprising as the original fees guide was drawn up by medical advisers to Blue Cross – predominantly surgeons – and has remained ossified in its thinking ever since.

Over the last few years there has been a merging of interests away from the complete separation of hospital fees (Blue Cross) and physician services (Blue Shield) as is the case in California, through many variations, to the combined plan such as the Blue Cross/Blue Shield Organisation in Michigan. It is difficult to decide whether there are any real advantages to the patient.

2. Commercial insurance companies are predominantly life insurance companies which use health insurance as a lever to get other business and are run on a profit-making basis. There are well over 1500 companies competing with each other, as well as with Blue Cross and Blue Shield, with only erratic control at state level. The main differences between the commercials and Blue Shield is that the former make a contract with the patient unlike Blue Shield where the contract is with the doctor. The doctor is, therefore, able to charge above the 'reasonable and customary' fee and the patient is responsible for the difference between this and the benefit payable through his policy. Unlike Blue Shield, where there is evaluation of the services provided by contract physicians, the commercials control costs by devices such as limiting the amount paid per day for in-patient hospital care, even though the patients are under the impression that they are fully covered, or they employ a large number of deductables for such things

as radiological and pathological procedures. The benefits and coverage provided by many of the smaller companies are so inadequate that it could well be asked why anyone insures with them at all. Probably the answer lies in the fact that the premiums tend to be lower and it is as much as many families can afford. It is significant that the majority of large industrial concerns insuring their employees on a group basis rarely use commercials (exception: John Hancock insures The Ford Motor Company) and it is the employees in small firms or individual patients who must pay their own premiums, who attempt to buy cheap medical insurance. The situation is finally made even more confusing for some patients as their medical coverage is often combined with some associated life insurance policy so that it is almost impossible to understand their entitlements – and then it is usually too late.

3. Prepaid plans, of which there are over 600, have a long history in the USA starting with the Roos-Loos Clinic in Los Angeles in 1929. This was followed during the 1930s by Group Health Association in Washington DC, Health Insurance Plan of Greater New York (HIP), Group Health Cooperative of Puget Sound, Washington and the Kaiser Foundation Health Plan in San Francisco. Such plans, which are organised by industry, unions or local communities, arrange with a group of physicians and hospitals to provide agreed medical benefits for their members and their families on prepayment of a fixed monthly premium. The difference between this type of plan and Blue Cross/ Blue Shield or commercial companies is that there is a specific contract between the patient and a particular group of physicians.

> It is important to emphasize that payment is usually made to a third party, i.e. a health plan, insurance company or foundation, and does not imply any particular organisational pattern for the providers of the medical service, or indeed for the manner in which they, as individuals, are paid for these services. As a matter of fact, however, most prepayment plans in operation today are integral parts of group practices. In prepaid group practice this prepayment is called 'capitation' and means that doctors and hospitals (providers), under contractual arrangements, receive single payment from the health plan for a specific period of time for an individual and, in turn, accept the responsibility for providing special services. (Shinefield and Smillie, 1973)

Public insurance

Public insurance for medical care is provided by the Medicare and Medicaid programmes which were passed by Congress in 1965 under Titles XVIII and XIX of the Social Security Act. They were intended to cover the over-65 years and the very poor. It is essential to understand the difference in historical background and philosophical approach as this may to some extent help to explain the attitudes of the general public and the profession to the two programmes. Medicare was the result of mounting public pressure to the plight of the elderly in trying to cope with the impossible costs of medical care. It was a social insurance programme, similar to the social security cash payment programme to which the worker became entitled through his personal payroll tax contribution while he was working. On the other hand, Medicaid was really an extension of state welfare programmes (which already had some federal support) for the very poor. In the minds of probably the majority of the general public, it is still considered as a charity programme although the Department of Health, Education and Welfare never thought of it as such. The American 'frontier spirit' of the survival of the fittest, that each man is responsible for himself, and that medicine is a consumer product for which everyone must pay something, made Medicare socially acceptable as everyone had already paid their payroll taxes. But Medicaid was different and, although many of the poor were felt to be unfortunate, most of the recipients were still considered to be 'typical welfare people' with all the implications of indolence and scrounging. Society at large did not, and perhaps still does not accept that these people are the collective concern and responsibility of the state.

In 1970, federal health expenditure accounted for $18.1 billion (9.2 per cent of total federal outlay) of which Medicare accounted for $7.1 billion (39 per cent) and Medicaid for $2.9 billion (16 per cent). In 1975, federal expenditure had risen to $35 billion (11.2 per cent of total federal outlay) of which Medicare accounted for $13 billion (37 per cent) and Medicaid $6.5 billion (19 per cent).

1. Medicare is a federal programme, administered by the Bureau of Health Insurance of the Social Security Administration with Blue Cross/Blue Shield and commercial insurance companies acting as intermediaries under contract with the Bureau of Health Insurance. There are two parts of the programme:

Part A: Hospital insurance programme to which everyone is automatically entitled. It is financed by the 1 per cent tax on salaries (payroll) with added contributions from general taxation. Coverage is not complete: for the first 60 days of any illness all costs are paid in full in an acute hospital, but there is no coverage for home nursing care and a patient must first be admitted to an acute hospital before benefits are payable in a nursing home. The patient is responsible for an initial deductable, equivalent to the average cost of one day's hospitalisation ($92 in 1975). From the 61st to the 90th day the patient must pay one-quarter of the deductable per day and thereafter at one-half of the deductable per day.

Part B: Supplementary Medical Insurance Programme (SMI). Patients must enroll and pay a premium of $6.70 per month (1976) and also pay the first $60 of any illness. After this the SMI reimburses at 80 per cent of 'reasonable charges' – i.e. what the physician usually charges or the current rate in the locality. The benefits provided include physicians' services, both on an in-patient and out-patient basis, including 100 visits per year plus X-ray, laboratory facilities, physiotherapy and speech therapy.

There is no coverage for eye or hearing testing, hearing aids, glasses, false teeth or prescribable drugs: this last exclusion is an extremely serious matter for a majority of the elderly. A further complication is now added as the physician can be reimbursed in either of two ways. First he can accept 'assignment' – by this he agrees to the 'reasonable fee' – and submit his account directly to Medicare so that the patient is not troubled or worried. Or he does not accept 'assignment' and can charge more than the 'reasonable fee'. He bills the patient directly who is then responsible for the additional cost. In both cases the patient is only reimbursed 80 per cent of the 'reasonable fee'. In fact, the number of doctors accepting assignment is steadily decreasing so that the elderly are increasingly liable for extra expenses. In 1976, it was estimated that 50 per cent of physicians accepted assignment.

It was the intention that Medicare should provide uniform benefits for all elderly people regardless of income or geographical location. How far have these aims been achieved? Certainly there is little doubt that the majority of the elderly find the regulations and form-filling exceedingly confusing, and that higher income groups benefit most because the exclusions (particularly prescribable drugs) and deductables are a considerable further expense.

With regard to geographical considerations, there are a number of complicating factors – physician/population ratios and whether the healthier and wealthier people settle in certain parts of the country – but some differences in benefits are clearly shown in Tables 13 and 14.

TABLE 13   *Medicare physicians and other Medicare service reimbursements and persons serviced by region: 1968*

	USA	Northeast	North Central	South	West
Persons receiving physician-reimburseable services per 1000 Medicare enrollees	387.8	397.0	358.0	368.6	476.4
Medicare reimbursement for physicians' services per person served ($)	198.16	209.37	178.01	192.21	213.13
Medicare reimbursement for physicians' services per person enrolled ($)	76.85	83.13	63.73	71.10	101.88

Source: *Medicare, 1968*, Section 1, Summary 1973, Tables 1.3, 1.5 and 1.6. Social Security Administration, office of Research and Statistics. Department of HEW

TABLE 14   *Physician/patient contacts 1968–9*

	Percentage of elderly persons seeing physician during year	Physician visits per elderly person per year	Physician visits per elderly person seeing physician
All areas	71.3	6.1	8.6
Northeast	72.8	6.5	9.0
North Central	68.8	5.6	8.1
South	71.5	6.0	8.4
West	72.8	6.7	9.3

Source: *Age Patterns in Medical Care, Illness and Disability, United States, 1968–1969*, Series 10, No. 70, Tables 9 and 15, National Centre for Health Statistics, Department of HEW

With regard to race, it has been estimated that in the South, where there are a higher proportion of negroes than in any other part of the USA, whites over 65 years receive 90 per cent higher Medicare reimbursements per person enrolled than do the over-65 years of non-white races. Theoretically the benefits are the same for all but the pattern of use varies.

Clearly Medicare provides only partial coverage and those that need the most receive the least.

2. Medicaid is the extension of an already existing welfare programme and is administered by the individual states (through the welfare departments in 42 and the health departments in 7). The federal government has no power to force the Medicaid legislation on the states and, in fact, in 1977 one state (Arizona) still had no programme. The cost is divided between state and local authorities with federal support on a sliding scale: 81 per cent for the poorest and 50 per cent for the wealthiest states. The intention of this financial arrangement was to give the greatest support where the greatest need existed – unfortunately the reverse has occurred. (See below.)

Eligibility is extended to the very poor (below poverty line), but many anomalies exist. When the legislation was introduced in 1965, it was stipulated that individual states could not reduce the level of welfare benefits already available so that inevitably the wealthiest states, such as California and New York, which already had the highest levels of welfare, would provide higher levels of Medicaid benefits than the poorer states – the maximum before, became the minimum afterwards. In addition, each state has the option to include or exclude the 'medically indigent' who are classified as having an income of less than 25 per cent above the poverty line: such families are considered too 'rich' for Medicaid and obviously are too poor to insure themselves privately. Further anomalies exist as the indigent cut-off point varies from state to state – for a family of four, $2200 in North Carolina to $5472 in Wisconsin – and again those in greatest need receive the least help. By 1977, over twenty states still elected not to include the 'medically indigent' in their Medicaid programmes. Finally the following group of poor are excluded: single individuals between the ages of 21 years and 65 years, childless couples and families whose head of the family is employed. As a result of these 'eligibility' regulations it is estimated that only between one-third and slightly less than three-quarters of the nation's poor in fact receive Medicaid.

What benefits are provided? If Medicaid is implemented it is obligatory for the state to provide hospital and physicians' services, skilled nursing home facilities, family planning, laboratory and X-ray facilities and the care and treatment of children up to the age of 21 years. All other types of medical care are optional. But, needless to say, limitations and complications abound. First, the number of days' hospitalisation per admission is restricted (anything between 10 and 30 days) as also are the number of visits to a doctor per year with great variations between states. Second, limited reimbursement rates of the 'usual and customary' fee for physicians' services are imposed (less than a half and sometimes as little as a third). This has inevitably resulted in many primary care physicians refusing to accept Medicaid patients who then have no alternative but to attend the emergency rooms of the nearest hospital. This policy has, in the end, cost very much more than if the 'usual and customary' fee had been paid to the doctor in the first place because the cost of emergency room care is at least three or four times as much. Another reason for refusing to accept Medicaid patients is the endless red tape and bureaucratic haggling over reimbursement, which may delay payments by six months and often a year. Inherent in the attitude towards Medicaid is the general belief that a number of patients are getting something for nothing, or even that many patients do not really deserve such help, and that a proportion of the medical profession are making an extortionate amount of money out of the system. It is true that a small proportion of doctors have set up groups which are known as 'Medicaid mills' in which there is as rapid a turnover of patients as possible – between 80 and 100 per day – and they are also accused of unnecessary referrals within the group for tests and examinations. Attempts have been made to curtail the activity of these 'mills' and it is easy to criticise them but at least these doctors are attending Medicaid patients who, in turn, strongly object to any threats of closure.

The original intention of trying to distribute Medicaid benefits equally throughout the country has had only very limited success both geographically and racially: this can be seen from Table 15.

The enormous differences in average Medicaid payments to poor families is in inverse relationship to geographical distribution of the poor – $50 per family in Mississippi and $1150 per family in California (Table 16).

Three states – New York, California and Illinois – with 24 per cent of

TABLE 15 *Medicaid payments for all medical services per re-cipient by race, region and residence, 1969*

		Payments to all ages ($)	
		White	Other races
Region			
	All areas	375.44	212.85
	Northeast	361.87	204.73
	North Central	448.52	249.46
	South	322.39	180.18
	Mountain	302.59	213.12
Residence			
	City 400 000 or more population	322.80	221.34
	Other SMSA*	425.96	227.54
	Non-SMSA	406.10	178.57

* Standard Metropolitan Statistical Area.
Source: *Medicaid Reports*, National Centre for Social Statistics, Department of HEW, 1973

TABLE 16 *Distribution of states by average medical payment per family, 1972*

Average health payment per family ($)	Number of states
Under 100	1
100–249	7
250–399	5
400–549	16
550–600	5
700–849	9
850–999	6
1000– or more	3

Source: Schulz, C. L., Fried, E. R., Rivlin, A. M. & Teestess, N. H., *Setting National Priorities: The 1973 Budget*, Washington DC, The Brookings Institution, 1972

the US population and 19 per cent of the poor, account for nearly 40 per cent of federal Medicaid payments. Conversely the South, with 40 per cent of the poor receives only 17 per cent of federal Medicaid outlay. Thus, despite the programme-matching formula, which provides a higher federal share to low-income states, there has been a transfer of federal revenues from low- to high-income states reflecting the higher income eligibility standards, richer benefits, and higher costs.

Medical manpower

Physician manpower statistics must be treated with caution as they are difficult to interpret and direct comparisons with other countries are almost meaningless for a variety of reasons.

First, there is no clear distinction between a specialist and primary care physician. According to the Department of HEW, general practitioners/family physicians, internists and paediatricians provide primary care; according to the AMA, gynaecologists should be included in this list, and unofficially it is acknowledged that psychiatrists, dermatologists and a wide variety of surgeons also provide some primary care. Patients can, and do, consult any specialist they wish and no constraints are placed upon this self-referral. It is accepted, both by patients and doctors, as a necessary part of the disorganised pattern of primary care. 75 per cent of all private (non-federal) physicians are office-based and of these 24.7 per cent are general practitioners/family physicians, 12.7 per cent are internists, 6 per cent are paediatricians and 7.4 per cent are gynaecologists, or considered in another way, 50 per cent of internists are office-based, 57 per cent of paediatricians and 72 per cent of gynaecologists (Table 17).

Second, osteopathic physicians are also concerned in first-contact care and are included in some statistics and excluded from others. In 1975, there were an estimated total of 394 400 physicians (active and non-active: federal and non-federal) of whom 379 700 had a degree of doctor of medicine and 14 700 had a degree of doctor of osteopathy. A final limitation in the absolute value of manpower figures is the new and increasing use that is made of medical auxiliaries – both physicians' assistants and nurse practitioners.

But a number of general trends and undisputable facts do emerge. There is no absolute shortage of physicians (Table 18), and health manpower legislation over the last ten years has produced a steady increase in the intake of medical students which will be reflected in the

TABLE 17   *Type of practice and primary specialty of active non-federal and federal physicians 1974*

| Primary specialty | Total active | Office-based | Hospital | | Others[a] |
			Training	Full-time	
Total physicians	330 266	205 955	59 022	36 261	29 028
GP/FP	69 445	51 029	8 445	5 294	4 677
Specialties:	260 821	154 926	50 577	30 967	24 351
Medical	90 519	50 853	20 325	9 948	9 393
Internist	51 752	26 213	14 823	5 599	5 117
Paediatrician	21 634	12 520	4 871	2 242	2 001
Surgical	105 870	73 677	19 558	8 299	4 336
Gynaecologist	20 987	15 187	3 455	1 373	972
Psychiatric					
neurologist	29 552	14 934	4 944	5 743	3 931
Others[b]	35 480	16 062	5 750	6 977	6 691

[a] Includes medical teaching, administration and research.
[b] Includes aerospace medicine, preventive medicine, occupational medicine, pathology, radiology and public health.
Based on: Roback, G. A. & Mason, H. R. (1975). *Physician Distribution and Medical Licensure in the US 1974*. AMA Centre for Health Services, Research and Development, Chicago.

1980s by a greatly increased number of qualified specialists. In 1974 there were 68 per cent more doctors than in 1951 and 18 per cent more than in 1968. In 1973–4 first-year students numbered 14 174, which was 25 per cent more than the number of students graduating in 1974. Certainly a ratio of 13 physicians per 10 000 population compares extremely favourably with any other developed country, particularly when it is appreciated that this figure only applies to those doctors who are in active patient care *outside* the hospital. The question is not now whether there are too few doctors, but whether in the 1980s there will be too many.

Brief mention must be made of foreign medical graduates (FMG) as approximately one-fifth of physicians practising in the USA received their medical school degrees from foreign medical schools. On 31 December 1973 there were 71 335 FMGs (excluding the 6325 of Cana-

TABLE 18   *Active physicians in relation to population 1950–74*

Year	Population in thousands	All active non-federal and federal MD	Physicians per 10 000 population
1950	156 472	208 997	13.3
1960	185 370	247 257	13.3
1968	201 787	296 312	14.7
1970	206 093	311 203	15.1
1974	213 219	350 609	16.4
		Providing patient care	
1968	201 787	238 481	11.8
1970	206 093	255 027	12.3
1972	209 979	269 095	12.8
1974	213 219	278 517	13.0
		Providing care in office-based practice	Population per physician
1968	201 787	180 991	1115
1970	206 093	188 924	1090
1972	209 979	198 974	1055
1974	213 219	203 943	1045

Based on: *Health Resource Statistics*, National Centre for Health Statistics, Department of HEW, 1975

dian medical schools). A total of 30 067 of the FMGs were hospital-based comprising 32 per cent of the total number of hospital-based physicians. A total of 27 270 of the FMGs were office-based comprising 13.5 per cent of the total number of office-based physicians (AMA, 1976). At the beginning of 1977 the federal government limited the entry of FMGs into the USA: how long this measure will be in operation remains to be seen.

If the purpose of medical education is to provide doctors who are able to meet the needs of the health service in which they are to work, then, even by the confused standard of the USA, there has been an over-production of specialists and a consequent imbalance between the number of general practitioners/family physicians and specialists. Between 1931 and 1974, general or family practitioners fell from 83 per cent of the total number of practising physicians to 18 per cent whilst specialists rose from 17 per cent to 82 per cent (Table 19). But the apparent almost total collapse of family medicine is misleading on two accounts. First, as has already been stated, primary care is carried out by specialists and second, throughout the late 1960s and early 1970s there has been a resurgence of interest in family medicine (Medical education, p. 265), which is just beginning to show itself in a reversal of the trend which has been taking place over the past 50 years or more: in 1974 there was an increase in the absolute numbers of family doctors (Table 20).

TABLE 19 *Distribution of non-federal physicians in patient care: 1931–74*

Year	Civilian population	MD in patient care Number	GP/FP in patient care		Specialist in patient care	
			Number	%	Number	%
1931	123 886 000	134 274	112 116	83	22 158	17
1940	131 658 000	142 939	109 272	76	33 667	24
1949	147 578 000	150 417	95 526	64	54 891	36
1960	177 472 000	165 844	74 553	45	91 291	55
1965	192 956 000	239 262	67 510	28	171 752	72
1970	203 046 000	255 027	54 098	21	200 929	79
1972	207 313 000	269 135	52 330	19	216 805	81
1974	210 600 000	278 517	50 935	18.3	227 582	81.7

Based on: *Distribution of Physicians in the United States, AMA. Population Estimates and Projections*, US Department of Commerce

Even so, in 1977, only about 26 per cent of office-based doctors were family physicians. Does this matter when, in the foreseeable future, internists, paediatricians and gynaecologists will continue to carry out a great deal of primary care? In fact, there is evidence that it is a matter for some concern, quite apart from the argument of whether a 'generalist' or 'specialist' is better equipped to deal with the ordinary day-to-day problems of first-contact care. Between 1930 and 1975, office visits increased from 50 to 75 per cent of all patient contacts, home visits have decreased from 40 per cent to under 3 per cent, hospital consultations either in the emergency room or out-patient department have remained fairly static at between 9 and 10 per cent, while telephone

TABLE 20   *Number of primary physicians: GP/FP internists, paediatricians (HEW category) with ratio of population per physicians*

	1931	1963	1971	1974
Physician category:				
GP/FP	112 116	68 091	49 528	51 029
Internist	3 567	21 144	23 829	26 213
Paediatrician	1 396	9 255	10 742	12 520
	117 079	98 490	84 099	89 762
Population in thousands	124 040	186 493	204 254	210 254
Ratio of population per physician	1060	1890	2430	2345

Source: *Physicians for a Growing America*, Washington DC. Public Health Service Publication No. 709, Department of HEW, October 1969. *Distribution of Physicians in the United States 1963, 1971 and 1974, AMA*

consultations have risen from almost nil to 12 per cent. Now 'the decrease in general practitioners is made more serious by the fact that they have customarily seen more patients than specialists and have worked longer hours. Although comprising only 28 per cent of all physicians in office-based practice in 1969, general practitioners were providing 61 per cent of all consultations, 82 per cent of all home visits and over half the telephone calls' (Parker, 1974). In 1977, there was no reason and no evidence to suggest that the situation had in any way changed.

The accessibility and availability of primary care physicians are influenced by a number of factors such as cultural differences which influence traditional patient habits and the acceptability rating by the patient, which are both difficult to quantify, but one of the most important and most easily measured factors, at least in a broad sense, is the maldistribution of doctors. Table 21 gives the latest readily available statistics: as yet it is too early to know if the increasing output of family physicians will have the desired effect.

Several interesting facts emerge from Table 21. Although there is a very wide discrepancy between the ratio of total physicians to population in the top and bottom states, the difference is very much less when only primary care physicians are considered. Even the worst state –

TABLE 21 *Number of physicians (non-federal in patient care) and primary care physicians (non-federal office-based general practitioner/family physician, internists and paediatrician) and ratio of physicians to population (per 10 000 population) showing the ten highest- and ten lowest-ratio states*

State	Total physicians			Primary care physicians					
	Number	Ratio	Order	GP/FP	Int.	Paed.	Total	Ratio	Order
DC	2 501	34.4	1	165	269	76	510	7.0	1
New York	36 370	19.8	2	4409	3530	1466	9 405	5.1	3
Massachusetts	9 825	17.1	3	1281	906	381	2 568	4.48	12
California	33 010	16.6	4	6388	3376	1422	11 186	5.6	2
Connecticut	4 985	16.3	5	588	547	245	1 380	4.5	11
Maryland	6 167	15.7	6	720	556	255	1 531	3.9	26
Colorado	3 318	14.8	7	575	296	173	1 044	4.66	8
Vermont	666	14.5	8	129	75	28	232	15.07	4
Rhode Island	1 318	14.2	9	183	136	71	390	4.21	17
Hawaii	1 009	13.7	10	182	105	76	363	4.92	5
Wyoming	301	8.9	42	120	23	6	149	4.42	15
Oklahoma	2 277	8.8	43	575	197	91	863	3.35	44
Idaho	625	8.6	44	248	49	28	325	4.46	14
N. Dakota	521	8.5	45	171	49	20	240	3.92	23
S. Carolina	2 160	8.5	45	620	149	96	865	3.39	43
Arkansas	1 589	8.2	47	556	111	49	716	3.70	34
Alabama	2 747	8.0	48	680	227	136	1 043	3.02	51
Alaska	214	7.5	49	72	20	15	107	3.75	32
Mississippi	1 652	7.5	49	539	106	77	722	3.27	47
S. Dakota	484	7.3	51	187	35	19	241	3.64	37

Source: *Distribution of Physicians in the United States*, AMA, Chicago 1972

Alabama – with 3.02 primary care physicians per 10 000 means one physician per 3311 patients. This figure is still well below the maximum allowable number of patients per general practitioner in the UK (3500) and is about the average per general practitioner in the Netherlands. Both these countries are considered to have a strong general practitioner service so that the USA cannot plead an excessive shortage of primary care physicians even if for geographical and logistic reasons these countries are not directly comparable.

These figures give only a crude indication of maldistribution and the position is in reality often far worse, as no account is taken of the differences within urban, suburban and inner-city areas. It is a well-known fact that more office-based specialists congregate near or around hospitals and that the majority of inner-city ghetto areas are almost completely devoid of private physicians' offices. The utilisation of medical services, which is a direct indicator of availability and accessibility decreases markedly with the distance the patient is from the nearest health facility. This is, of course, most starkly seen in developing countries (p. 334) and in the UK attempts are made to build health centres within the 'pram-pushing distance' of the main population centres. In the USA many studies have shown that distance, time and the ability to find or afford public transport or a taxi have the anticipated effects on primary care.

> Many people, in all social strata, will put off seeking care until their disease is far advanced or incurable. Some, especially among the poor and the ill-educated, do not take advantage of care that is available to them. As distance increases the services used – especially preventive ones – tend to decrease. The '$10 sick' in the Los Angeles suburb of Watts refers to the fact that getting to a county hospital across town takes hours on the bus. To avoid such a trip requires $10 for the taxi. Only when one is really sick is the trip made. A somewhat similar case study shows that in the Bronx in New York City, the infant death rate jumps 100 per cent within five miles, going from north to south. The reason is sad but simple. The south-east Bronx is inhabited mainly by blacks and Puerto Ricans. Although excellent clinics are open for pre-delivery and infant care, it takes several hours and several bus fares for a woman to visit one of them and, lacking a baby sitter, she probably had to drag her other children with her. The northern Bronx, on the other hand, is largely white Jewish and health conscious. There women go routinely to their private physicians for the same service. (Andreopoulos, 1974)

The '$10 sick' refers to 1968, but the principle remains the same in 1978.

During the 1950s and 1960s the rapidly declining number of general practitioners was only partially compensated for by the increase in the number of internists and paediatricians since much of their time was spent in hospital practice rather than in primary care and certainly there was no reliable information about how much of their time was actually devoted to primary care and how much time was spent in hospital practice, and there was a marked reluctance for them to settle in rural or inner-city areas. Therefore, in response to this shortage of primary care physicians, interest was suddenly awakened in intermediary medical personnel and medical auxiliaries. Two approaches are in evidence at the present time.

Physicians' assistants

In 1965, Duke University Medical School, North Carolina, started a two-year course to train personnel to work under the supervision of doctors. One of the next pioneering schemes was in the University of Washington, Seattle, and by 1971 there were 39 programmes involved in the training of physicians' assistants or 'medex' (as they are called in Seattle): by 1977 there were between 70 and 80 programmes. Initially, recruitment came through discharged medical-corps men from the armed forces, but this has changed and young men and women are now applying directly after finishing their 12 years' high-schooling.

Training is 'doctor-orientated' and is divided into Group A who are trained as generalists to help with family medicine, and Group B who are more technically educated in order to help in specialties such as ophthalmology, surgery and anaesthetics. In family medicine the functions vary according to the situation in which the assistants are working but, basically, these involve routine medicals, including insurance and employment examinations, the diagnosis and treatment of a wide variety of minor ailments (a comprehensive range of drugs is prescribable without a doctor's supervision), follow-up of hypertensives and diabetics and the initial treatment of traumas, including suturing, and simple fracture work.

Nurse practitioner

Recruitment takes place entirely from the ranks of registered nurses of which there were almost 1 500 000 in 1977: it is estimated that about 50 per cent are unemployed. The registered nurse's training is a three-year course and a further one year is necessary in order to qualify as a nurse practitioner. Unlike the physician's assistant training, a much greater emphasis is placed on preventive medicine, particularly in paediatrics: this last training was pioneered at the University of Colorado and later in the medex programme in Seattle.

The acceptability rating of both physicians' assistants and nurse practitioners is generally high amongst patients, particularly in rural situations where there has never been any medical care previously, and would appear to depend to a very large extent on the attitude of the medical profession in each locality (Lawrence, 1977). At the present time physicians' assistants are tending to work alongside private physicians while nurse practitioners are beginning to practise independently in rural areas, or in public health clinics or 'free clinics' in the cities.

Many doctors are naturally reluctant to be responsible for physicians' assistants and nurse practitioners when they work at a distance in a 'satellite' situation and are, therefore, unable to supervise their work closely. The mounting malpractice suits which are now a feature of the American medical scene, are a real fear to doctors. In the state of Washington, where nurse practitioners are working independently and in isolation, there is considerable interest, and not a little concern about their legal position: as yet no nurse has been brought to court for negligence. When this does happen, will it affect the recruitment for this type of work? Many physicians' assistants are also reluctant to work in isolation as they feel insecure and consider that too much clinical responsibility is placed upon them. It is important that these difficulties are resolved as they could well minimise the usefulness of these auxiliaries, particularly in rural areas.

The National Health Service Corps which was initiated and funded by the federal government in the early 1970s with the intention of directing health workers into rural areas, has partially succeeded. A further new avenue of attack against under-doctored areas was introduced by the passage of a new law in 1976 by which National Health Service Corps scholarships are awarded to medical students, in return for which they agree to carry out three years' work after qualification in those areas of the country where the federal government sees the greatest need: compare rural areas in the USSR and Eastern Europe.

Primary medical care

Primary care in the USA mirrors in many respects the strengths and weaknesses of society itself: energetic, hardworking, unorthodox and devoted to the concept of pluralism; on the other hand lacking in organisation, misdirecting its energy into improving what is already excellent and ignoring what requires attention, aware of scientific medicine but neglectful of the demand for social change, confusing the need for some alteration in the delivery of health care with the fear of control and government intervention. The different methods of organising primary care are too numerous to describe in detail and only the main patterns will be discussed.

1. Private physicians

This is still the main point of entry and accounts for between 60 and 80 per cent of all first-contact care (Table 22).

TABLE 22   *Percentage of medical care provided by private physicians according to age, family income and place of residence, 1970*

Age	Family income	Central city	Other urban	Rural
0 to 17	Low	26	57	64
	Medium	64	78	74
	High	77	82	81
18 to 64	Low	41	65	68
	Medium	62	75	72
	High	73	75	75
65 and over	Low	60	76	72
	Medium	77	80	80
	High	73	78	80
All ages	Low	41	67	68
	Medium	64	76	73
	High	74	78	78
All ages	All incomes	61	75	73

Source: *Health Service Use. National Trends and Variations 1953–1971*, (HSM) 73–3004. National Centre for Health Services, Research Development October 1972. Department of HEW

Primary care is carried out by three different categories of doctor: family physicians; internists and paediatricians – 'specialoid' physicians (Fry, 1969);* and highly trained specialists. The patient must decide to whom he or she should turn for first-contact care and the problems and difficulties associated with this arrangement have been discussed in Chapter 2 (p. 18). All three groups are 'office based' but may work in a wide variety of circumstances: solo practice, small groups and large multispecialty clinics of up to 50 physicians (Tables 23 and 24).†

TABLE 23 *Physicians in group practice (three or more physicians)*

	Number of groups	Number of physicians	Percentage of all active physicians
1946	368	3 084	2.6
1959	1546	13 009	5.2
1965	4289	28 381	10.2
1969	6371	38 834	12.8
1975	8483	66 842	23.5

Note. 1959, 1965, 1969 and 1975 include single-specialty, multi-specialty and groups of family physicians.
Source: *Bureau of the Census and Statistical Abstract of the United States 1971*, US Department of Commerce, Washington DC 1971, No. 534, p. 149. 1975 figures: *Profile of Medical Practice*, AMA, Chicago 1976, pp. 11 and 13

* A specialist is a physician who (*a*) has received further training in a special field and (*b*) then continues to perform his tasks and role within this limited field. A 'specialoid' is a physician who is either (*a*) a non-specialist who seeks to carry out a specialist role, or (*b*) a specialist-trained physician whose main function is to carry out primary medical care, thus limiting his ability to maintain and use his specialist skills.
† Group practice is the formal association of physicians. It may be composed of a single specialty or of multiple specialties; it may operate on a item-of-service or a prepaid basis (Piore, 1975). According to the AMA, three or more physicians formally organised to provide medical care, consultation, diagnosis and/or treatment through the joint use of equipment and personnel and with the income from medical practice distributed in accordance with methods previously determined by members of the group (AMA, 1976).

TABLE 24 *Distribution of physicians in group practice 1969 and 1975*

Number of physicians in group	Number of groups	
	1969	1975
3–4	4139	4437
5–7	1315	2284
8–15	616	1148
16–25	154	326
26–49	97	187
50 and over	50	101
Total	6371	8483

Source: *Profile of Medical Practice*, AMA, Chicago 1973, p. 32; 1976, p. 11

According to an AMA survey in 1975, group practice is rapidly becoming a major form of medical practice in the USA. Since 1969, the number of groups has increased by 33 per cent coupled with a 72 per cent increase in the number of group-practice physicians so that at the end of December 1975, 23.5 per cent of all active non-federal physicians were in group practice. For the purpose of analysis and comparison, medical groups are classified as either general practice, single specialty or multispecialty. Groups with 75 per cent or more of these physicians concentrated in the same specialty are considered single-specialty groups; otherwise they are classified as multispecialty groups. General practice accounts for 11 per cent of groups and 6 per cent of group-practice physicians, single specialty for 54 per cent of groups and 35 per cent of physicians and multispecialty for 35 per cent of groups and 59 per cent of physicians. Almost four-fifths of the groups (6721), accounting for 42 per cent of physicians (28 398), are composed of 7 or fewer physicians. The greatest concentration of physicians in general practice and single-specialty groups is in groups with 7 or fewer physicians. The reverse is true for multispecialty groups in which almost one-third of the physicians are in large groups (i.e. 50 or more physicians). There are no general practice groups with 50 or more physicians (AMA, 1976).

A small study in Washington County, Maryland (Rabin & Spector,

1976) which looked at the total work load in a small county, showed some interesting facts about the difference in the amount of primary care provided by family physicians, 'specialoids' and specialists (Table 25). Only 23 per cent of all the work could be considered secondary care, so inevitably internists and paediatricians provided a large proportion of primary care, but what was surprising was the extent to which medical and surgical sub-specialties were also very much involved. This surely must cast considerable doubt on whether this is an efficient and effective means of organising health care; whether it is a rational way of employing such highly trained personnel and whether it is possible for specialists and super-specialists to remain clinically competent if they are involved so little in secondary and tertiary care. The point was even more forcibly highlighted when an independent panel of doctors decided that of all the primary care provided almost 50 per cent could have been done equally well by medical auxiliaries and that they could have made a considerable impact on a further 43 per cent of the work; in fact, only 8 per cent

TABLE 25   *Volume of care, seen by specialty: two consecutive weeks (June 1974)*

Specialty	Volume of care as percentage	
	Primary care	Secondary care
Primary care specialists		
Family physician	97	3
Specialoid		
Internist	89	11
Paediatrician	100	0
Sub-total	96	4
Non-primary care specialties		
Medical sub-specialties	58	42
Obstetrics/gynaecology	88	12
General surgery	52	48
Surgical sub-specialties	34	66
Emergency room	93	7
Sub-total	57	43
Total	77	23

Source: *Washington County Auxiliary Care Survey*. Contract No. NO1–MB–44172. Bureau of Health Manpower, Department of HEW, March 1976

required the sole attention of a doctor – far less a specialist. While it is not suggested that the findings of such a small study can be applied to the whole country, there is nothing to indicate that the same principle does not apply.

The majority of physicians organise their work by appointment, usually giving 15–20 minutes per patient; a 4–6 weeks' waiting time for non-urgent consultations and routine examination is not unusual. But, according to the AMA, the situation is very different and the average waiting time for an appointment is 7.3 days with variations between specialty and type of practice. Obstetrics/gynaecology has the highest waiting time, with 17 days, paediatrics is next, with 8.9 days, then internal medicine with 8.4 days and general practice lowest with 4 days (AMA, 1976). Home visits are declining and 'out of hours' and weekend cover varies considerably: in rural areas, particularly, individual doctors or small groups work on a rota system while in urban areas increasing numbers of doctors are just unavailable and patients have no alternative but to attend the emergency room of the nearest hospital.

Facilities are excellent, both for diagnosis and treatment. Many doctors provide their own radiological equipment for chest and skeletal X-rays while the more complicated procedures are referred to a specialist radiologist or sometimes to the nearest hospital. In addition, small laboratories, staffed by a technician, carry out simple routine blood tests, bacteriological cultures and urine analysis with the more complex investigations being sent to a private laboratory. It is normal practice for the larger groups or clinics to have full radiological and laboratory facilities (even a brain-scanner). Physiotherapy is arranged privately on an item-of-service basis and patients may attend directly or by referral through a physician.

The staffing is certainly adequate and depends on the size of the office or group involved: nurses, sometimes with physicians' assistants and/or nurse practitioners; in addition, often full-time laboratory and radiological technicians, receptionists and a large number of clerks who are responsible for filing notes but, more particularly, are involved in the endless paper work and accounts associated with an item-of-service payment and the complexities of private insurance, Medicare and Medicaid.

Few studies have been carried out in the USA regarding the pattern and content of work in primary care, and research into morbidity and prevalence of disease has been almost exclusively confined to hospital medicine. But recently, with the renewed interest in family practice, data are beginning to accumulate in many departments of family medicine. A recent study comes from the Medical College of Virginia representing the most significant step to date towards the definition of the content of family practice and makes a quantum jump towards new knowledge in this area. It reports the occurrence of over half a million patient care problems presented over a two-year period in the practices of 118 family physicians and family-practice residents throughout Virginia. Urban, suburban and rural practice settings were studied and teaching and non-teaching practices were compared (Marsland, Wood & Mayo, 1976). But the survey has certain limitations in that it is impossible to relate the problems to any particular defined population at risk. Lack of access to primary care, either through inadequate insurance or perhaps physician maldistribution, merely emphasises the difference between the demands of some and the unmet needs of others. Demand depends first on a recognition that medical attention is required, which in turn depends on the education, social and cultural background of the patient. But, most important of all, in order that this demand should be satisfied, the patient must be able to find and afford a doctor. Therefore it should not be assumed that demands, which are then translated by the doctor into a clinical problem, are necessarily related to the needs of the community. But even accepting these limitations there are great similarities in the diseases encountered, when compared with the findings of the Royal College of General Practitioners in the UK. The major differences are the 'routine medical check up' (over 8 per cent in the USA and less than 1 per cent in the UK) and the frenzied management of such conditions as hypertension, diabetes and obesity in the USA. If, on the other hand, the USA were compared with the USSR, Finland or Sweden, these differences would be less noticeable. A further interesting comparative study between general practice in the USA and the UK comes to the rather sombre conclusion that neither group of doctors can be particularly happy with the results. The English and American ill patients do not appear to be very different in that their age structures and percentages of acute and chronic illness they present are similar. The differences are apparent when the general practitioner appears on the scene. American doctors are more orientated towards a ritualistic clinical approach leaning heavily on investigation and hospital support. Their system must be expensive. English doctors seem to operate at a less definite level of diagnosis (Marsh, Wallace & Whewell, 1976). There is little to suggest that the common diseases of primary care fare any better in the USA than in the UK, but it can be stated with absolute certainty that because of the fee for item of service and the almost inevitable consequences of over-investigation and over-treatment the cost of care is considerably and unnecessarily more.

2. Health Maintenance Organisation

Health Maintenance Organisation (HMO) legislation was passed by Congress in 1972 following the Health Maintenance Act of 1971 (HR11 728). The name is confusing and the idea was not new; in reality it was a political gimmick of renaming an old style of delivering health care by prepaid group practice which originated over fifty years ago. In the late 1960s and early 1970s, the enthusiasm and interest of the federal government in HMOs was directly related to the rapidly rising costs of medical care and motivated by the belief that only within the organisational framework of prepayment (The HIP, the Group Health Cooperative of Puget Sound and the Kaiser Foundation Health Plan) could costs be controlled and reasonably effective primary and secondary care be provided.

Prepayment involves a fixed monthly payment by the patient for himself and his family (known as a capitation fee) to a particular health plan in return for which agreed medical services are provided both on an in-patient and out-patient basis. Doctors who are employed by these health organisations agree to provide their services on a salaried basis. Numerous studies, both from university departments of public health and from the Department of HEW have shown that, compared with the usual 'fee for item of service' of private physicians and hospitals, there were fewer operations performed, hospital admission rates were lower (even by as much as 50 per cent) and, perinatal and infant mortality rates were improved, so that, as well as apparently providing improved care, the cost was considerably less. Subsequently it has been demonstrated that well-organised multidisciplinary clinics using the conventional item-of-service payment can reduce hospitalisation just as effectively as prepaid groups.

The most famous prepaid health plan is the Kaiser-Permanente in California, subsequently renamed the Kaiser Foundation Health Plan in 1952. In 1977, it had an enrolment of 3 200 000 patients, covering California, Oregon, Colorado, Ohio, Washington State and Hawaii, and provided 58 clinics and 23 hospitals throughout these regions. Some prepaid groups do not have their own hospitals and are responsible under the contract with the patient for organising any necessary hospitalisation. The staff are predominantly specialists and super-specialists with the result that many resent the considerable amount of time spent on primary care. In the future, according to the medical founder of Kaiser, it is hoped to recruit as many family physicians as possible so that a more rational use may be made of the highly trained specialists (Garfield, 1977). The plan provides for 24-hour cover but, owing to the size of each clinic, only a token attempt is made at continuity of care.

Contrary to popular and widespread belief, multiphasic screening, which is such a well-known feature of Kaiser, was not really intended to detect early illness, but was an attempt to regulate the flow of patients. It had been found after many years' experience that the 'drop-in' service although it provided immediate care, was unsatisfactory both for the patient and the doctor and provided little more than 'emergency room' care. Patients must wait two months for a non-urgent appointment and probably six months for a routine health check. Clearly this was again most unsatisfactory so it was felt that a reform of the organisation was needed to cope with the increase in volume of patients and the change in the character of demand which is inevitable if medical care is 'free' – i.e. no charge at the time of consultation. Patients have been found to fall into four categories: well, worried well, early sick and sick (Garfield, 1970). Multiphasic screening distinguishes these groups and was an experiment to try to improve patient care so that they could be seen more quickly. Whether it is cost-effective has yet to be proved conclusively but the next step forward was the use of paramedical staff rather than doctors in the initial screening procedures. A recent report from the Department of Medical Research, Kaiser Foundation Research Institute and Permanente Medical Group, Oakland, states

> the medical care delivery system involved the entry of patients through a paramedically staffed health evaluation service that effectively separated patients into three basic health status groups – the well and worried well (68.4 per cent); the asymptomatic sick (3.9 per cent) and the sick (27.7 per cent) – a process that permitted matching

the needs of each group with appropriate services. The system achieved increased physician accessibility to new patients by 20 times, reduced the waiting time for new appointments from six to eight weeks to a day or two, saved physician time and costs for entry work up to 70–80 per cent, reduced total resources used throughout the year by $32 500 per 1000 entrants and proved very satisfactory to patients and generally to staff. (Garfield *et al.*, 1976)

What have been the most significant achievements of an organisation such as the Kaiser Foundation? It provides broader benefits with less 'out of pocket' expense than the usual Blue Cross/Blue Shield plans: the patient knows where he can find 24-hour cover: reduction in hospitalisation has been achieved. In addition, it provides 'one-stop shopping' which Americans appear to appreciate and value. Also, if the new medical care delivery system were widely introduced it would improve the long waiting time which is a feature of the American medical scene. For the doctor there is an immediate steady income with retirement and long-term disability benefits. Immediate capital expenditure is not a problem and he does not spend two to three years building up his practice. He may enjoy the atmosphere and clinical stimulation of working with a group of colleagues surrounded by excellent facilities.

But what are the criticisms? The most serious concerns the policy of patient recruitment. 90 per cent of patients enrol through their company or union and often the entire monthly premium is paid by the employer as a negotiated part of wage bargaining. The worker and his family are now covered for medical care. But if he should become ill or have an accident and lose his job, then automatically the contract with the prepaid group ceases. Consequently, if he, or the remaining 10 per cent (usually self-employed) wish to apply for acceptance they must first undergo a vigorous medical examination and they are turned down if there is any suspicion of ill-health. But it is untrue to say that HMOs only succeed because they look after the young and healthy; rather it is because if a patient becomes ill enough to lose his job, or has some chronic, often not very serious, illness and cannot enrol on a group basis, then there is no way in which he or his family will be accepted. In other words, every means is used to exclude those patients who are likely to be in need of the most medical care. Patients also feel that the atmosphere is too similar to a hospital out-patient department; that there is no continuity of care or flexibility in the choice of doctors. Private physicians and the Blue Cross/Blue Shield organisations also say that there is a built-in incentive for the doctors to do as little as possible in the way of investigation and treatment so that costs are kept to a minimum and profits are high – these are distributed amongst the staff at the end of the year as a form of bonus. To counter this argument, prepaid group practices say that patients are free to leave (and very few do) or bring a legal action for negligence/malpractice.

Another type of prepaid group is the medical foundation which is usually sponsored by the county or local medical societies. The best known are at San Joaquin County and Sacramento, California and in Portland, Oregon. The basic principle of prepayment with no additional fees for an agreed set of benefits is similar to organisations such as Kaiser or Puget Sound but, unlike them, medical foundations do not have their own particular clinic or hospital; they do, however, have a greater degree of flexibility in that patients are free to go to any doctor's office or group practice which has a contract with the medical foundation. Where such foundations have been set up, over 90 per cent of doctors sign up each year for membership. Success depends on strict adherence to fee schedules, agreed benefits and cooperation between doctors.

The Health Maintenance Act stipulates certain strict criteria on any newly formed HMO before any financial support is forthcoming from the federal government. Four principles are involved: (1) an HMO is an organised system of health care which accepts the responsibility to provide or otherwise assure the delivery of (2) an agreed upon set of comprehensive health maintenance and treatment services for (3) a voluntarily enrolled group of persons in a geographic area and (4) is reimbursed through a pre-negotiated and fixed periodic payment made by, or on behalf of, each person or family unit in the plan. The problem arises in connection with the term comprehensive, which in effect means preventive, diagnostic, curative *and* rehabilitation services, including mental health, alcoholism and dental care for children. It is of interest to note that the Kaiser Foundation, upon which much HMO thinking was modelled, still does not qualify for financial assistance from the federal government because it fails to encompass all the federal guidelines: it excludes alcoholism and dental care!

In 1970, the Department of HEW announced its intention to support HMOs so that by 1980 perhaps between 80 and 90 per cent of the population would be covered in this way. In 1973, the law was further strengthened when it was made mandatory for all employers of 25 or more workers to offer the choice between an HMO, if it was available in the area, and the insurance cover provided by Blue Cross/Blue Shield or commercial insurance companies. Furthermore, there should be no restrictions devised by the local medical societies to prevent the setting up of an HMO: one common restriction was to refuse hospital privileges to those doctors working in an HMO. Why is it then that by 1977 there were still only just over 200 HMOs covering about 4 per cent of the population and that they made so little impact on primary care? Certainly the law appears to have been drafted badly with the fatal combination of modest financial support, plus burdensome regulations as compared with the usual private insurance. Mental health care, dental care for children, treatment for alcoholics, 24-hour cover and 'open enrolment' for a month for any patient, however ill or chronically disabled, without similar constraints on the private practitioner is hardly likely to succeed. In spite of federal support, the initial financing of an HMO is extremely precarious, particularly as they are at a disadvantage with the private sector. The premium for an HMO is usually greater than those for Blue Cross/Blue Shield or commercial insurance (between $8 and $10 more per month in 1977) and this may be sufficient to deter people from joining, particularly if they are fit and well or have to pay the whole premium themselves. Even if the patient joins on a group basis through his firm and the employer pays $50 out of the $70 per month (in 1977), as the premiums increase with inflation so the amount the individual must pay also increases. Finally, HMOs are still primarily concerned with those people employed in industry and have not focused on the problem of the poor urban areas.

3. Neighbourhood health centres

The prototype for this concept of health care started after the First World War with community centres which gave care to mothers and young infants, advice on nutrition and the immunisation of children. They gradually disappeared and were not considered again until urban and ghetto riots in the mid 1960s. In response to this social upheaval, the federal government, through the newly formed Office of Economic Opportunity (OEO) which was directly responsible to the President, financed the first neighbourhood health centre (NHC) in

December 1965. It was initiated by the Tufts University School of Medicine and was placed in a poor area in Boston (Columbia Point), Massachusetts with a population catchment area of about 6000 people. Congress directed the NHC programme 'to assure that such services are made readily accessible to the residents and are furnished in a manner most responsive to their needs and with their participation'. Patient participation has been a feature of the organisation of NHC – to many patients and doctors an important step forward but to others a warning sign of 'creeping socialism'.

It was hoped and assumed that the NHC would affect the overall health delivery process and improve the standard of primary care in poor urban areas. By 1977, there were over 300 NHCs spread across the USA, but only covering about 1 per cent of the population. The intention was to provide extended office hours from 08.00 hours to 20.00 hours with, if possible, a full-time salaried staff mainly of general practitioners, but by the late 1960s they took whatever physician was available whether full-time or part-time. Each centre has a small laboratory and simple X-ray equipment. Initially the majority of the patients received welfare allowances which subsequently became Medicaid. The remainder consists of those who receive Medicare and those families who do not qualify for Medicaid and yet cannot afford private health insurance.

Even though NHCs have done something to help urban areas where previously there was no medical care at all, their effect has been disappointingly limited and all the initial high hopes have not been fulfilled. Why is this? There are a number of reasons: first, in 1971/2 the federal government dismantled the OEO and transferred all NHCs to the Department of HEW. This, together with the effects of mounting inflation and relative economic stagnation, caused financial support to become unstable and unpredictable. Second, the image has naturally grown up that NHCs are only for the poor and medically indigent with the consequence that there is a distinct possibility that they have already, or will in the future reinforce segregation and the production of two levels of medical care: of course, some care is better than none at all! Some way must be found of encouraging everyone in an area to attend the local NHC, but the stigma of welfare is difficult to throw off. Third, difficulties have been experienced in recruiting doctors, not because of poor pay, but because of the type of patient and the type of illness encountered as well as the general level of unemployment and poverty of these patients with its inevitable social malaise and even physical danger and violence. Fourth, 'organised medicine' in the form of local medical societies has refused hospital-admitting privileges to those doctors working in NHCs and this has been a serious deterrent.

4. Free clinics

These started in the late 1960s and were an emotional response, catalysed by feelings of guilt, amongst many young medical students and young doctors who were concerned about the underprivileged groups in the inner-city ghetto areas, and felt that a fundamental alteration in the organisation of health care was needed. Primarily they were concerned with homeless young people, alcoholics, drug addicts and all those who felt alienated from society. Doctors and nurses gave their services free, but it was never possible to make a fundamental impact on the basic problems of providing primary medical care and, in 1977, free clinics provided less than 0.5 per cent of care. But, in spite of their quite obvious limitations, particularly financial, in many areas free clinics are still a viable entity forming the only means of contact between estranged groups and the medical profession. In certain states and counties the success of free clinics has encouraged local government to give them financial support, and some nurse practitioners feel attracted to this type of work.

5. Emergency rooms

These are increasingly being used as a way of entry into the medical system (Table 26). By 1977, it was estimated that about 10 per cent of all primary care visits took place in the emergency room although the variations were enormous: from almost 100 per cent in some inner-city areas, where the only options are for the patient to use either the emergency room or out-patient department, to less than 1 per cent in some rural and affluent suburban districts.

The increasing use of both emergency rooms and out-patient departments is the direct result of poor primary care, and should in fact be looked upon as a crisis or emergency in the health care delivery system. The reasons are well known and may be summarised briefly as follows:

(a) Inability or unwillingness on the part of the patient to have a personal doctor due to poor insurance coverage, lack of doctors in

TABLE 26   *Number of visits or admissions to hospital (in thousands) USA 1955–70*

	1955	1970	Percentage increase
Emergency-room visits (1000)	10 466	42 693	308
Out-patient visits (1000)	53 594	124 288	132
Hospital admissions (1000)	19 101	29 252	53
Visits or admissions per 1000 persons			
Emergency-room visits	6	21	250
Out-patient visits	33	61	85
Hospital admissions	12	14	17

Source: School of Public Health, Department of Medical Care Organisation. *Medical Care Chart Book.* University of Michigan 1972, p. 198

low-income areas and the high mobility of population, leading to a poor doctor/patient relationship.

(b) Inability or unwillingness on the part of doctors to be available at nights and weekends and their refusal to do home visits. With the increase in the number of specialist physicians who provide primary care there is an unwillingness on their part to accept responsibility for any condition outside their own particular field of interest.

(c) An increasing lack of confidence on the part of many doctors to treat a patient without the back-up facilities of the hospital. In parallel with this is the belief of many patients that only in hospital can expert and appropriate treatment be given.

(d) A hospital is always open – 24 hours a day – and this availability will increasingly be used, particularly now that all private physicians use appointment systems which are often inflexible and lead to long waiting times.

The utilisation of the emergency room has been well documented (AMA, 1976) and there is a consensus of opinion from a large number of surveys that at the very most 20 per cent of visits could be considered as 'true emergencies' and many would put the figure as low as 10 per cent. A generous view was put by the physician in charge of a large emergency department when he said that 90 per cent of patients may have acute symptoms, but at most only one-third are true emergencies (Luria, 1977). It has also been noticed in those hospitals which previously existed in a vacuum of primary care that, as soon as NHCs were set up, there was a considerable drop in the emergency-room attendances.

How appropriate is the emergency room for dealing with the relatively minor and chronic conditions of general practice? It is less than satisfactory for a variety of reasons: there is no continuity or support, comprehensive care is out of the question and no-one is ultimately responsible for the overall care of the patient. Finally the poor and inadequately insured families, in fact those who need a continuing and comprehensive service the most, are not surprisingly using the emergency room in the most inappropriate manner (Table 27).

TABLE 27   *Percentage distribution of emergency-department visits in five socio-economic areas by whether or not the visit was classified as an emergency. Rochester, New York, 1968*

	Social class:	5	4	3	2	1
Bonafide (%)		28	28	34	39	40
Not emergency (%)		72	72	66	61	60

Source: School of Public Health, Department of Medical Care Organisation. *Medical Care Chart Book.* University of Michigan 1972, p. 200

But the emergency room as a form of primary care is here to stay – in every country in the world; and in the USA, unless there is some dramatic and unlikely influx of private physicians and a rapid increase in the number of NHCs in the urban ghetto areas, they are likely to become the only form of primary care for a large section of the population. There is, therefore, an urgent need to reassess and alter the organisation and staffing of these departments so that a more tolerable and satisfactory pattern of care evolves, both for the patient and the doctor. Two new trends are emerging: one is the use of paramedical staff (physicians' assistants or nurse practitioners as an initial screen), and the second is the development of a new specialty in emergency care with its own Board Certified training and examinations. It is too early to know whether such a specialty will maintain the interest of doctors over their whole career.

Finally, hospitals have an obligation to improve their emergency-room organisation if only because 18 per cent of patients are admitted as in-patients, which produces a further steady source of income.

6. Out-patient departments (OPDs)

These provide another means of access for some patients into first-contact care, although their use by the patient and their function from the hospital's point of view are quite different from that of the emergency room. This can be understood from the following figures: 95 per cent of all hospitals have emergency rooms giving them a steady and increasing source of income; 100 per cent of university hospitals and 75 per cent of medical-school-affiliated hospitals have OPDs, while in non-teaching hospitals it is only 12 per cent. The OPD is seen primarily as a source of teaching material for medical students and only in a minor role as a service for the surrounding community.

Patients reach the OPD in a variety of ways: first, they may be referred by their private doctor for a specialist opinion; second, they may be referred within the hospital from the emergency room; and third, they may attend without any referral as in the emergency room. Inevitably the OPD is staffed by specialists and super-specialists who cannot and do not provide good primary care. Compared with the emergency room, which is open 24 hours a day, their accessibility and availability is poor, while, in addition, all consultations are by appointment so that the waiting time is in weeks and not just hours as in the emergency room. Although not comprehensive, the OPD can provide supportive and continuing responsibility for the follow up of some diseases even if long-term care for the patient and the family is out of the question. OPDs appear to provide more primary care than emergency rooms (Table 26), but these figures must be treated with great caution as there is no way of knowing what percentage of patients come without referral (primary visits) and what percentage are referred either from their own doctor or the emergency room (secondary visits).

7. Community hospitals

These are defined by the AMA as hospitals that are non-federal, short-term and general (although including orthopaedic and maternity). The Hospital Survey and Constitution Act – the Hill–Burton Act 1947 – resulted in the building of many new hospitals all over the country, particularly in rural and semi-rural areas. Throughout the depression of the 1930s and during the Second World War, hospital building had virtually ceased so that there was a tremendous need at this time. Unfortunately the Hill–Burton Act made no effective stipulations regarding regional planning or defining their function and role. By 1977 there were 5891 community hospitals of which 50 per cent had less than 100 beds, and it had been apparent for some years that with some planning they could provide a network of primary care facilities.

> Almost everybody lives within the reach of a hospital and that is where many are turning for medical care and advice they cannot find elsewhere. Thus there are two chief reasons to look to the community hospital for improvements in the organisation and delivery of primary care. First it is in a strategic position to marshall manpower and other resources and to enlist the support of many elements in the community to deal with the problem. Second the community hospital has already become a major source of such care in almost every corner of the land. Admittedly these hospitals, once chiefly for the care of inpatients, the acutely ill and the indigent, have by default rather than design become significant providers of those ambulatory and related procedures that make up the bulk of services to which we give the name of primary care. (Piore, 1975)

There are about as many variations in the way community hospitals can organise themselves to provide appropriate and adequate primary care as there are hospitals, but two main patterns are developing.

First, a specific department of primary care, which is given comparable status with the other clinical departments, is formed in the hospital and made responsible for the better use of the emergency room. Another method is for the responsibility to be spread amongst a number of physicians so that there is a wide variety of entry points for the patients: this is more confusing and less satisfactory for the patient.

Second, is an organisation which is almost unique in the USA in that it involved deliberate and rational planning and made the fundamental decision to separate primary, secondary and tertiary care, and then insisted that primary care was organised in the community, secondary care in the hospital and tertiary care referred elsewhere. Such an institution is the Hunterdon Medical Centre, Flemington, New Jersey. At the earliest stages in planning (1946) the then-revolutionary decision was formally taken that family physicians should provide primary care and that they should have admitting rights consistent with their medical competence and preference in medicine, paediatrics and obstetrics. The specialist staff were and are full-time and salaried and are used entirely in a consultative and specialist capacity, only seeing patients after referral by the family doctor. It was felt important to have some academic blessing and the hospital has always been affiliated with a university – first with New York University and, since 1972, with the New Jersey College of Medicine and Dentistry at Rutgers: all the full-time specialists and some of the family doctors have university appointments. At the present time, third-year medical students do clerkships in the major specialties and there is a flourishing Family Practice Training Programme over a period of three years.

The population covered is 75 000, the hospital has 200 beds and there are 38 full-time specialists and 38 full-time family physicians who work in solo, group practice or in four family health centres, two of which are staffed by salaried physicians attached to the hospital, while the other two have been built by the Hunterdon Medical Centre in areas of the county which previously could not attract doctors; the physicians rent the premises. One interesting feature is the emergency room of the hospital in which only 15–30 per cent of visits are for primary care as compared with the usual 80–90 per cent: this surely is a reflection on the satisfactory level of care provided by the family physicians in the community. Although the vision of this remarkable project was in no way influenced from the other side of the Atlantic it is worth noting the similarity between it and the Dawson Report produced in the UK in 1920 (p. 41).

What are the reasons for the undoubted success of Hunterdon and the fact that it has never been reproduced? First, it was started in a vacuum with no specialists and poorly distributed general practitioner services so that there was little entrenched medical opposition and no conflict between general practitioners and specialists. Second, and equally important, because the specialists are full-time and concerned only with secondary care there has been no rivalry between specialist and family physicians. Such a situation is unusual, although obviously not unique. Third, it has unfortunately remained an isolated but although much admired institution because very little was published about its success until recently (Curry *et al.*, 1974). The final reason, and most important of all, has been the powerful leadership, vision and tremendous hard work of the original lay Chairman of the planning committee, and subsequently of the Medical Centre, until he retired in 1976.

8. Community mental health centres

These were introduced in the early 1970s and are entirely federally funded. The intention was to redirect the emphasis in psychiatric care away from the large state mental hospitals towards community and ambulatory care. They are staffed by both full- and part-time psychiatrists and psychiatric social workers and have proved partially successful – at least in the primary care context. Many family physicians feel they serve a very useful purpose and remove much of the burden of behavioural/psychological/family/sexual problems away from them: on the other hand, this is yet another fragmentation of first-contact care as liaison is often poor.

Note. Primary care is also provided through the Indian Health Service, the veteran associations and the armed forces, but they will not be considered in the book.

Hospital service and primary care

In 1974, there were 7123 hospitals in the USA with a wide variety of ownership – public, private (including religious), profit-making and non-profit-making – with no discernible pattern of organisation or planning. Nothing has changed since the following was written in 1969:

> the US hospital services are still organised in a *laissez-faire* and independent fashion. A lack of co-ordinated planning in the past, in spite of the terms of the Hill–Burton Act, has resulted in the irregular distribution of hospitals and even in certain areas a degree of competition for patients between them. Hospitals have tended also to become 'status symbols' for a community with the result that there are many small hospitals with superfluous resources. There is no simple recognisable pattern of American hospitals. They cannot be graded according to population served or size or roles because there is so much overlap. (Fry, 1969)

The problem is as much philosophical as anything else because planning inevitably involves organisation which in turn implies some control which at the moment is a complete anathema to the medical profession and probably to the majority of the general public as well. Until it is accepted that every hospital should serve a specific purpose and its function should be defined according to the level of care it is providing – either secondary or tertiary – there will continue to be a wasteful, extravagant, disorganised and uneven hospital service. The epidemic spread of such items of equipment as brain-scanners, the presence of departments of nuclear medicine in 40-bedded rural community hospitals, the insistence that surgery by family doctors should be continued even when there are specialist surgeons near at hand, the building of expensive and large laboratory facilities in small communities or the unwillingness of specialists to refer certain procedures (for example hip replacements, cardiac surgery and neurosurgery) to their super-specialist colleagues – such examples are the essence of the American system.

According to the American Hospital Association, out of a total of 7123 hospitals 5891 are short-term, acute, general or community hospitals with a total of about 900 000 beds, which represents a slow, but gradual increase in the number of beds over the last 15 years. But, as 30 per cent of all hospital admissions are now in the over-65-years age group, it is in the province of skilled nursing and particularly the nursing homes that the greatest development has taken place: theoretically, in the former the patients require some nursing and medical attention while in the latter only custodial care is necessary. As in all countries, such a clear demarcation is no longer possible and with the phenomenal increase in the number of psycho/geriatric cases with or without other organic disease, it is extremely difficult to find suitable accommodation for the elderly. There are now over one million nursing-home beds, almost all of which are run privately on a profit-making basis, and there has of necessity been a merging of functions between the skilled nursing faculty and the nursing home. Local family doctors (or internists) provide the medical cover on a part-time basis for the great majority of these institutions.

In all hospitals, except public and university, there is open access to any physician who wishes to apply for admitting privileges, and provided he has passed the appropriate examination and is a certified Board Member of the specialty concerned, he is given these privileges. The implications of this are obvious: in urban areas many doctors have the right to treat patients in any number of hospitals, while in rural areas there are almost automatic admitting rights to the local hospital, even if the physician may be considered unsuitable. The quantity of surgery performed by general practitioners is steadily declining and is virtually confined to remote rural areas where there is often no alternative. In the university medical schools, particularly the more prestigious ones, very few family physicians are allowed to treat patients in the hospital although the situation is naturally different for those internists, paediatricians and obstetricians who may be spending a considerable amount of time in primary care.

A more detailed and coherent account of the relationship between the primary care physician and the hospital service is impossible, partly because of the lack of data, but also because the spectrum of opportunity is so diverse. Nevertheless, this brief survey does show the strengths and weaknesses of American medicine which are an inevitable consequence of a free-enterprise system without organisation and planning.

Medical education and primary care

The conflict between the specialist and generalist and the profound and lasting effect of the Flexner Report have bedevilled American medicine and its attitudes to medical education for the last 60 years. The attitude of the general public has been ambivalent; on the one hand decrying the gradual demise of the general practitioner whilst on the other hand insisting on seeing a specialist on the slightest pretext. The situation has been further complicated by extreme competition between specialist and generalist, by the assumption that the extravagant production of specialists can go on for ever, and by the apparent unwillingness of the medical profession to see that a referral system between doctors can only benefit the patient.

In 1913, the American College of Surgeons was formed, followed in 1915 by the College of Physicians. In 1920 the AMA, through its Council on Medical Education, formed 15 specialist committees in order to organise and develop further postgraduate training; these were the predecessors of the Specialty Boards of the 1930s. Repeated efforts to form a Specialty Board for general practice were thwarted and it was not until 1945 that the AMA agreed to form a separate section of general practice. Immediately following the end of the Second World War specialists became highly organised, highly esteemed by the general public and much more highly paid than their general-practitioner colleagues. These facts are mirrored in the residency training programmes for surgery: 808 in 1940, 4000 in 1950, 22 000 in 1952, 30 000 in 1957 and the incredible total of 45 000 in 1970. Procedure-orientated insurance with the consequent high earning capacity of surgeons, plus the irresponsibility of the medical profession have produced these extraordinary figures.

But general practitioners were slowly becoming organised and accepting their own deficiencies in training and performance, so that, in 1947, the American Academy of General Practice was founded by a group of doctors from within the AMA, and committees (or chapters) were set up in every state in the land (compare the following countries: Canada, p. 294; the Netherlands, p. 121; and the UK, p. 50). During the 1950s and 1960s, attempts to revive general practice appeared to be failing to the extent that, in 1968/9, only 4 per cent of medical graduates planned to enter general practice. According to the Centre for Health Service Research and Development, AMA, between 1968 and 1972 the number of office-based primary care physicians (general practitioners, internists, paediatricians and obstetricians) fell from 31.5 per cent of all active physicians to 28.4 per cent, while the number of hospital-based and office-based specialists (excluding general internists, paediatricians and obstetricians) increased from 51.1 per cent to 53.4 per cent. During this time, the number of primary care physicians increased by 1237, while that of hospital-based specialists, super-specialists and office-based physicians increased by 22 851. Certainly there was cause for concern for those who were interested in producing a more satisfactory and rational form of primary care.

In 1957, the Association of American Medical Colleges composed of deans of medical schools and academic physicians combined with the AMA and the Academy of General Practice to recommend a two-year training programme for general practice: its first real recognition as a specialty and a tremendous step forward. During the early 1960s, politicians, the general public, medical students and certain sections of the medical profession, were experiencing a dissatisfaction with the organisation of medicine and the obvious defects of primary care, and two important reports were initiated by the AMA to look into these problems: the Mills Report Commission in 1963, followed in 1964 by the Willard Committee Report, which both came to the same conclusion – that there should be a move away from the myopic Flexner standpoint. It was appreciated that a more broadly trained physician was needed to cope with the basic medical requirements of the majority of the population. During this time the American Academy of General Practice (renamed in 1969 American Academy of Family Physicians) was still pressing for Board Certification, and this was eventually granted in 1969 by the Council of Medical Education of the AMA; the first examination in family medicine taking place in 1970. The second Carnegie Commission reported in the same year and differed fundamentally from the first Carnegie Report (Flexner) of 1910. They recommended that there should be an emphasis on the training of generalists, with medical education being partially removed from the university and placed firmly in the hands of community hospitals with an associated emphasis on the behavioural sciences rather than pure science. In addition, a considerable increase in the number of medical schools was recommended.

What has been the result of all this activity and these recommendations? Between 1968 and 1974, 19 new medical schools were opened (Table 28) and by 1977 there were 120 medical schools of which 80 had

TABLE 28 *Increase in number of medical schools and students (excluding osteopathic schools and osteopathic graduates)*

Academic year	Schools	Students		
		All years	First year	Graduates
1954–5	81	28 583	7 104	6 977
1963–4	87	32 001	8 772	7 336
1967–8	95	34 538	9 479	7 973
1973–4	114	51 073	14 185	11 544

Source: Council on Medical Education. Education number of *JAMA*, 231, Supplement January 1975 (also prior annual issues)

family medicine programmes (for postgraduates). By 1978, it is estimated that 16 000 students will graduate per year and about 2000 will enter family medicine (about 12.5 per cent). In 1962, only 6 training programmes for general practice existed in the whole of the USA; by 1969 there were 30; by 1972, 133; by 1975, 259; and by 1977, 340. In accordance with the second Carnegie Commission, 40 per cent of programmes are centred on community hospitals, or, if they are not available, use is made of selected multispecialty group practice. Although tremendous progress has been made in postgraduate training, medical schools remain stubborn and reactionary in their attitudes to the undergraduate curriculum and in 1977, of the 120 medical schools only 30 have provided any introduction into family medicine for their students.

The federal government appears determined to come to grips with the problem of the overproduction of specialists and the production of more primary care physicians. The Health Manpower Bill 1976, stipulates that the capitation payment for each student which the federal government grants to all medical schools is to be tied to an agreement that each school will guarantee that, by 1978, 35 per cent of all graduates will enter primary care; by 1979, it will be 40 per cent; and by 1980, 50 per cent. The success of this bill, of course, depends on the definition of primary care and whether the agreement can, in fact, be implemented and, if not, whether the federal government cuts off the capitation payment. The Association of American Medical Colleges has persuaded the government that university departments of internal medicine, paediatrics and obstetrics/gynaecology are intensely interested in primary care, but in reality this sudden change of heart would appear to be connected more with the fear of losing the capitation payment than with any genuine interest in primary care. Certainly the government should insist that the existing training programmes are altered away from the production of super-specialists (particularly in internal medicine) before they accept the advice of the Association of American Medical Colleges.

The question remains: will the increase in the number of family physicians help the problem of primary care in the areas where the maldistribution problem is greatest – rural and inner-city areas – or will they merely increase the quality of medical care for the middle classes in suburbia? It is too early to know, but reports from medical schools are favourable (Curry, 1977), and a survey of 562 graduates carried out by the American Academy of Family Physicians is of considerable interest as it shows that, of the 516 graduates who responded, 47 per cent are working in populations of less than 30 000, which suggests that family medicine graduates are practising in areas of real need (Table 29).

Personal assessment

It is customary and fashionable in some quarters to blame most of the defects of health care in the USA on the medical profession. Such an interpretation is only partially true and takes a simplistic view of the situation, thus avoiding some of the more complex and wider issues. The USA proudly and rightly claims to be a classless society, but from

TABLE 29   Summary of distribution of graduated residents (1965) – by community size
Total graduates surveyed – 562
Total responses   – 516 (92 per cent)

Population of community	Number of graduated residents	Percentage of graduates entering practice	Percentage of responding graduates
Smaller than 5000	73	17.3	14.2
5000–15 000	106	25.1	20.5
15 000–30 000	61	14.5	11.9
30 000–100 000	59	14.0	11.4
10 000–500 000	76	18.0	14.7
Over 500 000	47	11.1	9.1
	422		
Others: Foreign, military	94		18.2
	516		

Source: *Proceedings of the Family Health Foundation of America*. Conference on Primary Health Care, Washington DC (1976)

this it must not be inferred that it supports a general philosophy of egalitarianism. In fact, the opposite would appear to be the case in economic, social, cultural and health matters, and the USA at least makes no pretence, is more realistic, less impossibly idealistic in humanitarian claims it cannot hope to fulfil than a number of its ideological opponents. In the capitalist world, equality cannot be distributed; privilege is a fact of life – as of course it is in the USSR (Van der Post, 1965; Kaiser, 1976; Smith, 1976) – and the inevitability of inequality in medical care must be accepted. The defenders of the present health care system (Schwartz, 1972) correctly proclaim that those countries which believe in egalitarian principles of health care have not succeeded; in the UK, the areas of continuing poor facilities and standards, associated with virtually no re-allocation of financial resources, have remained almost unchanged since the inception of the National Health Service in 1948, while in Norway, Sweden and Finland, so great is the gap between theory and reality in urban areas that private medicine is the only satisfactory form of primary care. Such criticisms are perfectly valid and strengthen the view that egalitarianism in health care outside the socialist world is merely an abstract posture which can never be accomplished. Furthermore, supporters of a free-enterprise system will say that at least their view is honest, even if unpopular, and perhaps even morally more defensible than promising a Utopia which can never be reached.

Therefore, any changes in health care which are advocated must be seen against this background: is medical care a privilege or a basic human right? American society, through Congress, must decide. It is an argument about moral value judgements but, whichever view is adopted, there can be no excuse for not attempting to improve the organisation of care and for maintaining a system which is manifestly failing a substantial minority and may well become too expensive for a decreasing majority. The profligate use of manpower and resources associated with a disorganised non-system of care is indefensible. What is crucial is whether the public has the confidence that the present medical establishment is willing to change or whether the alternative of large-scale federal involvement is more likely to produce the desired results.

The USA remains the only major industrialised country in the world without compulsory health insurance, and it has been recognised by some politicians, patients and doctors that reform of health insurance is one of the first priorities in any legislation to improve health care – both at the primary and hospital level. Compulsory insurance with an extension to protect those not already covered as well as coverage for catastrophic illness, may be introduced by the present administration. What form it will take can only be speculative. National Health Insurance, federally funded and modelled on the UK has been advocated (or threatened) for the last decade, but as yet no decision has been taken. *

Certainly extension of private insurance (Blue Cross/Blue Shield and a limited number of commercial companies, with safeguards and controls decided by the federal government but administered by the states), with income-related premiums shared between employer and employee and private insurance encouraged at the top end of the income scale, would seem to suit the American need for diversity and choice and be preferable to a centrally imposed bureaucracy. In addition, somehow the stigma attached to Medicaid must be removed and this will involve some government involvement with federal/state

* For a clear, concise, comprehensive account of the inadequacies of Health Insurance, the rationale for National Health Insurance and the options for Congress, see Fox (1977).

financial support for the poor, but organised within the restructured insurance system. Next, a re-orientation of insurance away from procedures towards consultative and preventive medicine as well as extension to cover visits to the doctor's office is essential if there is to be an improvement in the availability of primary care.

Defenders of the present insurance arrangements reiterate that most Americans have reasonably good coverage including most in-patient services. Furthermore catastrophic coverage is expanding rapidly and lifetime limits below $50 000 are becoming increasingly rare. It is said that if the 'average' American could not obtain coverage then National Health Insurance would have already been introduced and passed by Congress. Such arguments are thoroughly unconvincing: first, only those who are wealthy enough can increase their coverage adequately and, second, the 'average' American excludes 20 million without any coverage and at least 40 million with inadequate insurance.

Both in primary and secondary care, unrealistic expectations of health have been placed before the general public. Patients have been led to believe that optimum care is synonymous with hospital care, that more tests, investigations and treatment must of necessity be better and that the more specialist-trained the doctor, the more likely it is that he will have a solution for their problems. Unnecessary investigation and treatment and the unjustified seeking for expensive cures for quite trivial illnesses is now a national phenomenon. How will it be possible to change patients' attitudes and re-educate two generations who in the last 25 years have come to regard this type of care as a necessity? How is it possible to re-educate the medical profession away from procedures and curative medicine when the financial incentive is to do more and more? Although this situation is partly physician-induced, it is by no means the whole story. The news media must accept some responsibility with their relentless focusing on spectacular therapy or the latest piece of sophisticated technology, while the legal profession, to a greater extent than in any other country, is involved in an enormous number of malpractice suits on behalf of patients, which inevitably has had an effect on patient management. To an outside observer, the blatant, almost unscrupulous, encouragement given to patients and their relatives by lawyers appears to be motivated more for their own personal gain than for any real sense of justice between patient and doctor. The fear of litigation inevitably plays a large part in inappropriate treatment, and particularly in over-investigation. It is to be hoped that sanity will eventually prevail and some way will be found to alter the whole mode of practice so that incentives are given both to doctors and patients to avoid unnecessary services and thus reduce medical costs.

It seems unlikely that in the foreseeable future there will be any radical change in the organisation of primary care. There may be a marginal increase in the number of HMOs, NHCs and large multispecialty group practices but, apart from the emergency room in inner-city areas and the probable increase in the use of medical auxiliaries, primary care will remain the province of private physicians working in small groups. The desire for a generalist physician has been voiced by patients, politicians and some members of the medical profession for many years and the recent interest in family medicine, shown both by young doctors and the federal government, has brought into focus the relationship between the internist, paediatrician and gynaecologist, on the one hand, and the new breed of family physicians on the other. At present the omens for family medicine seem good, but it is too early to know if the problem of physician maldistribution can be permanently solved, or if the patient will change the habits of a lifetime and choose the services of a family physician rather than a 'specialoid' primary physician. Patients will need to see clearly the advantages of a family physician compared with his internist or paediatric colleague. It must be remembered that the original reason for the growth in the number of internists and paediatricians providing primary care was the poor standard of general practice. The most that can be expected from the renaissance of family medicine is that in rural, semi-rural and, to a lesser extent, in some suburban areas the family physician will become the physician of choice but, for the majority in the vast urban areas, his influence will be marginal and primary care will remain predominantly in the hands of 'specialoid' physicians.

If the standard of primary care depended on original and independent thought, on stimulating and unconventional ideas, on a general disdain for orthodoxy, on flexibility and experimentation, on a distrust and fear of bureaucratic inertia, on hard work, boundless energy and a desire to 'get things done', then the USA would lead the world. But health care, particularly primary care, is a product of the social and political environment of any country. It is constrained and influenced by the mentality and philosophy of both patients and doctors. Here lies the basic problem for the USA.

9

AUSTRALIA, NEW ZEALAND AND CANADA
by Eric Gambrill

Introduction

Australia, New Zealand and Canada together represent the countries of the old, i.e. white, British Commonwealth. Culturally and historically they share a common heritage, with the majority of their inhabitants either recently migrated from Britain or descended from first generations of British immigrants.

Because of this shared background it was inevitable that social and political developments in all three countries would proceed along broadly similar lines. However, each of these countries has its own unique mixture of geographical, climatic and population factors and these, together with differing internal pressures and outside influences, have served to produce subtly different approaches to the provision of health and social services.

Australia and Canada are both vast countries, encompassing large areas of desert or mountains, with a minority of their population spread sparsely over most of the terrain, and a concentration of their population in the cities (Table 1). New Zealand is a much smaller country, unaffected by the fierce heat of Australia or the severe cold of Canada, but occupied by a small, sparse population who are increasingly concentrated in the metropolitan areas. Australia and New Zealand are relatively isolated in the South Pacific while Canada is adjacent to the powerful influence of the USA.

All three countries share a democratic tradition, with a federal structure preferred in Australia and Canada and a unitary structure in New Zealand. Similarly, all three countries have a capitalist economic system, modified by varying degrees of state control and involvement in each country. They have in common a free and critical press, active and powerful trade union organisations and sophisticated legal systems. The general standard of living is high in all of these countries and their future economic potential almost unlimited.

Health expenditure as a proportion of GNP is high and increasing (Table 2) and combines government spending, private insurance payments and individual contributions in varying degrees, a mixture

TABLE 1 *Distribution of population, 1970*

	Percentage distribution	
	Urban	Rural
Australia	83.4	16.6
Canada	76.3	23.7

Source: *UN Demographic Year Book*

TABLE 2 *Health expenditure as a percentage of the GNP*

	1960	1970	1973
Australia	4.6	4.9	5.6
Canada	5.3	6.8	7.1 (1971)

Source: *UN Demographic Year Book*

TABLE 3 *Distribution of doctors and nurses, 1972*

	Doctors per 10 000 population	Habitants per doctor	Nurses per 10 000 population	Habitants per nurse
Australia	12.7	790	9.7	1030
New Zealand	11.8	850	74.9[a]	130
Canada	15.0	670	15.0	670

[a] Number of nursing certificates issued annually: may not all be practising.
Source: *WHO Statistics* and *Fifth Report on the World Health Situation 1969–72*, Geneva 1975

similar to that used in most Western European systems of health care (see Chapter 4). The supply of doctors and nurses is generally adequate (Table 3) but there are considerable problems in the distribution of skilled health personnel.

In terms of the usual comparative statistics related to health care (Table 4) all these countries lie in the middle rank of the advanced industrial nations, approximately level with the UK and other EEC countries, behind the Scandinavian countries, but ahead of the USA and the nations of Southern Europe.

TABLE 4   *Health indices, 1972*

	Infant mortality (per 1000 live births)	Neo-natal mortality (per 1000 live births)	Maternal mortality (per 1000 live births)	Life expectancy	
				M	F
Australia	16.7	12.0	0.1	68 approx.	74 approx.
New Zealand	15.6	10.1	0.2 (1971)	69.2	74.8
Canada	17.1	11.9	0.2	69.3	76.7

Source: *WHO Statistics* and *Fifth Report on the World Health Situation 1969–72*. Geneva 1975

AUSTRALIA

Introduction

The continent of Australia has an area of about three million square miles, approximately equal in size to the USA or Europe. One third of the continent consists of an enormous arid desert and another third has very little rainfall and is semi-arid. The climate varies from tropical in the north to temperate in Tasmania.

As a result of these extraordinary geographical features most of the country is very thinly populated and the total population is under 13 million. Paradoxically, Australia, with its vast land area, is probably the most highly urbanised society in the world with 83 per cent of the people living in cities. Moreover, all the major cities, with the exception of Perth in Western Australia, are situated along the eastern and south-eastern seaboard.

Up to the end of the Second World War the population was over-
whelmingly of British origin, but since that time the acceptance of
refugees and an energetic immigration policy has increased the proportion of immigrants from the rest of Europe, both west and east.
Italy, Greece and Malta, in particular, have provided many new
Australians. The age structure of the population is weighted towards
youth with almost a third of the population under sixteen and less than
10 per cent over 65.

The Commonwealth of Australia was founded in 1901 by the federation of six states, Western Australia, South Australia, Tasmania,
Victoria, New South Wales and Queensland, each of them originally
separate British colonies. Although the agricultural sector is still an
important part of the economy, it no longer holds a pre-eminent
position. The last thirty years have seen considerable development of
Australia's enormous mineral potential and of secondary industry.
The economy boomed in the late sixties and early seventies and the
people of Australia currently enjoy one of the highest standards of
living in the world.

Health and social security

In 1905, Australia became one of the first nations to introduce
social security legislation and the basis of a welfare state, and there is
now comprehensive provision of pensions for the aged and chronic
sick, family allowances and unemployment benefit. The federal government has a Repatriation Department, headed by a Cabinet Minister, which provides an extensive system of health and social security
benefits to ex-servicemen and their families. Each state makes provisions under Workmen's Compensation Acts for people injured at
work.

The history of the development of government-supported provision
for health care in Australia is one of continual turmoil between the
medical profession and governments of varying political complexions.
In the late 1940s the Labour government's plans for a health service
were bitterly resisted to the extent that the profession contrived to have
the employment of doctors by a National Health Service declared to be
a form of peacetime conscription and therefore unconstitutional!

Eventually, in the 1950s, the Liberal–Country-party government
implemented compromise proposals whereby hospital charges and
medical fees, both inside and outside hospital, were partially reim-

bursed by a combination of voluntary insurance and Commonwealth government support. Medical staff in hospitals treated patients in 'private' or 'intermediate', i.e. semi-private, wards on an item-of-service basis and patients in 'public' wards without fee and without payment from the hospital. Because of this charitable element in their work they were known as 'Honoraries'. Except in Queensland, it was necessary for the patient to pass a means test or to be in receipt of a state retirement or invalid pension in order to qualify for treatment as a 'public' patient. In Queensland, 'public' wards had long been open to any resident and the public hospital doctors were salaried on a sessional basis. General practitioner services to 'pensioners' and 'repatriation patients', i.e. ex-servicemen (*vide supra*), were provided by a voucher system, with the doctor claiming concessional fees from the Commonwealth government. In addition, a pharmaceutical benefit scheme was introduced whereby a limited range of drugs was made available at nominal charge.

By the mid 1960s, the problems inherent in these rather complex arrangements were becoming increasingly acute and in 1968, the Nimmo committee was established in order to investigate the situation. The multiplicity of voluntary insurance companies, each offering varying rates of contribution and reimbursement, were incurring very high overheads and the patients were having to find an increasingly large proportion of sharply rising medical and hospital fees from their own pockets. Many services were not covered at all, including home nursing, physiotherapy, optometry and dentistry. In this situation many general practitioners were carrying bad debts of up to 20 per cent of nominal income.

Legislation in 1970 (Australian Govt., 1970), following the report of the Nimmo committee, endeavoured to overcome some of these problems by introducing the concept of the 'most common fee'. The intention was that, provided the doctors charged the most common fee for any given service, the amount the patient would have to pay would be nominal. Again, there was bitter opposition from the medical profession, especially the general practitioners, who felt that the new fee schedules, introducing the concept of a different and higher benefit for certain procedures when carried out by a registered specialist, mitigated against the interests of the general practitioners. Indeed, in 1971, at least one-third of general practitioners were charging more than the most common fee for surgery (office) consultations and home visits.

The relative failure of the Nimmo committee reforms led to increasingly critical press campaigns and with the election of the first Labour government for nearly 25 years, in 1972, the stage seemed set for a major confrontation.

'Medibank' was to be the new, comprehensive, tax-financed, health care plan for Australia, featuring equal services for all, irrespective of means. It was envisaged that patients would opt for free hospital care in public wards by salaried specialists although retaining the option of private treatment at greater cost. General practitioners were encouraged to save overheads and simplify administration by billing Medibank direct for fees and accepting 85 per cent of the agreed tariff, as in the Canadian model, but this was strenuously opposed by the professional organisations as an attempt to make the doctors accept a government fee schedule. Instead, general practitioners have preferred to continue to send their bills to the patient, leaving the patient to claim reimbursement from Medibank.

Since the election in 1976 of a more conservative government, legislation has been introduced to levy a specific new tax to finance the scheme and the higher income earners have been allowed to opt out. The situation remains extremely fluid with neither the profession, the patients, nor the government completely satisfied.

Primary medical care

Unfortunately, the great confrontation over money has served to cloud and confuse the more basic issues of the role of the general practitioner in modern Australia.

In 1947, 79 per cent of all medical practitioners were in general practice. By 1965 this figure had fallen to 44 per cent and by 1976 to 39 per cent. It has been estimated that each general practitioner now cares for more than 2000 patients. There appears to be a rising demand for service, from 2.5 doctor/patient contacts per annum in 1955 to 4.2 doctor/patient contacts per annum in 1970. The average workload varies from 136 doctor/patient contacts per week in Tasmania to 172 doctor/patient contacts per week in Queensland (Ryan, 1972; Medimail, 1976; RACGP, 1976). Working-time for a general practitioner appears to average about 50 hours per week, excluding time 'on call' (Australian Medical Association, 1973).

The average age of general practitioners is also rising and is now over 50 years; there are problems in the recruitment of general practitioners in spite of the expectation of high financial reward (Ryan, 1972). No doubt the position would be much more serious were it not for the large number of immigrant doctors, especially from the UK and Eastern Europe, who have entered general practice in Australia over the past 30 years. One of the major factors in the relatively poor level of recruitment to general practice of native-born doctors appears to be the uncertainty which many established general practitioners feel about their future role in the provision of medical care. Traditionally, the Australian general practitioner has been a man for all seasons and all reasons, involved to a considerable extent in hospital work, performing minor and sometimes major surgery, anaesthesia and obstetrics. About 20 per cent of general practitioners hold a higher qualification in some specialty (Farrar, 1977). As the numbers of specialists increase and extend their range beyond the capital cities and as the differential fee schedules discourage general practitioners from performing technical procedures, the general practitioner sees his role in this field diminishing. The patients' expectations are changing too, and increasingly they seek specialist care. However, referral by a general practitioner is required in order to claim full reimbursement of fees.

While the population is still predominantly young, nearly 10 per cent of Australians are now over 65, and the burden of chronic illness and geriatric care is increasing. Faced with this situation the general practitioner sees his role in long-term and continuing management of these problems becoming greater. The prospect does not greatly appeal to the traditional general practitioner and there has been little development of, or appreciation of the need for, the team approach to primary health care. Thus, the Australian general practitioner feels himself to be losing one role without fully accepting a different and more relevant role, especially in the urban setting.

Rural practice

Primary care in the most isolated areas of the country is provided by the widely known Royal Flying Doctor Service, which is now largely a misnomer since the doctor gives advice over the radio-telephone and visits outlying clinics, while it is normally the nursing sister who actually flies out to bring the more seriously ill patient in to the base hospital. This service is totally salaried. In Queensland and Tasmania the state governments are responsible for small hospitals staffed by salaried district medical officers who provide primary care in some rural areas.

The isolated rural general practitioner has become increasingly rare since, with the improvement in roads and transport facilities, and the great reluctance of any doctors to take up these posts, the tendency has been for rural doctors to group together in the small country town and for the patients to travel to them. This provides the doctor with professional aid and support, thus allowing him to develop an interest in surgery, anaesthesia and obstetrics, which are particularly required in these conditions, and which may be practised with reasonable facilities within the community hospital. The emphasis on technical medicine and the opportunity to pursue specialist interests makes these jobs particularly attractive to doctors trained in a surgical specialty who have been unable to find a specialist niche in an urban area of Australia or in the UK.

Most of the community hospitals provide basic pathology and X-ray facilities or these may be provided by the doctors themselves on their own premises. Contrast radiography or more sophisticated investigations may require a journey of up to 200 miles to the base hospital. Depending on the interest and the degree of training of the rural general practitioner, he may tackle any procedure for which he considers himself capable. There is no system of accreditation or graded privileges as in Canada and the system therefore demands a good deal of ethical restraint and self-knowledge by the doctor in regard to his own capabilities. Procedures up to and including cholecystectomy, hysterectomy and lower segment Caesarian section are performed regularly by country general practitioners, and they also undertake a good deal of trauma surgery. More complex cases of non-urgent surgery, especially malignant conditions, are usually referred to the surgeon at the base hospital or to the teaching centres in the capital cities. However, base-hospital surgeons are increasingly visiting outlying community hospitals to undertake this type of work.

Because of this emphasis on hospital work and technical skills, there tends to be a lack of interest in non-surgical conditions and especially in the psychological, social and community care aspects of general practice. This is not because there is no requirement for these services in rural areas, but rather that the outlook and temperament of the doctor, the pressure of work, and the relatively poor facilities available within the community, militate against any effective developments.

The community nursing service is patchy, depending as it does on voluntary nursing services and a few public health nurses. Because of the vast distances it is not feasible for the doctor to undertake home visiting, except within the town itself.

In spite of the attractive and responsible conditions for practice in the country towns, it has proved increasingly difficult to attract doctors, especially Australian graduates, away from the urban areas. The reasons given are many, but high on the list must be the relative cultural deprivation for the doctor's family, together with the intense heat, the dust, the swarms of insects, and the degree of isolation. Locums are difficult to attract and out-of-hours duty is frequent and onerous. A vicious circle has been created, in which poor recruitment has led to a considerable degree of overwork for rural general practitioners, leading to some doctors returning to urban areas to practise as general practitioners or take up a specialty, and many others declining to leave the city at all.

Urban practice
Traditionally, the urban and suburban general practitioner has had an approach to general practice which is similar to that of his rural brother. However, the increasing pressure upon him from patients presenting with more vague and ill-defined complaints relating to stress and ageing, together with the increased availability of specialists, and official encouragement to refer patients to them, and a progressive restriction of access to the large hospitals, have all combined to produce a sense of uneasiness about his future role (RACGP, 1976).

Traditional solo practice is still common in the urban areas. It is estimated that 75 per cent of metropolitan general practitioners use deputising services to provide cover at night and at weekends and most of the others take part in rotas so that solo practice is an acceptable way of life (Farrar, 1977). There is, of course, no contractual requirement for the doctor to be available to his patients out of hours and no continuing legal responsibility, so that many patients have become accustomed to using the casualty department for urgent consultation and, indeed, as the sole source of primary care in some of the inner-city areas. Group practice has been slow to develop but it is increasingly popular among the younger graduates and probably 30–40 per cent of urban general practitioners now work in groups (Farrar, 1977). The facilities available are superior and the standard of premises, normally purpose-built or adapted, is higher in group practice than in solo practice.

Nurses are employed by the majority of groups of general practitioners but often their functions could be performed just as well by a receptionist or clerk. Infant welfare clinics are operated by the individual states and municipalities, using specially trained nurses, and there are home-nursing organisations in most urban areas. However, cooperation and coordination with general practitioners is almost completely lacking, and the concept of the primary health care team has been slow to develop. In recent years the Commonwealth government has offered increasing financial assistance to home-care services, including home nursing, meals on wheels and the provision of aids. There are a few experimental schemes such as that organised in Melbourne at Monash University, where comprehensive home-care services are provided. Community health centres providing comprehensive and multidisciplinary care were a feature of the health planning of the new Labour government in 1972 and a token number are now in operation. The provision of nursing-home facilities for the chronic sick and geriatric patients is good and is based largely on government support for private nursing-home fees. A doctor's certificate is required each month to confirm the need for nursing-home care and higher fees and reimbursements are provided for patients needing intensive nursing care. Staffing does not appear to be a problem in these units and a system of state regulation and inspection maintains standards.

The urban general practitioner can arrange pathological and radiological investigations for his patients either through the relevant specialists in private practice or through the hospital service. He has access to the many private hospitals in the cities, some of which are profit-making and some of which are run as non-profit-making charities, often by religious orders. He also has access to the suburban state hospitals in which up to 40 per cent of staff may be general practitioners, but not to most of the large teaching institutions (Farrar, 1977).

The range of his work is likely to be similar to that of his counterparts in urban practice in New Zealand, Canada and the UK, with the emphasis on respiratory, cardiovascular and psychological problems. The care of well patients, including immunisation, contraceptive advice and insurance examinations, accounts for 12 per cent of the total workload (RACGP, 1976). A number of multiphasic screening units have been established in the major cities, but there is no tradition of the general practitioner performing routine screening examinations as is commonplace in North America.

Domiciliary obstetrics is virtually unknown and, since there is no provision for shared care, an increasing number of urban general practitioners are totally relinquishing their role to the obstetricians. Older general practitioners and those with surgical qualifications still do a significant amount of surgery in urban areas and many general practitioners give anaesthetics on a regular basis.

Training

Departments of community medicine or community practice have been established in all universities which contain a medical school, enabling the undergraduates to have some contact, however brief, with general practice.

The development of postgraduate training for general practice was initially rather slow, but the 1972 Labour government encouraged and financed the Royal Australian College of General Practitioners' (RACGP) Family Medicine Programme. This is confined mainly to the young graduate and Commonwealth funding is in the vicinity of $A5 million annually. The Family Medicine Programme is intended to provide a flexible and relevant course of study lasting up to five years, with the young doctor alternating between hospital posts and short spells in various practices for the first three years, and then working for two years in selected training practices. There is no government subsidy involved during the final two years' experience. It is envisaged that most new graduates entering family medicine after 1980 will have passed through a partial or complete training programme.

Continuing education by means of refresher courses is popular. In NSW the state government pays an annual grant of $A12 500 to the NSW Faculty of the RACGP to employ a part-time postgraduate Fellow whose job is to determine as far as possible the educational needs of established general practitioners within the state (Farrar, 1977).

A correspondence course, emphasising self-audit, called 'Check Programme' is used, particularly by those practitioners who wish to sit the College examination. This qualification, the MRACGP, is stated by qualified observers to be approximately equivalent in standard to the British MRCGP and Canadian MCFPC.*

There is no likelihood in the foreseeable future that either adequate postgraduate training or the passing of an appropriate examination will become a mandatory requirement for a doctor wishing to provide general medical services in Australia.

NEW ZEALAND

Introduction

New Zealand principally consists of two islands, North Island and South Island, lying south-east of Australia, 1300 miles across the Tasman Sea. The total area is a little over 100 000 square miles, slightly larger than Great Britain, but the population is less than 3 million.

The climate of North Island is subtropical with lush vegetation while South Island is temperate, with the Southern Alps and the Canterbury Plains as its main geographical features.

The small population is roughly 90 per cent European and about 10 per cent of Maori and Polynesian origin. Most of the Europeans (98 per cent) are of British stock and strong ties still exist between New Zealand and the UK. Over 70 per cent of the population live in urban areas and this proportion is increasing.

New Zealand is still a predominantly agricultural economy and a primary producer, although secondary industry is developing in the urban areas. There are no great extremes of poverty and wealth and the overall philosophy tends towards egalitarianism, in the framework of a mixed economy. The average standard of living is comfortably high, but the New Zealand economy has not expanded so dramatically as that of neighbouring Australia.

Health and social security

New Zealand led the world in making medical, hospital and allied benefits available to all through the passing of the Social Security Act, 1938. This same Act provided comprehensive age, unemployment and sickness benefit and in 1941 the General Medical Services (GMS) and Pharmaceutical Benefits Scheme commenced.

* MRACGP, Member of the Royal Australian College of General Practitioners. MRCGP, Member of the Royal College of General Practioners. MCFPC, Member of the College of Family Physicians of Canada.

The Department of Health administers the provision of health care through four divisions: of Hospitals, of Clinical Services, of Nursing and of Mental Health. The Division of Clinical Services is responsible for promoting primary medical services, pharmaceutical benefits, the provision of artificial aids, laboratory and X-ray facilities, physiotherapy and maternity services among many other functions.

The New Zealand health scheme is financed out of general taxation. All services in public hospitals are free of charge to the patient and specialists providing medical services within the public hospitals are full-time or part-time salaried employees. However, many specialists treat patients privately in private institutions, facilitating free choice of specialist and avoiding the waiting list for admission to the public hospital.

The original intention was that the cost of the primary care services should also be borne entirely by taxation, and that general practitioners would become salaried employees. This was bitterly opposed by the medical profession, so that a system of item of service arose, with part of the cost, originally about two-thirds, being paid by the state and the rest borne by the patient. The state contribution, the GMS benefit, remained at the same level for many years and gradually came to represent less than one-third of the usual fee. Following increasing public dissatisfaction the schedules were brought up to date in late 1974, so that, while 'ordinary' patients still have to pay the bulk of the consultation fee out of their own pocket, the 'special group' patients, including dependent children, pensioners and the chronically ill, are asked to pay little or nothing directly to the doctor.

Primary medical care

The general practitioner is considered to be the hub of the New Zealand health care system. There are a little over 1200 general practitioners actively engaged in practice, of whom about 350 practise in rural or semi-rural areas. The proportion of general practitioners as a percentage of doctors in private practice and as a percentage of the total on the medical register has declined considerably over the last 25 years and the average general practitioner is now responsible for well over 2000 patients. It is known that the average general practitioner renders about 7500 services a year, or 150 services per week. In 1973, the total number of general practitioner/patient contacts worked out at 3.9 per head of population per year (NZ Govt., 1974).

The general practitioner, whether he works in a rural or an urban area, provides primary care in his surgery (office) or in the patient's home and sees a similar spectrum of disease to his opposite number in Australia, Canada and the UK. He is able to mobilise various community services such as district nurses, meals-on-wheels, home aids, social welfare workers, physiotherapists and some occupational therapists. These services are usually based on the public hospital. He may refer his patients for a specialist opinion at the public hospital or privately if the patient prefers. Laboratory services are free to the patient, as also are X-ray facilities at the public hospitals.

Rural practice

A few remote and sparsely populated areas are served by salaried medical officers and the patients are entitled to free medical attention and drugs.

Designated rural-area doctors practise as any other general practitioner in New Zealand but, by virtue of working in an area declared rural by the Minister of Health, i.e. having a total population of less than 5000 in the locality, he becomes eligible for certain benefits. These include an assisted passage scheme for doctors from the UK, free housing and surgery accommodation in some instances, a bonus of 10 per cent on GMS benefit and 25 per cent on GMS mileage payments, a special fee for telephone consultation, a subsidy for the employment of a locum, a rural practice grant to junior medical officers and the ability to count this area of private work as a qualifying period for postgraduate bursary. These bursaries provide financial help towards continuing postgraduate education both within New Zealand and abroad.

These incentives to rural practice were introduced in 1969, but probably the most important of all was the introduction of a registered nurse subsidy, enabling the doctor to employ a nurse to work alongside him in his rooms and to visit on his behalf the housebound elderly and chronic sick. The subsidy is made up of 50 per cent reimbursement of an approved salary, and fees for each visit made by the nurse, or by 100 per cent reimbursement of the nurse's approved salary. Thus it is similar in concept to the UK scheme whereby general practitioners are reimbursed 70 per cent of an approved salary scale for nurses and administrative staff employed, up to a maximum of two full-time equivalent employees per doctor. The nurse fulfils a role similar to some practice nurses in the UK, but not as extensive as that of the nurse practitioner in North America. Where they are available there would also be district nurses undertaking home nursing, public health nurses and nurses sponsored by the Plunkett Society, a voluntary agency with government support, who have a particular role in the care of well-babies. (See UK, p. 37.)

Although the country is thinly populated, the standard of roads and transport facilities is high, so access to the base hospital is rarely too difficult in case of emergency. Small public community hospitals are usually available in these rural areas, but it is unusual for the general practitioner to undertake surgery to any extent.

Urban practice

Most New Zealand general practitioners fall into this category, since the process of urbanisation is affecting even this predominantly agricultural country. While solo practice is still the norm, there is an increasing tendency for general practitioners to work together in groups from purpose-built or adapted premises. The concept of primary care is still very much doctor-orientated and the development of the team approach is in its infancy. However, following the success of the registered nurse subsidy in rural areas, the scheme was extended in late 1974 so that an increasing number of general practitioners employ a practice nurse. Relationships with other nurses working in the community vary considerably from area to area, but are rarely close enough to constitute a primary health care team. Emergency work is usually arranged within a group or on a rota between solo practitioners. Urban general practitioners do not normally look after their own patients in the public hospitals, but they do have access to the private hospitals (Anyon, 1976).

Health centres, as envisaged in New Zealand, are places in which primary care is administered by a team under the direction of the general practitioner. The medical profession is now tending to look toward state-financed centres rather than private centres, although state loan finance is available for the latter. However, because of the cost of construction and operation of these centres and the inherent conservatism and dislike of too much state involvement by the general practitioner, it seems unlikely that any rapid development will occur.

The composition and number of members in the team has not yet been agreed, but it has been suggested that the basic requirements, in addition to a group of general practitioners, are registered nurses,

social workers, physiotherapists, and possibly occupational therapists, plus clerical and managerial staff. In future, it is envisaged that
district nurses, who are employed by hospital boards, and public and
industrial health nurses from the District Health Office will be housed
under the same roof. The development of the team concept is highlighted in the recent White Paper, *A New Health Service for New Zealand*,
but implementation of this document may be deferred by the new
government (NZ Govt., 1974).

Training

Medical students studying at both of the two medical schools
in New Zealand are required to spend a compulsory period of four
weeks in general practice. However, there are no fully developed
departments of general practice within the medical schools as yet.
Specialised postgraduate training for general practice is still in its
infancy but the scheme for registrars in general practice is expanding in
spite of difficulties arising from the attachment of registrars within the
present item-of-service structure. Continuing education for primary
care physicians is conducted primarily at base hospitals throughout
the country. The courses are arranged by the various postgraduate
medical societies or the New Zealand College of General Practitioners,
often jointly.

CANADA

Introduction

Canada is the second largest country in the world (the largest
being the USSR), with an area of 3.9 million square miles. It extends
from the 49th parallel in the south to the Arctic in the north, and from
Vancouver in the west to St John's, Newfoundland, over four
thousand miles to the east. The summer climate is temperate, except in
the Arctic region, but the winters are severe, especially in the prairies
and the north.

The total population is now more than 22 million and over 90 per
cent of Canadians live within 100 miles of the border with the USA.
Over 70 per cent of the population live in urban areas with the greatest
concentrations of population in Toronto and Montreal in south-
eastern Canada. The two main ethnic groups are the British who
account for nearly one-half of the population and the French who

account for one-third. The rest of the population is made up of other European nationalities, together with a small number of Asians, Negroes and native Indians and Eskimos.

Canada is extremely rich in mineral resources and is also a major industrial and trading power. The *per capita* income is one of the highest in the world.

Health and social security

By 1960, Canada and the USA remained the only developed countries in the world where the provision, or at least the financing, of health services for large groups of the population was not considered to be a responsibility of the state. In the 1930s, legislation had provided for unemployment insurance, retirement pensions and allowances for children. After the war, voluntary medical and hospital insurance plans became available and over 50 per cent of the population had some degree of cover by 1957.

The Hospital Insurance and Diagnostic Services Act of 1957, which all provinces had implemented by 1961, provided for the federal government to share with the provinces the cost of providing specified hospital services to insured patients, and now covers 99 per cent of the population of Canada. Hospitals in Canada are mostly operated as voluntary, usually non-profit-making agencies. Consequently, provincial and federal government control is indirect, through the provision or withholding of capital grants and reimbursements. As a result, coordinated development of hospital provision has been slow.

In 1962, Saskatchewan implemented a controversial compulsory medical-care insurance plan which provoked a famous doctors' strike but, with this sole exception, major developments in medical-care insurance had to await the report of the Royal Commission on Health Services in 1964, which recommended the initiation of a universal and comprehensive health insurance scheme for Canada. The Commission also made recommendations regarding financial and organisational aspects of the health services complex. This was a watershed in the development of health-care financing in Canada. Beginning in Saskatchewan in 1962 and ending in Quebec in 1970, all provinces have introduced comprehensive government insurance schemes. The pattern varies from one province to another. In some provinces the services are financed out of general reserves, in others via compulsory insurance plans. The federal government contributes to the provincial costs on a matching basis, and exercises control by providing financial support only if the provincial plans fall within the recommended guidelines. Most provinces make provision for welfare recipients and the elderly to receive prescribed drug benefits, dental services and some other health-care benefits in addition to physicians' services and hospital care.

For all other patients the plans pay for all physicians' services and hospital services, but not for drugs prescribed outside the hospital and not for dental care. The physician may choose to send his bill direct to the insurance plan, in which case he is usually paid 85–90 per cent of the standard fee, or to the patient, who reclaims from the plan. Provincial fee schedules are drawn up by the provincial medical associations and are then negotiated with the provincial government. As seems to be the pattern in all fee structures, the schedules are unduly weighted towards surgical and other technical procedures and against time spent in consultation, examination and counselling (Collyer, 1975).

Primary medical care

The provision of actual services by the government is limited to comparatively small groups for whose health services the federal government has assumed responsibility. The federal government thus provides services for registered Indians and Eskimos, for certain categories of seamen and immigrants and for members of the armed services and veterans. Many primary care doctors in very isolated areas work as salaried employees of third-party institutions and agencies.

The present provision of primary care services is mixed. In small towns and rural areas, family physicians often provide all services including surgery, obstetrics and anaesthesia. In urban and suburban areas, primary care is also provided by paediatricians, obstetricians and internists. The relative proportion of specialists and general practitioners providing primary care varies greatly across Canada. However, it is true to say that the bulk of primary care in Canada is in the hands of the general practitioner and that the proportion is increasing.

There are now over 35 000 active civilian physicians in Canada including interns and residents. Well over one-third are located in Ontario, which has the lowest population/physician ratio in Canada of 591. Thus Canada has a good supply of doctors by world standards. However, urban areas have a disproportionate supply of physicians compared with the rural areas, a situation which is aggravated by the fact that rural physicians are generally older and have less logistic support in terms of auxiliary personnel and facilities. Canada has over 80 000 qualified nurses and is also well supplied with hospital beds, having about 200 000 beds of all types available, i.e. over 9 hospital beds/thousand population.

The Royal Commission on Health Services reported in 1964 that the average working week of a general practitioner was 52 hours, with a doctor/patient contact rate of 159/week. Of these consultations, about 14 per cent were home visits, about 60 per cent office or surgery consultations and the remainder hospital visits. The average size of practice was about 1700 patients at risk. The time spent per office call was about 15 minutes, and the average number of doctor/patient contacts per patient per year was 4.18. In 1967, an unusual community-owned group practice employing salaried doctors reported 2000 patients per doctor. Each doctor averaged 148 patient/contacts in a 45.7 hour working week, spending 10.9 minutes with each patient (Wolfe & Badgely, 1972). Collyer, in 1975, reported an estimated doctor/patient contact rate per annum of 2.5–2.9 in a suburban practice with 81.5 per cent of contacts in his office, 1.5 per cent in the patient's home, 2 per cent in the emergency department, and 15 per cent in hospital (Collyer, 1975).

Rural practice

In the very sparsely inhabited Northwest Territories and the Yukon, the federal health department maintains nursing stations staffed by trained lay dispensers and has developed family medical packs for families and small bands of people who have no regular contact with the established services. Parts of the Arctic are visited annually by a ship carrying medical supplies and personnel. There are plans to cover the Arctic northern territories by flying circuits which would also provide for regular visits by professional personnel to the various outlying settlements.

Many of the smaller townships have great difficulty in attracting doctors and dentists to work single-handed and the small cottage hospitals in these areas are disappearing. The tendency has been for services to become centralised in the larger country towns, with the development of better transport and ambulance facilities, travelling clinics and strategically located group clinics. However, the problem as yet remains unresolved.

General (family) practice

There are many varieties in the pattern of practice in Canada, and the situation is changing rapidly. Solo practice is still the norm in many areas, even though the doctor may work in a medical arts building with other general practitioners and specialists, with ready access to pathology and radiological facilities. In small towns group practices are more common, often including one or more certified specialists and providing all services at the local hospital. Large, multi-specialty clinics, employing up to 100 doctors, with or without general practitioners, are found in some urban areas, particularly in the west. In addition to the doctor-sponsored groups and clinics, industry and government have in a few instances attempted to promote independent clinics with limited success (Rice, 1977). In several provinces, notably Quebec, plans have been proposed which include the provision of community health centres for the provision of primary health care by multidisciplinary teams.

The general practitioner's routine office work is similar in content to that of his counterparts in the UK or Australia, except that there is a much greater concentration on screening and preventive care in Canada, as in the USA. Around 20 per cent of his working time is spent in performing routine check-ups on healthy adults, an activity which consumes professional time and resources and is generally of unproven benefit. Telephone consultations also have an important place in the doctor's day and Collyer spoke to 68 patients by telephone in a sample week (Collyer, 1975). Emergency care is provided out-of-hours either by rota, within a group or among solo practitioners, or by hospital emergency departments. Indeed, the Canadian general practitioner increasingly uses the emergency department of his local hospital as a convenient and well-equipped consultation point. There is no legal obligation for the doctor to be available to his patients at any time.

Primary care is rarely practised today from the general practitioner's home. Most doctors work from purpose-built or adapted premises, either privately owned or rented. The general standard of accommodation, equipment and facilities is high.

The traditional role of the nurse in Canadian general practice was that of receptionist, telephonist, and performer of minor nursing duties such as injections and dressings. New concepts of the nurse's role in general practice have been much discussed and include: (1) the physician associate – working as a colleague and complementing his role in such areas as health education, disease prevention, well-baby and ante-natal care. This role would seem to be equivalent to that of the health visitor and the midwife in British terms, and (2) the physician substitute – replacing the physician as the primary contact with the patient but working under his supervision. This role would appear to be more akin to that of some practice nurses in the UK, the nurse practitioner in the USA, or the *feldscher* in the USSR (McWhinney, 1972).

The specific role required of the nurse will obviously vary according to the number of physicians available and the community in which she works. A programme for training physician substitutes was pioneered at McMaster University, Hamilton, Ontario by Professor Spitzer and his colleagues (Spitzer *et al.*, 1973, 1974).

Because of the emphasis on office consultation and hospital work and the decline of home visiting, and because there has been inadequate insurance coverage until recently, the facilities available for care in the community have been limited and patchy. Home-care schemes are being promoted by numerous voluntary health agencies, for example the Canadian Heart Foundation, the Canadian Cancer Society, and the Canadian Arthritis and Rheumatism Society. These services provide meals-on-wheels, nursing services, chiropody, physiotherapy and social support. Other agencies, mostly private and non-profit-making, are organised to provide certain types of service such as home nursing.

An interesting development is the institution of organised home-care plans which coordinate and make available to the patient and his physician the services of several agencies serving the community, including nursing, home-making, therapies and social services. These plans are organised either within the community or by a hospital to facilitate earlier discharge and appropriate after-care. They have particular value for the aged and the chronic sick and represent an important development in health care outside the hospital setting.

It is usual in Canada for a general practitioner to have admitting privileges in at least one hospital, even in a teaching hospital if he is a member of the teaching staff. On appointment to the active staff, the practitioner becomes entitled to general practitioner privileges, as defined by the hospital, and also becomes a member of the hospital department of family medicine. Membership in the department carries certain duties and responsibilities including committee work and administration. In city hospitals, the general practitioner can usually admit patients to the medical and paediatric wards and perform normal obstetrics and minor surgical procedures. It is usual for consultation with a specialist to be mandatory in defined circumstances and the committee structure monitors notes and records to see that the requirements have been complied with. In smaller towns and rural areas it is much easier for general practitioners to obtain surgical and obstetric privileges and to undertake major surgery.

In the days of voluntary insurance, coverage was often provided for reimbursement of the costs of care within hospital but not outside. This important factor, together with the decline in home-visiting and the relative lack of community facilities, resulted in many patients being admitted to hospital who could have been managed at home.

The system of medical audit operative in the hospitals did not prevent this waste of resources and it is only now, with government footing the bill, that serious attempts are being made by the administrators to encourage the substitution of low-cost community care for high-cost hospital care.

The traditional work-pattern in Canadian general practice is for the doctor to spend the morning in hospital work and the afternoons and some evenings in his office. However, the increasing demands of office practice are leaving less time for hospital work, the growth of specialisation in hospital means that more patients are referred, and urban traffic problems make travelling from office to hospital more difficult. A minority of general practitioners are now beginning to opt out of hospital practice entirely.

Education and training
The first departments of family medicine in Canada were established in 1967 and since that time there has been considerable development. All 16 medical schools now have family practice teaching units, which are model group practices providing a setting for research and for undergraduate and postgraduate teaching. This implies that all physicians wishing to practise family medicine in the community will be required to have undertaken specific training at a postgraduate level. The province of Ontario has intimated that medical schools should aim for 50 per cent of their graduates to become family physicians.

The Candian College of General Practitioners, formed in 1954, was initially active in promoting continuing education for general practitioners. Prior to 1966 the only formal training available for a general practitioner was the two-year rotating internship provided by a few hospitals, but then the College, together with the respective universities, jointly pioneered training programmes in London (Ontario) and Calgary. These programmes were of three-year duration following graduation and consisted of work in a university teaching practice as well as certain hospital departments. These pioneering efforts became models for the development of similar programmes in other universities, although there has been some pressure for the course to be reduced to two years.

The Canadian College of General Practitioners was renamed the College of Family Physicians of Canada in 1968 in order to emphasise the change of role which the College perceived, stressing the continuing care of family groups rather than the episodic care of disease episodes suffered by individual patients. In 1969, the College established its examination for certification in family medicine. Candidates must have completed three years of residency training in an accredited programme or have been in family practice for a minimum of five years. Outside observers have suggested that the standard of the examination is approximately equal to that of the Australian MRACGP and the British MRCGP.

COMPARISONS, EVALUATION AND CONCLUSIONS

Primary medical care

It is evident that the bulk of primary care in all three countries is in the hands of the general practitioner or family physician. Because of the historical background and the geographical isolation of many of these general practitioners until comparatively recent times, traditional general practice was dependent on the omnicompetent doctor, able and willing to turn his hand to medical, surgical and obstetric emergencies alike, with little or no help from specialist colleagues. From these historical traditions have developed attitudes and habits of work which have carried through to the increasingly complex and urbanised societies into which all three countries have developed.

Hospital work

One of the most important consequences of these traditions has been the great emphasis on the role of the general practitioner within the hospital, with a consequent denigration and relative demotion of his role in comprehensive community care outside of the hospital. This emphasis is seen most markedly in Canada and least in New Zealand. Other factors have conspired to emphasise the importance of the hospital role in the eyes of the general practitioner, not least the fee structures, which in every case emphasise the rewards for technical and surgical procedures rather than consultation, communication and general care. The training of medical students, in these three countries as in most others, is predominantly in hospitals, by hospital doctors, on hospital patients, and leads to the attitude that 'real medicine' can be practised only in the hospital setting. Until recently, especially in Canada, some patients were insured only for hospital care and this has led to the tradition of frequent admissions for the investigation and management of conditions which are usually managed in the community in other countries. Consequently, large numbers of hospital beds have had to be provided at great cost, and even these rich nations are beginning to reconsider their priorities in terms of hospital provision.

Further problems have arisen with regard to doubts about the ability and training of general practitioners to perform satisfactorily by modern standards in the increasingly technical fields of surgery, obstetrics and investigative medicine. It is my impression that surgical rates for operations such as tonsillectomy, appendicectomy and even hysterectomy are high in Canada and Australia by world standards. Evidence from the USA shows convincingly that an item-of-service system leads to surgical rates for these common operations which are more than double those on matched groups of patients looked after by a prepaid group practice. There is in Canada, at least in the urban areas, a reasonably effective system of peer review of clinical notes, tissue committees and the other paraphernalia of an audit system, but in Australia little or no control is exercised beyond the professional conscience of the individual doctor. It would seem that strict and limited licensing of privileges is mandatory if the quality of care is to be safeguarded.

While the need for a good deal of involvement in hospital work is an obvious necessity in the rural areas, it may be questioned whether concentration on this aspect of the general practitioner's work to the detriment of other requirements is appropriate in the growing urban areas, where easy access to specialist opinion and advice is the norm. Obviously the patient benefits from continuing contact with his own doctor while in hospital and this aspect is to be encouraged, but general practitioners engaged in specialised procedures need to have suitable training and enough continuing experience in order to remain competent. Otherwise they must be prepared to relinquish responsibility to the appropriate specialist when required.

Surgery (office) work and home visiting

It is fascinating to note that the volume of weekly work and the average number of doctor/patient contacts per annum in these countries is very similar, probably around four per year in primary care. The frequency of conditions diagnosed is also very similar, with far greater differences between individual doctors, particularly with regard to their perception of psychological problems, than between countries. The only major difference is in the much greater incidence of routine examination for screening purposes in Canada. In this respect Canadian doctors and patients behave more like Americans, whilst Australian and New Zealand doctors and patients behave more like the British. It is interesting to speculate why this should be so. Canada has been strongly influenced by the USA in many aspects of life, and Canadian doctors and patients seem to have adopted this American habit of screening rather uncritically. However, the principles of indiscriminate screening are increasingly being questioned in academic circles and opinion is moving towards positive health education and a more selective screening process. In all of these countries respiratory, cardiovascular and rheumatic conditions predominate, with psychological and social problems assuming an increasing importance.

Most general practitioners operate an appointment system and in all countries some patients complain that they are not able to be seen when and where it suits them. The habit of visiting patients in their homes has declined markedly in all three countries, but again in this respect Canada is more like the USA with many general practitioners refusing to visit under any circumstances. Instead, the emergency room of the local hospital has become a convenient meeting place for doctor and patient. This has certain advantages in terms of technical equipment and convenience for the doctor and may be positively beneficial in the acute case, but it is not appropriate for the continuing care of chronic conditions.

Emergency care out-of-hours is provided either by the general practitioners themselves, alone or in a group or rota, or increasingly by impersonal deputising services and junior staff in accident and emergency departments in the urban areas.

The lack of any administrative requirements for continuity of care or availability of the general practitioner is a defect of the system of primary care in all three countries, especially in urban areas.

The team and community care

While reports and official publications from all three countries have stressed the increasing inability of the general practitioner working alone to provide for all the needs of his community, the team concept of primary health care has been very slow to develop. However, the general practitioners are beginning to work in groups and to enjoy the benefits of professional cooperation and mutual education, and in Canada there have been some important experiments in defining the role and effectiveness of the nurse practitioner. Reimbursement of the salary of an attached nurse in New Zealand has been a great success, and the recent White Paper encourages closer working relationships with other community nurses. Nurses working in primary care in Canada and Australia are too often employed in a clerical and reception capacity and their nursing expertise is largely unused. They rarely leave the practice premises and play little part in the nursing care of patients at home. Contact between the general practitioner and the few community nurses who are available is often poor, and home-care facilities are not well developed. As the costs of hospital care rise there will no doubt be increasing pressure to provide alternative community facilities.

In all three countries there is little idea among general practitioners of the part which a trained social worker and community psychiatric nurse could play in managing the problems unearthed in primary medical care and, except in a few exceptional academic settings, co-ordination and cooperation with these workers is minimal.

While the development of community health centres providing comprehensive medical, nursing and social services from shared premises has been advocated in all three countries, there are major obstacles in the way of further development. First, the cost of such facilities is very high if provided out of the doctor's own pocket, and the medical profession in each country is suspicious of working from rented premises owned by the government. Second, the item-of-service system tends to discourage the doctor from sharing his work with other professionals, and third, to work effectively in a group setting with other professionals requires attitudes and methods of training which are foreign to doctors trained in the traditional manner to function alone.

Education, training and research

There has been increasing interest taken in the problems of primary care in many countries, and Canada, Australia and New Zealand are no exception. Most undergraduates have some exposure to general practice and to community medicine and in Canada, particularly, departments of family medicine have exerted increasing influence on the undergraduate curriculum. In Australia and New Zealand these influences are, as yet, rather limited.

Postgraduate or specific vocational training for all potential general practitioners has been accepted in principle by the academic bodies of general practice in all three countries, and the medico-political associations have come round to acceptance of the concept. In Canada, the programmes are based almost exclusively on the university departments of family medicine, while in Australia and New Zealand there are relatively few problems in devising the hospital components of the training but, until recently, little finance has been available for the payment of general practitioner trainees while gaining experience in practice. However, the Australian government has now made considerable sums of money available for the development of postgraduate education in general practice.

All three academic bodies of general practice, the CFPC, the RACGP and the RNZCGP,* conduct examinations for membership or certification which appear to be of a roughly comparable standard, but in none of these countries is either vocational training, the passing of an examination, or membership of an academic body, a requirement to practise primary medical care. The tendency in continuing education

* CFPC, College of Family Physicians of Canada. RNZCGP, Royal New Zealand College of General Practitioners.

has been for general practitioners themselves to play an increasing part in the organisation, administration and learning content of courses provided. Nevertheless, the tradition of didactic teaching of technical medicine by hospital specialists dies hard.

A few practitioners have produced research work of quality from primary medical care in all three countries and the academic bodies are active in correlating the work which has been done and stimulating further research and experimentation (RACGP, 1976; CFPC).

Finance and payment systems

Payment of general practitioners by an item-of-service system is the norm and some of the problems associated with this system have been outlined previously. National, state or provincial governments bear the bulk of the cost and are becoming increasingly concerned at the open-ended nature of the financial burden in a situation where neither provider nor consumer has any interest in keeping costs down, Because these are all rich countries the cost has been acceptable up to the present but, increasingly, governments and insurance agencies are questioning how long the free-for-all can continue. In Canada, provinces such as Ontario have established a ceiling on doctors' earnings from health insurance sources, and other provinces have taken to publishing statements of the annual payments received by individual doctors in the local press. In Australia, it has been avowed by opponents of the scheme that Medibank will bankrupt the country, and in New Zealand the White Paper talks of the need to control costs and assure value for money.

Since the profession in all three countries is extremely resistant to any change in the method of payment, it may be confidently predicted that this will continue to be a major source of conflict. It is interesting that in Canada, which was the latest of the three nations to develop government-financed health care, the doctors have accepted the principle of directly billing the health insurance plan, whereas in Australia and New Zealand, with longer established schemes, the doctors generally maintain the tradition of sending the bill to the patient.

The future

While the future of the general practitioner or family physician as the chief provider of primary medical care in all three countries seems assured, it seems equally certain that he will need to change his training, his role and his expectations if the needs of the population he serves are to be met.

The patterns of disease and the demands of the patients are changing in all developed countries. There is less emphasis on the acute illnesses, where episodic and hospital care is often appropriate, and more emphasis on preventive care, the long-term management of the chronic degenerative diseases and problems arising from psychosocial breakdown which require care in the community and a broader approach than that provided by technical, scientific medicine.

The public, the press and their political representatives are already aware of these needs and will exert increasing pressure on the medical profession to meet them. It seems likely that methods of payment will be modified or even radically changed, with increasing resources being made available for the development of primary health care teams based on community health centres. It is likely that there will be less emphasis on the role of the general practitioner in the hospital, although this will remain important in Canada and rural Australia.

All three countries have had problems in bringing primary care services to their rural areas, but these seem to have been largely overcome in New Zealand. In Canada and Australia it seems likely that there will have to be increased incentives for doctors to practise in these areas. These may be financial, organisational or linked with undergraduate scholarships and postgraduate training.

While problems remain, the strong traditions of general practice in these three countries provide a sound base for the development of the newer concepts and the wider horizons of the family physician.

10

JAPAN

Japan lies at the edge of the Asian continent. It consists of a group of four large islands and many smaller ones, stretching from north to south for just over 2400 miles and separated from the USSR, China and Korea by the Sea of Japan. The main island is Honshu and it is about the same size as the UK, or just smaller than the state of California, although only 20 per cent is habitable. The population, which is ethnically homogeneous, is about 103 million. It is estimated by the Institute of Population Problems of the Ministry of Health and Welfare, Tokyo, that by 1985 the total population will be 120 798 000, of which 9.5 per cent will be over 65 years of age compared with 7.0 per cent in 1970. Like most countries in the world, there has been considerable migration from rural to urban areas since the Second World War: the proportion of inhabitants in urban areas increased from 56.3 per cent in 1955 to 72.2 per cent in 1970. There were 118 900 physicians in 1970 (of which 11 319 (9.5 per cent) were female), giving a ratio 1 doctor to 860 population. There are no reliable figures available for the number of doctors concerned solely with primary care.

The development and organisation of medicine in Japan today appears, to the Western observer, to be haphazard, muddled, even chaotic. Although there is some truth in these impressions, it is not an entirely fair assessment of the situation, though possibly an inevitable one to an outsider on account of the unique nature of Japanese traditions, culture and society. The development of health services throughout the world has been influenced by historical, social and political factors, and Japan is no exception: in fact this applies more to Japan than to any other country under detailed consideration in this book. Without this background knowledge, unless one is Japanese or has lived in Japan, it would probably be beyond the capacity of most people to understand the present organisation of medical care.

History of Japanese medicine

Until the middle of the nineteenth century, there was almost no exchange of ideas or people with the outside world – at least the Western World. Certainly since the ninth century, when first Nara and then Kyōto were made the capital of Japan, she has remained isolated, independent and remote. There has been no migration of people and they have maintained their own customs, traditions and language for over a thousand years with practically no interference from outside influences. Before this, Buddhism came in AD 538 from India via China and Korea, and the language was developed from that of the Chinese mainland.

Medicine has followed the same pattern – 'traditional medicine' influenced mainly by India, China and Korea. It is true that in 1543 the Portuguese Catholic missionaries reached the southern part of Japan and introduced some aspects of Western medicine, but on a very limited scale. Following this, in 1639, there was a period of 250 years' absolute isolation when foreigners were forbidden to enter the country. The Dutch traders at Nagasaki were an exception, and they were allowed to continue their work. From this small centre of influence, Dutch medicine persisted, but it only affected a small number of patients and doctors in the Nagasaki region. Thus, by the time of the Meiji Restoration in 1868, knowledge of Western medicine was almost non-existent. There were a few exceptions, such as the importation of smallpox vaccine by a Dutch physician named Mohnike in 1849 and the eventual setting up of the Okamagaike Vaccination Centre in 1857 by a number of Japanese doctors trained in the 'Dutch School'. The centre was highly successful and in 1861 was renamed the Western Medical Institute. In 1858, a Dutch naval surgeon, J. L. C. Pompe van Meerdervoort, came to Nagasaki and taught medicine to any students who chose to attend his lectures. This was the origin of the medical faculty of Nagasaki University. The Tokingawa (Eido government), having maintained a state of isolation for nearly 250 years, found difficulty in continuing this policy because of outside pressure from Western countries, and also because the population became aware of the defects of a feudal system. In 1868, the old regime was overthrown, and was followed by the Meiji Restoration in which the government intended to modernise Japan – a far-reaching programme which included the Westernisation of medicine, mainly in the German tradition. In 1874, a new law was passed concerning the medical services; there was to be a complete transfer from 'traditional' to Western methods and, in fact, a prohibition was placed on the traditional style of practice. The urgency with which everything was done can be seen by the fact that, in 1869, Tokyo Medical School was founded, immediately followed in 1870 by the Osaka Medical Faculty, and by 1878 most of the prefecture governments had set up hospitals which were functioning partially as teaching hospitals. Financial difficulties, however, led to the closing of most national hospitals by 1887, forcing doctors to set up private hospitals. This really is the origin of some of the problems in the hospital service in present-day Japan, more particularly when it is realised that no hospitals existed before 1868. The first signs of the government taking an interest in the organisation of the nation's health was in 1872, when a new medical section was set up at the Ministry of Education. In 1875 it was transferred, but not upgraded, to the Ministry of Home Affairs, and remained there for more than fifty years. As so often happens, not until there was a threat and danger of war was more definite action taken and a separate Ministry of Health and Welfare was created in 1938.

The disasters of the Second World War reduced Japan to ruins, both physically and morally. In the re-establishment of medical services which followed, for obvious reasons the traditions of Germany were discarded, with the important exception of medical insurance. A new foreign influence – the USA – took over.

Medical insurance and method of payment

During the Meiji Era (1868–1912) there was unprecedented modernisation and economic development, with all the social changes and tensions which accompany such rapid industrialisation. In addition, urbanisation and the movement of workers and their families gave rise to a growing discontent. This was not a problem peculiar to Japan, but perhaps it was more noticeable, as the changes which took place here occurred within a few decades and not over a much longer period of time as in Western Europe or the USA. The idea of 'free medical care' for those who could not afford to pay for treatment was introduced in 1910 by the Emperor Meiji, who said, 'We are most seriously concerned over the situation in which the poor people who cannot afford a medicine die before their time. So, desiring as we do to provide public welfare by serving out medicine and giving medical treatment to the poor, we wish to apply the money from a private purse to this purpose.' But this has not been fully achieved, even today.

Since 1910, many laws have been introduced to try to improve the quality of life. The first health insurance legislation was passed in 1922: unfortunately, the law could not be enforced because of the Tokyo earthquake in 1923, and benefits were first paid out in 1927. The four main points of the health insurance law were:

(*a*) It covered illness, childbirth, injury and death.

(*b*) It applied compulsorily to all covered by the Factory Law and to other low-income workers.

(*c*) Contribution costs were borne equally between insured and employer. The insurance agents were the government and health insurance societies approved by the government.

(*d*) Benefits applied only to the insured and not to his family.

However, fewer than two million people were in fact covered in 1927. The law has been frequently amended since then, and the present one, passed in 1959, stipulated that everyone had to be covered by 1961. Thus, nearly forty years after the original law of 1922, the final goal was achieved: a comprehensive health insurance system. But full insurance cover must not be confused with full financial cover for the patient and his family, because each separate insurance scheme varies considerably, both in contributions and benefits. According to a survey in 1970, 88.8 per cent of patients attending hospitals and clinics had their medical expenses covered by some form of health insurance.

In the same year, the statistical department of the Ministry of Health and Welfare estimated that the financing of the health service was derived from three sources in the following proportions: compulsory insurance 67.8 per cent, central taxation 11.1 per cent and private payment 21.1 per cent. The benefit rates, as already stated, vary enormously, and those workers attached to the largest trade unions are looked after very well. At the moment, large companies (employing over 1000 people) provide extra health facilities to make up for any deficiency there might be in insurance coverage. Almost one-third of the working population are covered in this way and the large unions are happy about what has been achieved for the workers, and naturally the government is happy about this state of affairs as it reduces the amount of money which needs to be invested in health services. But what of the other two-thirds of the population who are not represented by the large trade unions? They have no influence and are largely ignored both by the government and their fellow-workers.

Demand, however, is growing from the public, from a few politicians and from many doctors working in the field of public health, for a free medical care plan. Over the last fifteen years, the growing problems of environmental pollution have been watched by the general public with fear, despondency and alarm. Nonetheless, it gradually became apparent that authorities could be influenced in such matters, and perhaps it was this atmosphere which encouraged doctors to insist that *'nanbyo* diseases' should be treated without payment. *'Nanbyo'* is the Japanese name given to all diseases in which the pathology and treatment is not clear, or the treatment is difficult, expensive or prolonged. An extension of this was the introduction in 1971, in five prefectures, of free medical services for all over seventy years of age and the very poor. The hope is that within the next decade this will cover all people over sixty-five years throughout the entire country.

Methods of payment

Doctors working in private clinics – the primary care physicians – are paid on an item-of-service basis by the patient, who receives some or all the money from the appropriate insurance scheme. The scale of fees is worked out between the medical profession, the various insurance agencies and the government, and is a constant source of irritation and friction to everyone involved.

Over-investigation is inevitable as a result of the item-of-service payment, and is freely admitted by many Japanese doctors, both in private hospitals as well as in private clinics. But the importance of prescribing, both as a method of payment for the doctor and as an expectation from the patient, is the biggest problem in relation to this aspect of primary care. There are over 20 000 prescribable drug preparations, all of which have a different item-of-service payment! The general feeling about the present insurance system, whereby a doctor's income depends so much on the drugs he prescribes, is that it is fundamentally wrong. Such a system inevitably leads to massive over-prescribing, for only in this way can a doctor maintain his income. The only lasting solution would entail a radical overhaul of the insurance payment system, and patients would need to be re-educated to go to the pharmacist for their prescription to be dispensed. At the present time, it is universal practice for drugs and medicaments to be issued by the doctors, and there is distrust of the pharmacist by the patient who traditionally has always received drugs from the doctor. Also, it is deeply ingrained in the Japanese culture and tradition that a doctor is always expected to provide medicine. It is of interest to realise that *'kusushi'* is the name for an old traditional physician, while *'kusuri'* is the modern name for a medicine or drug. Another factor which perpetuates the system is the fact that if the doctor prescribes something, but it is dispensed at the chemist, then he receives only a token payment.

Many people believe that a greatly increased fee for consultation with less emphasis on the item-of-service payment for drugs and investigations would help. This might well apply to X-ray and laboratory over-investigation, but the question of separating doctor and pharmacy is much more complex and seems to be a particularly Japanese problem related closely to their culture and traditions. The difficulty is that, by and large, patients are happy with the present arrangement whereby drugs can be procured from the doctors and would resent a second visit to the pharmacist. This high use of drugs is a definite barrier to progress in the field of primary care.

Primary medical care

Before describing the basic organisation and structure of this aspect of the health service, it is necessary to clarify certain definitions:

Clinic: An office or consulting room in the community, usually run by one or two doctors, where patients are seen for diagnosis and treatment. Clinics can be with or without beds and by definition in Japanese health statistics, a clinic with twenty beds or more is considered as a hospital.

Health centre: A building owned by the prefecture or designated city government (i.e. local authorities) in which very limited care and guidance in health, sanitation, health education and preventive medicine is practised.

The patient's first contact with a doctor is carried out in one of three different situations:

(*a*) A private clinic, with or without beds, run by a doctor with some specialist training, most commonly in internal medicine or paediatrics (Table 1). There are very few government-owned clinics (Table 2).

(b) An out-patient or casualty department of a hospital.

(c) A health centre staffed either by a public health doctor or a part-time clinic doctor.

There are no general practitioners (except in rural areas), in other words every doctor working in the community has a specialist interest

TABLE 1 *Number of clinics, according to specialty, with or without beds, 1970*

Type of Clinic	Total clinics		Clinics without beds		Clinics with beds	
	Number	%	Number	%	Number	%
Medical specialty:						
General medicine	37 375	54.2	26 803	68.4	10 841	36.3
Paediatrics	4 057	5.9	2 869	7.1	1 118	3.9
Surgical specialty:						
Obstetrics and Gynaecology	6 734	9.8	360	0.9	6 374	21.3
General surgery	5 947	8.4	818	2.1	5 129	17.1
ENT	3 725	5.4	1 705	4.4	2 020	6.8
Ophthalmology	3 596	5.2	2 339	5.9	1 257	4.2
Orthopaedic	1 834	2.7	216	0.5	907	3.1
Others	4 729	8.3				

Source: Department of Public Health, Osaka University Medical School

TABLE 2 *Ownership of clinics, 1970*

	Number of clinics	Percentage of total
Private	60 638	88.3
Religious organisation	3 931	5.7
Local government	2 715	4.0
Red Cross, various insurance agencies	846	1.2
Government	567	0.8

Based on data from: Department of Public Health, Osaka University Medical School

and does not consider himself to be a generalist. Although many clinic doctors think of themselves as family doctors (Takemi, 1970a), in the densely populated urban areas this does not appear to be the case. Patients are free to attend any doctor and there is no registration of patients.

Since 1955, there has been a steady increase in the number of clinics (and the figures for 1970 are shown in Table 3), but there has been a decrease in the number of younger doctors setting them up because of the trend to work longer in the hospital service in order to gain more experience. When it is considered how poorly junior hospital doctors are paid, and that there is nothing in theory to prevent a doctor setting up his clinic immediately after qualifying, this trend is greatly to the credit of the younger doctors. Clinic doctors show no signs of developing group practices or even partnerships (Table 4) and the great majority are in single-handed practice (Table 6).

TABLE 3   *Clinics in Japan, 1970*

Type	Number
Clinics without beds	39 156 (56.8%)
Clinics with beds	29 840 (43.2%)
1–9 beds	20 774 (30.1%)
10–19 beds	9 067 (13.1%)

Based on data from: Department of Public Health, Osaka University Medical School

TABLE 4   *Medical staffing of clinics*

Type	Staffing
Clinics without beds	87.3% by one doctor
	8.9% by two doctors
	3.9% by three or more doctors[a]
Clinics with beds	81.2% by one doctor
	14.0% by two doctors
	4.8% by three or more doctors

[a] These figures never include more than two full-time doctors, the others being part-time.
Based on data from: Department of Public Health, Osaka University Medical School

Medical clinics are very well equipped – too well equipped, some would argue – as far as diagnostic and therapeutic facilities and equipment are concerned (Table 5). A wide variety of surgical procedures – gastrectomy, cholecystectomy, hysterectomy, caesarian section – are carried out in surgical clinics in urban areas by primary care physicians.

TABLE 5   *Clinics concerned with medical specialties*

Equipment	Number of clinics	Percentage of total
X-ray unit for diagnosis including contrast medium	35 142	71.3
ECG	33 825	68.6
Fundus camera	5 140	10.4
Gastroscope	3 559	7.2

Source: Department of Public Health, Osaka University Medical School

One of the major problems in primary care is the extreme shortage of paramedical staff – nurses, midwives, health visitors, secretaries and receptionists (Table 6).

Most doctors organise their work with consultations between 09.00 and 12.30 hours, home visits between 15.00 and 17.00 hours and a further consultation session from 18.00 to 20.00 hours. The number of patients seen varies between 60 and 180 patients per day, with home visiting kept to a minimum, rarely more than six. It is generally recognised that the consultation rate in Japan is high (15 per year) compared with any other country. Morbidity is notoriously difficult to define and classify, often depending more on patients' expectations and demands and doctors' susceptibility to different forms of patient pressure, than on accurate diagnosis. There is nothing to suggest that Japan suffers from a higher morbidity than other countries, so why is the consultation rate so high? Some possible explanations are given, none of which is related to increased morbidity.

First, many patients attend for minor conditions of eyes, nose and throat, and are asked to return on successive days for treatment. It is estimated that 30 per cent come into this category. Without being unduly cynical, it would seem that the method of payment encourages such attendance patterns, rather than decisions being made on purely clinical considerations.

Second, injections (both intravenous and intramuscular) are given frequently, and it is illegal for them to be given by anyone else but a doctor, i.e. a nurse can give them only under direct supervision. They are used commonly in such conditions as colds, upper respiratory infections, gastritis, lumbago, hypertension and liver disease.

TABLE 6 *Staffing of clinics*

Staff	Number of staff	
	Clinics with beds	Clinics without beds
Doctor (full-time)	1.1	1.0
Doctor (part-time)	0.2	0.3
Registered nurse[a]	0.4	0.3
Practical nurse[b]	1.0	0.3
Nurse aid	1.8	0.8
Midwife	0.1	0
Pharmacist	0	0.1
Clerical staff	0.8	0.4

[a] Registered nurse has a 3-year training, after 12 years' full-time education
[b] Practical nurse has a 2-year training, after 9 years' full-time education
Based on data from: Department of Public Health, Osaka University Medical School

Third, because there is no separation of the doctor and the dispensing of medicines, and the method of payment encourages over-prescribing, an increase in the consultation rate is the result. It is quite common for a physician to dispense vitamins for months at a time, and each prescription counts as a patient attendance.

Local medical associations

Over the last fifteen to twenty years, there have grown up, throughout Japan, local medical associations composed of doctors practising in a particular area. The intention was to aim at total participation of all branches of the profession, but unfortunately in many areas only clinic doctors have become involved. This situation has arisen because of the mutual suspicion and antipathy between salaried hospital, public health and clinic doctors. Although not primarily interested in academic standards or responsible for them, such medical associations in some way resemble the colleges and academies of general practice that have sprung up all over the world in recent years.

The aims of these medical associations fall under six main headings:

(a) To improve communication between members and foster mutual understanding between all sections of the profession, in the belief that, if doctors know each other personally, then cooperation is much more likely.

(b) To improve educational standards, by arranging lectures, hospital visits and discussion groups.

(c) To set up diagnostic centres with X-ray and laboratory facilities, so that there is more rational use of equipment. This is considered to be group practice, Japanese style, and is as far as it is likely to develop in the foreseeable future (Takemi, 1970b).

(d) To bring pressure on the government and colleagues to improve the organisation of medical care by providing emergency centres for Sundays, holidays and perhaps, ultimately, for nightwork.

(e) To organise a pension scheme.

(f) To try to change the insurance schemes, so that less of a clinic doctor's income depends on excessive prescribing of drugs.

Diagnostic centres

Although it is important for doctors working outside hospitals to have access to modern diagnostic and therapeutic facilities, for over 70 per cent of doctors to possess their own X-ray equipment must constitute a great waste of resources and increase the likelihood of poor standards of X-ray interpretation, particularly of contrast media studies. This realisation has led to the establishment of diagnostic centres whose aims include the centralisation of X-ray and laboratory facilities and work, thus reducing the large capital outlay for each practitioner and at the same time rationalising the use of such expensive equipment. This would raise diagnostic standards by enabling doctors to discuss the interpretation of X-rays and laboratory tests. In many centres it has now been found possible to employ a radiologist from the local hospital, who comes once a week to read and report on the films.

Most doctors who have access to these centres agree that they have resulted in more-accurate X-ray findings, have enabled laboratory tests to be carried out more quickly, and have, of course, widened the scope of investigation compared with that which was carried out previously in an individual practitioner's clinic. Some centres have included beds – to be used for investigation purposes only. One of the most important considerations when setting up a diagnostic centre is that it must be convenient for the patient, who is accustomed to receiving consultation, investigation and treatment under one roof.

Emergency services

The question of who is responsible for providing care for patients out-of-hours, at night, and on Sundays is causing considerable anxiety in Japan today. Ordinary consulting hours usually finish between 18.00 and 20.00 hours, and most clinics are closed on Sundays and public holidays. This problem did not arise until the mid-1950s; before that, there was a high ethical standard and sense of responsibility amongst clinic doctors, and the majority provided emergency services.

But gradually, over the last twenty years, the pattern of life has changed for both doctor and patient. This does not imply a drop in ethical standards, but rather that the attitude of society as a whole has altered. Doctors, who for the most part work in single-handed practice, are no longer prepared to be on duty seven days a week and at night – in the same way that their patients are demanding a shorter working day. As has already been seen, this is not a unique Japanese problem, and few countries have found a satisfactory solution. The problem is most acute in densely urbanised areas where there has been a gradual deterioration of the doctor/patient relationship, partly because of the stresses of everyday living and partly because universal insurance has created greater expectations from the patient, which the doctor is unable to fulfil within the present primary care organisation – or lack of it. There is no registration of patients, and clinic doctors are under only nominal legal responsibility to provide a 24-hour service. If a patient becomes ill on Sunday or at night, there are two options open to him: first, he may contact a clinic doctor, whose response will depend on whether he knows the patient; if he does, then he may provide some treatment, or at least help to arrange admission to hospital. There is no financial incentive for doctors to provide night care, as the fee is only twice the normal daytime consultation rate, which in any case is low. To stave off unnecessary night calls, many doctors try to educate patients in what to expect when young children are taken ill. Others arrange with the relatives of ill-patients special signals on the telephone: it sounds haphazard, but appears to work! The second alternative is for the patient to dial the emergency ambulance number, '119', and it is then the responsibility of the ambulance service to arrange hospital admission.

In order to try to produce a rational answer to this problem, local medical associations are trying to persuade the national or prefecture governments to build emergency health centres, covering perhaps a population of up to 200 000, for use on Sundays or public holidays – as yet there are no plans for nightwork, but this is also very much in the minds of many doctors. It is envisaged that they would be staffed both by hospital and clinic doctors, depending on the local circumstances.

Throughout the country, the ambulance service is run by the fire service, and is not connected with the Ministry of Health. All fire stations contain an ambulance as well as fire engines. In Tokyo, with a population of about 12 million, there are 120 sub fire stations, each with three or four engines and one ambulance. This gives a ratio of only one ambulance per 100 000 people, which is grossly inadequate by any standards. The ambulance is manned by a driver and crew of three, all of whom receive a short training in accident, emergency and first-aid work. Three teams per ambulance work eight-hour shifts round the clock. The ambulance service covers traffic and industrial accidents, home accidents (although by law it is the responsibility of the individual to deal with these) and acute illness, referred either by a clinic doctor or patient. Approximately half of all calls come direct from the patient, a large percentage of which are paediatric emergencies.

Many problems are associated with the emergency and accident service. A report on 6 December 1972 in the *Japan Times* showed that ambulances were being used five times more frequently in 1971 than in 1962, owing both to increased accidents and the fact that neither clinic doctors nor hospitals are willing to accept out-of-hours responsibility. Only 50 per cent of cities, towns and villages are served by ambulances, although 80 per cent of the total population is covered. In some large cities, for instance Osaka, emergency medical service information centres have been organised to deal with calls where hospital accommodation cannot be found by the ambulance crews.

Medical education and primary care

In 1972, there were 59 medical schools, of which 26 were national, 8 prefecture and 25 private. Students apply for admission after three years at secondary school and three years at high school. There is far more competition for national and prefecture schools because fees are low; entry to a private school depends as much on the parents' income as on academic standards.

On completion of a six-year course, students sit a national examination for MD. This is under the control of the Ministry of Health and Welfare, while training is supervised by the Ministry of Education. Compulsory one-year internship was abolished in 1968, and doctors now spend on average twelve years in further training before leaving hospital to set up private clinics in the community. Although such a degree of commitment to gaining postgraduate experience is indeed praiseworthy, many would question the appropriateness of this further training in relation to primary care.

In 1971, a committee was set up by the Ministry of Health to consider the question of increasing the number of medical student places, either by the expansion of existing schools or by building new ones. During their deliberations, two fundamental questions had to be asked in connection with any future planning! 'What is a good medical education?' and 'What is a good teaching hospital?' Answers must be found to these questions if Japan is to overcome the obvious defects of its present system, mesmerised as it is with technology, and suffering from a complete lack of training in community-based medicine. Although the principles involved in such changes are gradually being accepted, by 1977 there had still been no fundamental alteration in medical training.

Personal assessment

Clinic doctors (primary care physicians) are extremely hard working and fiercely independent. They fear any interference with clinical freedom, and are suspicious of any directions from the Ministry of Health and Welfare, which they believe will inevitably bring increased bureaucracy and no benefits either to themselves or their patients. Their apprehension about the Ministry of Health and Welfare is probably justified, for at the present time it has no positive or worthwhile plan for the future organisation of the health service. But this independence is in many ways an illusion which only creates and perpetuates a 'treadmill' existence for the doctor: cooperation between doctors should not be confused with interference from outside.

Even if group practice is considered to be unacceptable and unnecessary to the Japanese style of medicine, surely the same cannot be said of partnership between two, or at most three doctors? The advantages of such an arrangement are well known: it allows holidays, time-off for sickness and postgraduate education; Sunday duty or even night-work can be arranged more easily. Such partnerships would help to lessen the feeling of professional isolation.

The standard of primary care is also influenced by the severe shortage of nurses and paramedical staff, and one of the most important aims over the next twenty years should be to increase the number of nurses, then define their function and role and use them within a reorganised system of first-contact care. Japan, amongst the major countries in the world, is alone in believing that primary care can be provided by doctors working in complete isolation without making use of the full potential of nurses, health visitors and receptionists.

The setting up of diagnostic and emergency centres should be encouraged, as should some solution to the problem of over-prescribing. In making such suggestions, it is necessary to remember that at present most patients appear to be relatively satisfied with the arrangement of receiving consultation, investigation and treatment at one and the same time, preferably within the same building, therefore patients and doctors would need to be convinced of the advantages of any recommended alterations.

Primary care cannot be considered in isolation from the rest of the health service, and without good secondary care in the hospitals, it will founder. A great many people – both in and outside Japan – would contend that the serious defects within the hospital service are yet another obstacle to improving not only the health service in general, but primary care as well. There is a poor distribution of hospitals, almost no grading according to function within regional, area and district levels, difficulty in staffing, much reduplication of activities between private and public hospitals, leading to gaps in health care and a foolish use of already scarce resources, and finally no regulation of specialists: all these things must be rectified.

The perennial question of medical education and postgraduate training for primary care physicians poses enormous difficulties. Every country is, or should be, striving to find an answer to this particular problem: Japan, as much as any country in the world, needs to break away from the shackles of medical technology, and focus its attention on the more mundane work of organising an adequate level of first-contact care. Medical education must be tailored to meet these needs.

It is difficult to be more conclusive about what can be learnt from the Japanese situation. Their culture, their style of life and their expectation from life are quite different from the Western World.

For these reasons, much that seems inappropriate to the Western observer may not, in fact, be so. But there would seem to be one lesson for every country: here in Japan the item-of-service payment in its most extreme form (with over 20 000 different payments for different medicaments) leads to excessive prescribing: for every 100 consultations, 220 prescriptions are given and 49 injections administered (Seki, 1972). Such a situation can only be an obstacle to good general practice.

Note: For further information about the Japanese Health Service, see my report to the Nuffield Foundation (Stephen, 1972).

11

DEVELOPING COUNTRIES

Poor health is a direct consequence of poverty and its attendant miseries and, in turn, poverty is accentuated by ill health. Poverty and health are, therefore, inextricably interwoven, so that it is impossible and pointless to consider the problems of health care in isolation.

What is the nature and extent of poverty in the developing world? Over the last twenty-five years, the WHO, Unicef, The World Bank, individual governments, university and individual research groups have revealed the magnitude of the situation. The Third World involves 75 per cent of the world's population and only 12 per cent of the world's wealth. In 1972, the average *per capita* income of advanced countries (including Eastern Europe and the USSR) varied between 1530 and 5590 US dollars, while that of the poor nations was between 80 and 880 US dollars (Table 1).

In most developing countries the situation shows no evidence of improvement – rather the reverse, as the gap between rich and poor nations widens – and the grinding, relentless circle of never-ending poverty seems likely to continue into the foreseeable future. This treadmill existence encourages an atmosphere of apathy and despair, with a further downward spiral both in human and economic terms. Although the political and economic reasons for this situation are beyond the scope of this book, on the ability to find a solution rests the ability of any country to provide even the limited resources necessary to finance, amongst many objectives, a basic health service (Table 2).

Features of developing countries
It is arrogant, incorrect and misleading to consider the 2600

318

TABLE 1 *GNP at market prices (1972), GNP per capita (1972) (GNP at market prices rounded to US$ tens of millions, GNP per capita rounded to nearest US$ 10)*

Country	GNP at market prices amount (US$ millions)	Average per capita (US$)
Asia		
Afghanistan	1 220	80
India	61 940	110
Iran	15 220	490
Nepal	950	80
Saudi Arabia	4 160	550
Thailand	8 340	220
Africa		
Ethiopia	2 140	80
Ghana	2 700	300
Kenya	2 050	170
Malawi	460	100
Nigeria	9 350	130
Sudan	2 030	120
Tanzania	1 580	120
Uganda	1 560	150
Zambia	1 730	380
South America		
Cuba	3 970	450
Costa Rica	1 150	630
Guatemala	2 340	420
Mexico	40 340	750
Panama	1 340	880
St Kitts, Anguilla	20	410
Developed countries		
Canada	97 080	4440
France	187 360	3620
Sweden	36 350	4480
UK	144 900	2600
USA	1 167 470	5590
USSR	377 700	1530

Source: *World Bank Atlas*: World Bank, Washington DC, 1974

TABLE 2   *Per capita government health expenditure in developing countries*

		Number of countries					
Per capita GNP ($)	Total number of countries	Less than $1.00	$1.01 to $2.00	$2.01 to $3.00	$3.01 to $5.00	$5.01 to $10.00	Above $10.00
Less than 100	12	9	2	0	1	0	0
101–200	15	7	3	4	1	0	0
201–300	16	0	4	5	5	1	1
301–600	14	1	1	3	4	4	1
601–1000	8	0	0	2	1	0	5
Totals	65	17	10	14	14	12	5

Source: *World Bank: Health Sector Policy Paper*. Washington DC, 1975

For comparison: *Per capita government health expenditure in developed countries (in US$)*

Country	Year	Health expenditure (US$)
Canada	1970	239.08
USA	1972	149.00
UK	1972	84.09
USSR	1972	53.35
Australia	1972	63.14
New Zealand	1972	108.48

Source: *World Health Statistics Report*, 1974, vol. 2; 1975, vol. 2

million people (who by the end of the century will have increased to outnumber the developed nations by four to one) who make up the developing world as a single entity. Each developing country – there are over 90 – has its own political, social and economic problems which are directly affected by the cultural, religious and tribal traditions and customs of its people. Notwithstanding this, there are a number of basic common manifestations of poverty which affect all these countries to a varying degree.

The realisation that poverty is not a problem of the whole population is perhaps the biggest surprise to the uninitiated Western observer. The glaring contrasts in living standards between the small, élite ruling class and the great mass of the people graphically demonstrate the indifference of men to the plight of their fellow human beings.

> In Latin America in the mid 1960s an estimated 40 per cent of the total of all incomes was received by the top 10 per cent of earners, whilst the poorest 40 per cent received only 10 per cent of the total. In countries such as Peru, Chile, Panama, Venezuela, the richest 5 per cent of the population received nearly forty times as much as the poorest 20 per cent. (OHE, 1972)

However much the rich nations may be made to alter and relax their attitudes to the inequalities of world trade in the hope of improving the economic prospects of the developing world, the great mass of people will not benefit, but only those who are in government or industry or own land, or the small educated professional classes. Unless these privileged groups are made by their own people to redistribute their wealth and alter the use and ownership of land and industry in a more equitable fashion, the ability of any country to achieve a self-sufficient economy is remote. Productivity and the GNP will, therefore, never rise above a subsistence level, and consequently the amount of money devoted to medical care will remain miniscule.

The lack of basic amenities is all too obvious in most rural areas: inadequate water supply, poor housing, primitive sanitation, over-crowding due to poverty combined with an uncontrolled birth rate and visible signs of malnutrition. Over the last 20–5 years there has been a drift to the cities in the hope of finding work. Young people, often the healthiest and most able-bodied, have been lured by the prospect of work, leaving a depleted labour force in the rural communities. Unfor-tunately, unemployment is as much part of the urban as of rural life, so that the increase in urban poverty can be seen in the dirt, squalor and overcrowding of the expanding shanty towns and slums on the edges of most capital cities. Furthermore, the social effects of unemployment and urbanisation – alcoholism (often encouraged by government-owned breweries and liquor stores), increasing incidence of venereal disease as well as increasing vandalism and violence – are as much a part of the Third World as of deprived areas in industrialised societies. The consequences of ignorance and lack of education (Table 3) com-plete an appalling picture of human misery and degradation. The magnitude of the problem is beyond the comprehension of most people, but to ignore it is a recipe for eventual disaster.

TABLE 3   *Percentage illiteracy*

Country	Illiteracy (%)
Africa	84
Asia	51
Latin America	27
Developed countries	3.5

Source: WHO Statistics, 1971

Basic medical problems

It is important to appreciate the demographic and socio/economic differences between the developed and developing world, since so many of the difficulties of providing health services, and improving levels of health, flow from these. Essentially it is a rural problem, in that 75 per cent or more of the population live in rural areas (Table 4). Certainly in the future the increase in urban populations will magnify the medical problems in and around the cities unless there is a dramatic change in the level of poverty and unemployment. The rate of population growth is difficult to forecast, but 10–15 per cent seems a likely figure (UN, 1971).

The distinctive age structure found in developing countries is caused by the high birth rates and high infant mortality rates associated with increased general mortality in all age groups, resulting in a diminished life expectancy (Table 5). Between 40 and 50 per cent of all deaths occur in the under-5-years age group.

This pattern is similar to the situation found in the developed countries during the nineteenth century, and it is in no way unexpected. The improvements in health which occurred in the Western World during the end of the nineteenth century and early part of this century were almost entirely brought about by greatly improved standards of living, associated with better nutrition, housing and sanitation. Later, inoculation and vaccination also proved to be important factors but, contrary to what the medical profession suggests, curative medicine played very little part until the advent of sulphonamides in 1935 and

TABLE 4   *Distribution of health personnel between rural and urban areas*

	Percentage distribution		
	Urban area		Rural area
	Capital	Total	
Africa			
Ethiopia 1972			
Population	4	5	95
Physicians	44	60	40
Medical assistants	14	16	84
Nurses and midwives	47	60	40
Ghana 1971			
Population	6	19	81
Physicians	33	62	38
Medical assistants	6	19	81
Midwives	21	39	61
Nurses	21	42	58
Kenya 1973			
Population	5	8	92
Physicians	56	77	23
Medical assistants	37	54	46
Nurses	48	75	25
Midwives	56	70	30
Lesotho 1971			
Population	2	2	98
Physicians	39	39	61
Midwives	28	28	72
Nurses	6	6	94
Nigeria 1971			
Population	2	21	79
Physicians	13	67	33
Medical assistants	0	51	49
Midwives	11	67	33
Nurses	13	58	42
Zambia 1971			
Population	4	6	94
Physicians	28	69	31
Medical assistants	12	25	75
Midwives	12	59	41
Nurses	21	55	45

TABLE 4   *Distribution of health personnel etc. (contd.)*

	Percentage distribution		
	Urban area		Rural area
	Capital	Total	
Asia			
India 1972			
Population	0	20	80
Physicians	0	70	30
Indonesia 1973			
Population	4	18	82
Physicians	27	76	24
Midwives	8	37	63
Nurses	13	48	52
Iran 1972			
Population	13	43	57
Physicians	44	87	13
Midwives	36	81	19
Nurses	55	99	1
Thailand 1970			
Population	6	13	87
Physicians	54	86	14
All nurses and midwives	22	57	43
Latin America			
Bolivia 1974			
Population	12	24	76
Physicians	20	90	10
Nurses	47	93	7
Brazil 1969			
Population	0	54	46
Physicians	0	95	5
Guatemala 1971			
Population	14	–	–
Physicians	85	98	2
Midwives	92	–	–
Nurses	77	–	–
Panama 1970			
Population	29	64	36
Physicians	67	95	5
Nurses	70	93	7

TABLE 4 *Distribution of health personnel etc. (contd.)*

| | Percentage distribution | | |
| | Urban area | | Rural area |
	Capital	Total	
Peru 1969			
Population	18	26	74
Physicians	62	79	21
Midwives	0	59	41
Nurses	0	80	20

Source: *World Health Statistics Annual* vol. 3, 1972 (published 1976)

antibiotics after the Second World War. Similarly, in the developing world the least important factor in improving the overall standard of health is curative or 'immediate' medicine.

Malnutrition, first and foremost, is the main cause of morbidity and mortality in developing areas since it seriously lowers the resistance to infectious diseases (bacterial, viral and parasitic), respiratory conditions, gastroenteritis, measles, pertussis, tuberculosis, tetanus, trachoma, malaria, cholera, yellow fever, hookworm, filariasis and schistosomiasis. What must be stressed is that illnesses such as non-specific diarrhoea, influenza and measles, which in developed countries are of minor importance, in the developing world often prove fatal; or at least accelerate the effects of malnutrition (Morley, 1973). The health of women of child-bearing age is generally poor owing to repeated pregnancies accentuated by infections and the lack of proper diet, by overwork and the inadequacy or absence of ante-natal care or anyone to attend during delivery (Table 6).

Clearly nutrition is of prime importance in the assessment of medical priorities. According to the United Nations' estimates, the desirable basic level of kilocalories is about 2500 per day: in the developed world the average intake is over 3000, while in the developing world it is just over 2000. Protein (both animal and vegetable products) intake should be kept at about 66.6 g weight per day: in the developed world it is nearly 100 g weight per day, while in the developing world it is between 50 g and 60 g per day, much of it being second-class protein. Such are the statistics, but in fact the position is almost certainly much more serious, since many governments are unlikely to broadcast the

TABLE 5   *Health indices in developing and developed countries*

Country	Crude birth rate	Infant mortality	Crude death rate	Life expectancy
Africa				
Congo	45.1	180	20.8	43.5
Egypt	37.8	120	15.0	50.7
Ethiopia	49.5	162	23.8	40.0
Malawi	47.7	148	23.7	41.0
Nigeria	49.3	150–175	22.7	41.0
Sudan	47.8	130	18.5	47.2
Tanzania	50.1	122	23.4	44.5
Uganda	46.9	160	15.7	50.0
Zambia	51.5	259	20.3	44.5
Asia				
India	41.1	139	16.3	49.2
Pakistan	47.6	130	16.8	49.4
Sri Lanka	28.6	50	6.3	67.8
Thailand	43.7	23	10.4	58.6
Latin America				
Bolivia	43.7	60	18.0	46.7
Brazil	37.1	110	8.8	61.4
Chile	25.9	71	8.1	64.3
Cuba	28.9	28	5.9	72.3
Guatemala	42.0	63	8.6	63.2
Peru	41.0	67	11.9	55.7
Developed countries				
Bulgaria	16.2	26	9.1	71.8
Japan	19.2	12	6.6	73.3
USA	16.2	19	9.4	70.4
USSR	17.8	23	7.9	70.4

Source: *World Bank: Health Sector Policy Paper*, Washington DC, 1975

true extent of their failure and the great differences between urban and rural populations.

The supply of clean water and the adequate disposal of sewage for all people by the end of this century remains one of the main aims of the WHO. More than 1000 million people living in rural areas do not have reasonable access to safe drinking water. This number is growing faster than safe water supplies can be installed (World Bank, 1976). Whether the WHO can achieve its aims remains doubtful, but neither these, nor improved housing, nor adequate food supply can be realised without fundamental changes in society. Self-sufficiency in agriculture must be encouraged, together with some chance of employment in urban areas with the purpose of increasing the productivity and wealth of these countries: of course, without an actual redistribution of wealth very little will be altered.

TABLE 6 *Percentage of deliveries attended by a physician or by a qualified midwife*

		In hospital	At home	Total
Bolivia	1971	5.5	12.8	18.3
Guatemala	1970	–	–	25.0
Peru	1971	15.2	–	–
Sudan	1971	–	–	10.0

Source: *World Bank; Health Sector Policy Paper.* Washington DC, 1975

Traditional Western-style medical services

The impact of conventional 'Western-style' medical education, medical care and planning in developing countries, with an overemphasis on doctors, hospitals and curative medicine, may well be judged by future historians as one of the most disastrous episodes in the history of medicine. The inevitability of failure until recently did not prevent the medical profession in developed countries from advising these policies, and neither did it prevent the medical profession in developing countries from readily accepting such advice. Both must accept responsibility for the misuse of very limited money and manpower. This advice has helped to produce a situation in which, according to the WHO, less than 15 per cent of the rural population and other underprivileged groups – slum and shanty-town dwellers – have any access to medical services. This has been graphically described:

> although three-quarters of the population in most countries in the tropics and sub-tropics live in rural areas, three-quarters of the spending on medical care is in urban areas, where three-quarters of the

doctors live. Three-quarters of the deaths are due to conditions that can be prevented at low cost, but three-quarters of the medical budget is spent on curative services, many of them provided at high cost. (Morley, 1973)

Even in an advanced country such as Sweden, with its high standard of living and egalitarian principles of health care, it is now recognised that a hospital- and specialist-dominated health service is inappropriate, does not serve the needs of the people and is too costly to finance. How much more does this apply to poor countries, where the building of hospitals as repositories of so-called 'high standards' of medical care has proved a ghastly mistake? (This does not, of course, apply to the privileged few, whose expectations are similar to those in the 'advanced' Western countries of the world.)

> The influx of Western medical technology is easy to criticise. It is frequently stated to have been the root cause of the present maldistribution of health care, and to have set the present attitudes to be found amongst members of the Third World medical profession. It is now enlightened to suggest that what 'they' want is increased emphasis on preventive medicine with training of some type of village-level doctors, mainly in public health, providing only a very simple curative service. Even if this approach is the correct one, it is unlikely that an effective change of this nature will actually take place without a similar alteration in emphasis within Western health care delivery systems. (Heller, 1976)

Thus the status symbols of modern curative medicine flourish – cardiac, neuro-surgical, renal transplant and radiotherapy departments – while common, preventable and easily curable diseases are allowed to fester in the midst of urban and rural poverty. It cannot be stressed too often that improvements in medical care are not prevented through lack of knowledge, but by the unwillingness and inability of the medical profession to implement present knowledge. The rigidity and traditional values of medicine are quite inapplicable to the problems of the Third World. Consider two aspects of Western medicine: hospitals and doctors.

1. Hospitals

The objections to using hospitals as the main facility of health care are simple and obvious. They are too expensive to build, too expensive to run, too greedy in engulfing medical and nursing personnel, they do not reach the population for whom they are intended and very often do not even attain one of the objectives for which they are built – namely to act as referral centres for special problems.

At the present time, the new University Teaching Hospital is being built in Riyadh in Saudi Arabia. It has every conceivable 'show piece' department to satisfy even the most technically orientated doctor, its cost is immense, its use is very limited and it cannot possibly benefit the majority of peasants and nomads. In Zambia, the new teaching hospital in Lusaka is still in the process of being built, and it has been estimated that 250 health centres could be built for the same cost. Furthermore, in Africa it has been found that the building of one health centre (plus beds) is equivalent to the cost of four beds in a teaching hospital (King, 1966). At Tamale in Northern Ghana, a new hospital has been built at the same cost as would be necessary to construct eighty rural health centres (OHE, 1972).

> In most low-income countries, hospital-based medical care systems are being established, or at least attempts are being made to establish them. However, in the absence of substantial income development, such hospital-based systems are making impossible the spread of essential health services to the mass of the population. It is not unusual for the capital costs of a large city or regional teaching hospital in Africa to be greater than the entire annual budget of the country. (Gish, 1971)

The idea that such centres of excellence act as referral centres for patients from many parts of the country has proved to be untrue. In the Malago Hospital in Kampala, Uganda, 88 per cent of all admissions were found to come from the Mengo district of Kampala within the immediate vicinity of the hospital (Hamilton & Anderson, 1965). In Ghana, at the Central Hospital in Accra, less than 10 per cent of the patients came from outside the capital. In the four other major hospitals in the country, only 20 per cent of the in-patients came from beyond the urban district surrounding the hospitals.

Good evidence has been provided from Tanzania showing the benefits of investing money in either health centres or hospitals (Table 7).

President Nyerere has perhaps summed up the views of many developing countries: 'We must not again be tempted by offers of a big new hospital with all the running costs involved, until at least every one of our citizens has basic medical services readily available to him.'

TABLE 7 *Comparison of rural health centres and district hospitals in Tanzania, 1971*

	Capital cost[a]	Running cost[a]	Out-patient visits	Admis-sions	Population coverage
200-bed hospital	6 000 000	2 060 000	400 000	9 000	10 000–30 000
15 rural health centres	6 000 000	2 250 000	1 100 000	15 000	300 000–500 000

[a] In Tanzania schillings (7 Tanzanian schillings = 1 US$).
Source: Gish, O. (1976). *Les carnets d'enfance*, No. 33, 44. Children's Fund, Geneva

2. Doctors

The need to rethink the use of doctors and the need for doctors in developing countries is based on simple, unassailable facts. They are too expensive to train in the numbers necessary to staff such health services; usually they are trained for the needs of people living in Paris, Melbourne or Chicago, and they congregate in urban areas where they can earn a reasonable living and practise the type of technological medicine for which they have been trained. To believe that doctors can even begin to solve the medical problems of rural populations is manifestly absurd and, in fact, in some countries there are not even enough doctors to staff the hospitals that have already been built (as has happened in the teaching hospital in Addis Ababa, Ethiopia). The extent of the problem can be gauged from the number of doctors and nurses available (Table 8), and, perhaps even more important, the maldistribution of personnel between rural and urban areas (Table 4).

In the developing world, young doctors are trained to the highest standards of specialised, scientific, Western-style medicine. From whatever viewpoint this is judged, it does little to help. For the young doctor it produces a feeling of frustration and despair, even anger, since he is quite unable to practise medicine as he has been taught, and he realises that his own country will never be able to provide even the simplest facilities and equipment which he has been taught are necessary. If he is aware of the needs of the rural population, he will be angry with the medical establishment for educating him in this way. The

TABLE 8 Distribution of physicians

	Physicians per 10 000 population		
Country	1950	1960	1970
Africa			
Ethiopia	0.08	0.10	0.13
Ghana	0.34	0.46	0.77
Kenya	1.00	0.94	1.28
Lesotho	0.39	0.51	0.38
Uganda	0.43	0.72	1.08
Tanzania	0.35	0.56	0.46
Zambia	0.59	1.05	0.74
Asia			
Afghanistan	0.13	0.25	0.49
India	1.71	2.08	2.08
Indonesia	0.15	0.21	0.36
Iran	1.31	2.45	3.03
Nepal	–	0.14	0.20
Sri Lanka	1.67	2.22	2.71
Thailand	0.77	1.29	1.25
Latin America			
Bolivia	2.41	2.34	4.35
Brazil	3.65	–	5.12
Chile	3.63	5.53	4.97
Cuba	9.72	9.68	8.67
Guatemala	1.70	2.35	2.76
Mexico	4.45	5.61	6.92
Peru	2.37	5.05	5.22
Developed countries			
Australia	9.84	13.27	–
Canada	10.19	11.00	14.56
Czechoslovakia	9.21	16.12	21.03
France	7.75	10.77	13.39
New Zealand	12.56	11.80	11.50
USA	13.26	13.39	15.78
USSR	13.08	17.99	23.78

Source: *World Health Statistics*, vol. 3, 1970 (published 1974)

conflicting opinions regarding medical education, with the traditional views of hospital-orientated medical care versus the aspirations of those who see the requirements of medical education in a wider context, have been well described (King, 1972).

What can he do? There are three options: emigrate to a developed country, remain in his own country to provide care for the privileged urban minority, or become a disillusioned and disgruntled doctor in the rural situation. The majority of patients, even in developed countries, are completely unaware of the requirements of a relevant medical education. The small proportion of the population who may regularly see a doctor are persuaded by the medical profession that a Western-style education is necessary in order to maintain 'standards', and so they naturally encourage and expect the present style of medical training to remain. For the governments who largely finance their education, the problem of emigration is serious and perplexing, but no-one should be surprised. It has been estimated that, in 1967, 11 per cent of Indian doctors were permanently working abroad; in the five-year period from 1962 to 1966, Pakistan lost 50 per cent of the total output from its medical schools; in Sri Lanka, with an output of about 250 doctors per year, in the year May 1971 to April 1972, 108 doctors left the country (Senewiratne, 1975). In Thailand, 67 per cent of doctors emigrate at some stage in their careers, although the permanent figure is estimated to be no higher than 4 per cent. Even so, the postgraduate experience, largely gained in the USA, is likely to benefit only the élite, urban classes. In Turkey, 17 per cent of the 22 per cent of Turkish doctors who emigrate do not return home (Committee on the International Migration of Talent, 1970), while Iran loses 25 per cent of its medical graduates (*Lancet*, 1973).*

The answer to this complicated, seemingly insoluble problem is far from clear: to maintain the *status quo* is irresponsible and perpetuates an intolerable situation, but to suggest that the solution will be found by merely altering the medical curriculum to meet the specific problems of a developing country is too facile an answer, and makes a number of unwarranted assumptions: first, that universities and medical schools will be prepared voluntarily to change their syllabus; second, that medical students who have been trained in this way will be prepared to live and serve in the rural populations; third, that the

* For a full annotated bibliography on this subject see DHEW (1975).

selection of medical students will be widened to include those from rural or poor urban areas – this, of course, presupposes a dramatic improvement in educational standards – and, finally, that revolutionary change in the structure of society will occur, and thus readily permit and encourage such alterations. In fact, revolution is the most likely possibility and has already taken place in China, Cuba, Vietnam, North Korea, Laos, Cambodia, Moçambique and Angola.

Primary medical care

At first sight, the principles of primary care in developing countries would appear, of necessity, to differ fundamentally from those of the developed world. This is not so, although the use of medical manpower and the organisation of facilities show a different emphasis. Certainly, as the problems are obvious and more easily definable than in developed countries, there is little excuse for continuing policies which cannot solve these problems. The Third World will remain poor in the foreseeable future, so they should not pursue policies which waste very limited resources. The medical profession must surely recognise that it will have to function within specific and very limited financial stringencies for many generations to come. Doctors, if they wish to provide a service which will help the majority of the population, must be realistic and accept that there will *never* be enough money to provide a Western-style health service, even if this is the correct solution to the problems of rural poverty. Directly leading on from this is the necessity to tackle the conflicting views of priorities – rural versus urban services, health centres and dispensaries versus hospitals, and medical auxiliaries versus doctors. In addition, attention must be concentrated on specific high-risk groups, such as mothers and children, on preventive medicine and public health measures, on health education and, probably most important of all, on nutrition.

The triad of basic requirements for primary care in developed countries has been discussed in Chapter 2. How applicable are these requirements to the developing world?

1. *Availability* and *accessibility* are obvious fundamental requirements, but their implementation by health planners and doctors depends on values often accepted only in theory and is difficult to organise in practice. Distance and logistics, not surprisingly, are the main problems. It is found that there is an inverse relationship be-

tween the use of hospital or health centre and the distance patients live from these.

> In a developing country, distance is a critical determinant of medical care, and it is widely realised that only those close to a medical unit can derive the full benefit from its services. While this may seem obvious, it is not generally appreciated just how inequitable is this way of distributing medical care. For example, it was found in Kenya that 40 per cent of the outpatients attending a health centre lived within 5 miles of it, 30 per cent lived between 5 and 10 miles of it and a further 30 per cent lived more than 10 miles away. It will be seen that approximately four times as many people came from each square mile within the 0–5 mile zone as came from one in the 5–10 mile zone. The same grossly inequitable distribution of outpatient services has also been found in Uganda in the study based on Mityama hospital. Here data were obtained from a hospital dispensary and an aid post, and it was found that the same principles governed outpatient attendances at all three of these units. (King, 1966)

In India, a study showed that 60 per cent of patients lived within one mile of a primary health centre (Roemer, 1972). The same principle applies to the frequency of attendance per patient. Transport and distance are, therefore, of prime importance and, just as in the planning of health centres in the UK it is customary to talk of the 'pram-pushing distance', so in the developing countries 'walking distance' is the deciding factor: generally 5 miles (two hours' walking time) is found to be the maximum for reasonable use of facilities.

2. In developing countries *acceptability* is of far greater importance than the *luxury of continuity* – in fact without it, no health service can hope to achieve anything.

The reasons which prevent or inhibit patients from using the available facilities vary from country to country, depending on religious, cultural and social factors, but reports from primary health workers in many parts of the world all tell the same story: that there are a number of common 'acceptability factors'. First, it is vital that cultural, language and tribal barriers should be bridged and fully understood, so that patients do not feel frightened and completely alien when visiting a dispensary or health centre. For this reason, it has been found that if primary health workers are chosen from the local community, then there is a greater chance of confidence and *rapport* developing between them and their patients. A doctor or other health worker imported from an urban or foreign environment with a different background and outlook, often not speaking the same language or dialect, may act as a considerable deterrent. There are, of course, exceptions, and the success of Christian missionary doctors in many parts of the world needs no elaboration. For instance,

> in Malawi, health services were largely built up by Christian missionary bodies with small financial resources but with a sense of dedication. To provide health services, they trained local medical auxiliaries under various titles and with varying degrees of preliminary schooling. In 1964, the government of independent Malawi inherited a situation in which it could only maintain the health services by continuing support to and cooperation with the Christian missions which provided health services and trained health staff at a very much smaller cost to the government than if it took over these services itself. (Stevenson, 1975).

In Tanzania, the Church, before and under successive colonial administrations, helped to develop the medical services. Since independence in 1961, the government of Tanzania and the Churches have collaborated in attempting to improve the health of the rural population. The integration of Church and state has not always been smooth, but at the district level much has been achieved. (Schulpen, 1975).

The community or village should not feel that health programmes and facilities have been imposed upon them, so local leaders therefore must be involved in decisions from the very beginning. The poorest communities, with inevitably the biggest health problems, are paradoxically those who are the least interested in health services. These people, who in the view of health planners and doctors are in need of most 'medical help', are more concerned with housing, employment, education, help with their agriculture and an adequate supply of food and a reliable water supply than with specific health matters. Equally, to the frustration, even irritation of many workers in the field, when it is perfectly obvious that simple public health measures would improve the general level of health to a satisfactory minimum level, it is to curative medicine that the villagers may be looking.

Too much must not be promised, as one of the recurring cycles in rural health care is the disillusion and apathy which follow the false hopes and unfulfilled promises of government agencies. Self-help and a feeling of personal responsibility always make a scheme more likely to succeed and, finally, a number of experienced workers state that free treatment may not be valued: in fact, if it is free, then it is assumed to be of poor quality (Mukerjee, 1975). Others would disagree and feel that, provided the health services are good and there is no financial barrier, then people readily use the available facilities (Banerji, 1973).

At the WHO Assembly in May 1975, priority was given to the promotion of primary medical care, and seven basic principles were set out.

(*a*) Primary health care should be shaped around the life pattern of the population it should serve, and should meet the needs of the community.

(*b*) Primary health care should be an integral part of the national health system, and other echelons of services should be designed in support of the needs of the peripheral level, especially as this pertains to technical supply, supervisory and referral support.

(*c*) Primary health care activities should be fully integrated with the activities of the other sectors involved in community development (agriculture, education, public works, housing and communication).

(*d*) The local population should be actively involved in the formulation and implementation of health care policies, so that health care can be brought into line with local needs and priorities. Decisions upon what are the community needs should be based upon a continuing dialogue between the people and the services.

(*e*) Health care offered should place a maximum reliance on available community resources, especially those which have hitherto remained untapped, and should remain within the stringent cost limitations that are present in each country.

(*f*) Primary health care should use an integrated approach of preventive, promotive, curative and rehabilitation services for the individual, family and community. The balance between these services should vary according to community needs and may well change over time.

(*g*) The majority of health intervention should be undertaken at the most peripheral, practicable level of health service by workers most suitably trained for performing these activities.

Is this merely a declaration of good intent by a well-meaning international agency? How realistic are any of these principles in the present political climate of most developing countries? Is it an established fact that most of the rural populations do not want curative medicine, hospitals and the technology of Western medicine? What evidence is there to suggest that the majority of health workers – either doctors or nurses – are anxious to implement these principles?

Alternative approaches to primary care

From many parts of the world, successful attempts are being made to overcome the enormous problems already described and to provide some health care for the rural populations. All these projects have involved the use of various categories of medical auxiliaries, not only in preference to doctors, but also because the alternative would mean no medical attention whatsoever. There is nothing new in this idea (p. 14), nor in the logical step in providing dispensaries and aid posts near to the people, rather than expecting them to travel long distances to the nearest hospital, nor in the principle that medical care should flow from the periphery to the centre. What is new, though, is the absolute and definite commitment to implement these ideas which have been talked about for so long. The objectives and organisation of a number of countries have been fully documented (Newell, 1975), and an evaluation of their success has also been made. Broadly, the countries fall into three overlapping categories:

(*a*) National change – revolution: China, Cuba, Vietnam, North Korea, North Vietnam, Tanzania, Laos, Cambodia, Moçambique and Angola.

(*b*) Extension of existing systems: Iran, Nigeria and Venezuela.

(*c*) Local community development: Guatemala, India and Indonesia (Djukonovic & Mach, 1975).

This is by no means a definitive list, and further examples come from as far afield as Java, Bangladesh, South Korea and Egypt.

In most developing countries there are two levels of medical auxiliary. At the first level, the auxiliaries, often with eight or nine years' basic education, followed by three years' special training, are employed in health centres serving populations of 25 000–40 000. They are involved in both preventive and curative medicine (including primary diagnosis and treatment, maternity supervision, sometimes involving Caesarean section, and also routine and emergency anaesthetics), and they acquire a remarkably high degree of skill. They work under the supervision of visiting doctors. At the second level, auxiliaries are recruited from the villages and are subjected to a short period of intensive training (often only 3 months). They usually work part-time in the village health post, carrying out their normal employment, generally as agricultural workers.

The best known and most widely studied country is the People's Republic of China (see Bibliography, p. 396), where the alleviation of poverty, the use of simple public health measures, the involvement of the people in self-help and the widespread use of the now famous 'barefoot doctors' has enormously improved the health of 500 million people. But two questions must be asked which in no way reflect on the success of China or any other country which is striving hard to overcome the problems of primary care. First, when the major health problems of infectious disease and those associated with poverty and underdevelopment have been solved, will these alternative methods of providing primary care be any more successful in dealing with the problems of heart disease, malignancy, the degenerative diseases of middle and old age, and the self-inflicted diseases of affluence? Second, will the medical auxiliaries, even though they are chosen from the local community, be content to remain in the villages? It appears that isolation, both professional and social, affects auxiliaries just as much as it does doctors, and they have a similar desire to go to the capital city or nearest town. Will they be content not to improve their medical skills and education by moving to the large urban hospital for further training? As yet, no-one can reply to these questions, but the answers will be awaited with great interest because, if these workers are to be the cornerstone of health services in most developing countries, certainly well into the twenty-first century, then the hopes of millions of people depend on the success of this policy.

Consideration will now be given to the organisation of primary care in two developing countries with certain similarities: Chile and Cuba.* They have similar population size and geographical location, and both have introduced some form of organised health service – Chile in 1952 and Cuba in 1959. But here the parallels end, and the effects of pursuing different philosophies of health care within a similar administrative structure will be seen clearly. Likewise, the impossibility of separating health care and politics is shown graphically.

CHILE
Chile stretches for two-thirds of the length of South America,

* I wish to state that my visit to Chile was originally arranged through Professor Hugo Behm, Department of Public Health, University of Santiago in April

banked on the one side by the Andes mountains, and on the other by the Pacific Ocean: about 2500 miles from north to south, and at its widest no more than 200 miles from east to west. Chile is separated from Peru by the Atacamá Desert, some parts of which have not seen rain in living memory and, although the southern tip is virtually uninhabitable, much of the southern half of the country contains magnificent farmland.

Chile has a population of just over 9.5 million, mostly concentrated in the large towns – Santiago (3 million), Valparaiso (1.5 million), Concepción (1 million) – producing the all too familiar problems of urban squalor (Table 9).

TABLE 9 *Total population in urban and rural Chile*

Year	Population				
	Total	Urban	(%)	Rural	(%)
1920	3 731 573	1 732 567	46.4	1 999 006	53.6
1940	5 023 539	2 639 311	52.5	2 384 228	47.5
1960	7 374 115	5 028 060	68.2	2 346 055	31.8
1970	9 726 277	7 489 297	77.0	2 236 980	23.0

Source: XIX Conferencia Sanitaria Panamericana. Ministerio de Salud Publica, Santiago, Chile, 1974

The people of Chile are racially homogeneous. The reason is that the mixing of Spanish and Indian blood occurred so long ago that the result is now apparent as a racial unity unique among South American countries. In addition, over the last 100 years, immigration has been severely restricted, usually to people of European stock, by successive Chilean governments.

Chile introduced a health service in 1954. It was the first country in South America to do so: in fact, there has been some form of modified health insurance since the early 1930s. This was very advanced social

1973, five months before the overthrow of President Allende. The purpose of the visit was to study the organisation of primary care, but it proved impossible to ignore the political nature of the problem. There was, and is, no intention of aggravating the political situation in Chile: merely to state the situation as I saw it. Professor Behm was arrested some months after the *coup d'état* and imprisoned for over a year: he was subsequently released and is now living in Costa Rica.

legislation, particularly in this part of the world, but not altogether surprising because Chile has had a long history of parliamentary democracy and has until recently enjoyed a far greater degree of internal stability than most of the rest of this vast sub-continent. This long tradition was tragically shattered by the overthrow of President Allende and his government in September 1973. Since that time, the country has been under the control of a military dictatorship led by Augusto Pinochet.

The structure and organisation of health services

Chile is divided administratively and from a health service point of view into 12 regions with populations of between 750 000 and 800 000, each containing at least one regional hospital with the usual specialist and super-specialist facilities. The regions are divided into areas, with hospitals providing general specialist services and, in turn, these areas are further divided into sectors. Administratively, and in basic regional organisation, Cuba and Chile are similar – at least in theory (p. 347). The director of the area, and also of the sectors within that area, is the chief doctor (specialist) of the area hospital: the implications of this appointment will be considered later.

The Servicio Nacional de Salud (SNS) is financed 75 per cent from direct taxation, 10 per cent through social security payments and 15 per cent by a variety of smaller means – cemetery tax and prescription charges. The service covered perhaps two-thirds of the population in 1973. At the same time, it catered for those people insured through the Servicio de Seguro Social (social security), about 45 per cent, and also for the low-income and unemployed categories, about 20 per cent, who were not eligible for any social security benefits (Kadt, 1974).

Because of the seemingly insoluble problem of inflation, these figures are changing. In December 1974, it was estimated that the number of workers insured through the Servicio de Seguro Social had decreased to 32 per cent, while the number in the lowest paid and unemployed categories had risen to 42 per cent, and there is no evidence to suggest that this latter figure is not continuing to rise. The social security organisation is complicated, with 39 different agencies which are hopelessly inefficient and administratively wasteful: in fact, 30 per cent of its income is dissipated in administration, and in 1967 there were 40 656 administrators as compared with 6487 medical professionals (Waitzkin & Modell, 1974).

In 1961, there were 4340 doctors, i.e. 5.5 per 10 000 population, and in 1970 the number of doctors rose to 6096, that is 6.27 per 10 000 population. The distribution of doctors is far from satisfactory. In 1970, the province of Santiago had 9.8 doctors per 10 000, while in the rest of the country the ratio was 3.8 (Ministerio de Salud Publica, 1974). In fact, these figures give a much better impression than the reality of the situation, as most of the practising doctors are concentrated in the large hospitals in Santiago, Valparaiso and Concepción, while the actual proportion of doctors involved in patient care, administration and research is not available. Reliable recent statistics, including the period of the Allende government (1970–3) are not available.

Primary medical care

The basic health unit is the sector, each with a population varying between 30 000 and 70 000. Medical care is provided by neighbourhood health centres or *consultarios*, and the hospital out-patient and emergency departments.

The doctor of first contact is a specialist, based on the area hospital. In principle, although not in reality, the *consultarios* are staffed by:

1. Specialists trained to work exclusively in the hospital environment, with no idea of or interest in the problems of primary care. They are employed on a salaried basis to work, in theory, six hours per day for the SNS – four hours in hospital and two hours in the *consultario*. In fact, those who do attend the *consultario* spend, on average, only four hours per week there, and a number do not attend at all. Most of their time is spent in hospital work, but poor pay has encouraged many doctors to spend even less than their allotted six hours per day on health service work, and to devote as much time as possible to private practice. It is not difficult to appreciate that the *consultario* service (primary care) suffers most of all, with many specialists not even fulfilling their very limited obligations. Quite apart from this, the other main, quite understandable reasons for not wanting to work in the *consultario* are:

(*a*) the very poor conditions and facilities;

(*b*) the poor professional status accorded to primary medical care both by the profession and the government;

(*c*) a fear that, as specialists, they are 'losing out' scientifically and wasting their time on trivial work.

2. Nurses, midwives and social workers who are in very short

supply while physiotherapists and occupational therapists are an almost unknown luxury.

3. Young doctors and medical students who spend a varying time in the *consultario* each week: this depends more on their sense of social and moral responsibility than on any encouragement from their senior colleagues or the present government. This scheme was initiated and strongly encouraged by the government of President Allende.

Most *consultarios* have no laboratory, X-ray, physiotherapy or ECG facilities. Specialists obviously do not want to work under conditions in which the lack of facilities and general organisation are so appalling. The area hospital is responsible for a number of *consultarios*, depending on the population and catchment area: for example, San Juan de Díos hospital in Santiago covers seven, each with a population of about 85 000. The staffing of the Consultario Andes was (in theory only): five internal medicine specialists (for example cardiologist, neurologist, nephrologist, but no general physician), five paediatricians, one obstetrician, one gynaecologist and one surgeon for two hours each per day. It was interesting and illuminating to discover on visiting the university hospital José Juan Aguire, with over 1000 beds, that it had no responsibility for any *consultarios*. This gives an immediate and correct insight into the attitude of the medical profession towards primary care. As in many medical schools throughout the world, students are unaware of the problems and opportunities of primary care, and the hospital staff are insulated from the real requirements of the health service.

The final obstacle to a rational *consultario* service is the fact that the annual budget for each area is designated to the area hospital. It is the responsibility of the director of the hospital (and his team of specialist advisers) to allocate funds. The result of this policy is self-evident – the *consultario* service is chronically starved of money.

Rural health service

It is extremely difficult to assess the situation in rural areas because there are so many conflicting reports. Certainly during the Allende period of government compulsory national service for all newly qualified doctors was started, and attempts were made to improve and increase the facilities and staffing of rural hospitals and clinics. A 'health train' also toured the southern provinces, and it is estimated that, in all, it treated 30 000 people (Waitzkin & Modell, 1974). Although some young doctors still work in the rural service (Stephen, 1974), there is no compulsory service, and consequently there has been a definite decline in the number of doctors serving in rural areas.

Politics and health care

From the inception of the health service in 1954, there was no attempt to provide a fully comprehensive service for the whole population – how could there be? The SNS was orientated towards curative medicine and the hospital service, and it was accepted that at least one-third of the population would pay their physician privately. As a direct consequence of this, it has been decided by successive governments that a substantial part of a doctor's income should come from this source. In the early 1960s, under President Frei, it was recognised that the SNS was failing in a number of directions. Gross under-financing led to an increase in private practice and the creation of separate services for railway workers, miners, the armed forces and white-collar workers. The SNS was unable to direct medical and nursing personnel away from the rich urban areas, particularly Santiago, to the poor rural and very low income shanty towns on the outskirts of all large cities. The gross imbalance between the hospital and *consultario* services was not redressed.

Under President Allende, the government tried to provide a comprehensive medical service for the entire population, and failed for a number of extremely complex political and economic reasons. The Unidad Popular government did make serious attempts to shift the emphasis away from the hospital to the *consultarios*, which was an entirely logical and essential step if there was to be any hope of improving the effectiveness of the service and the health of the low-paid and unemployed. As well as this, several programmes were started in an attempt to improve the distribution and quality of care. There was also official government recognition of the importance of improving the standard of housing, sanitation and nutrition, with great emphasis placed on the diet of children and pregnant and nursing mothers (Waitzkin & Modell, 1974). To be fair and accurate, it must be pointed out that the distribution of extra powdered milk was started in 1958–9, initially to children up to one year and to pregnant and nursing mothers: what President Allende's government did was to increase the age range of the children and try to provide for a more comprehensive distribution.

President Frei's administration first suggested making the SNS more democratic; it remained for President Allende to implement these changes. A government decree of September 1972 set out plans for three new organisations to improve representation and participation, following the example of Cuba (p. 350):

1. *Consejos locales de salud* (local health councils), were formed, both at *consultario* and hospital level: each included representatives of unions, women's organisations, schools and health workers.

2. *Consejos partarios de salud* (executive councils of health) were formed, again both at *consultario* and hospital level, under the chairmanship of either the director of the hospital or *consultario*: their twelve members were chosen half from local representatives and half from health workers. There is some dispute as to whether these committees were merely a sounding board for political indoctrination, or whether they did in fact make people more aware of the difficulties of providing health care, and prepare them for an active and more mature role in the field of primary care (Kadt, 1974). Some proposals were definitely implemented: for example, one university teaching hospital in Santiago responded to the demand for increased staffing at *consultario* level by sending out physicians (Waitzkin & Modell, 1974).

3. *Responsables de Salud* were also formed. They were modelled on the Committee for the Defence of the Revolution, as in Cuba. They worked in close cooperation with the *consultarios*.

In retrospect, it seems that the Responsables de Salud were the most effective of the three committees, and did work of positive value – perhaps because they were given direct responsibility for advising about feeding, sanitation and general health education, including vaccination and inoculation programmes. The military junta under General Pinochet have disbanded all three committees.

Another change in the structure of the SNS, brought about by the Allende administration, was the training of medical auxiliaries to work in the countryside and shanty towns, carrying out preventive medicine and health education. This was, in the context of a developing country, an obvious, rational and necessary solution to the acute manpower problem.

Unfortunately, President Allende met two formidable obstacles to his health policy. First, the economic plight of his country gradually increased and finally became uncontrollable. This made it impossible to carry out many reforming plans and rendered impotent the new social awareness of the health authorities. It was no use setting up *consultarios* if, in practice, they had no facilities – sometimes not even running water. Such a situation only led to despondency and disillusion, the danger of which has already been referred to (p. 336). Second, he was opposed by most of the Chilean medical profession, who interpreted his ideas to improve the primary care services and his attempts to change the maldistribution of doctors and resources as a Communist threat – an infringement of their personal liberty. Such an attitude was entirely predictable and would almost certainly be the response of most doctors in the non-Communist world.

In the years since the *coup d'état* in September 1973, what has been the present government's thinking on health policy? By December 1974, the Ministry of Health had intimated (and this has since been confirmed) that it wanted an alteration in direction of the SNS. It is the present government's policy to 'diversify the cost of the SNS' so that the burden on central taxation can be reduced as much as possible. This is to be carried out by:

(*a*) Encouraging private medicine and insurance coverage as in a free market system.

(*b*) Strengthening the individual health services (miners, railway workers and armed services) by encouraging the key industries to build their own *consultarios* and to pay the doctors higher wages than the SNS.

(*c*) Encouraging 'Sermena' (National Medical Service for Employees: white-collar workers) to extend its influence and coverage.

This stimulus to private medicine, with the continuing and inevitable underfinancing of the SNS in current expenditure and capital outlay, will make the gradual collapse of the SNS almost inevitable. Three levels of care will follow from this policy. First, the SNS, providing limited and increasingly inadequate care for patients who cannot afford private medicine, or are unable to insure themselves – this is an increasing proportion of the population as inflation escalates and unemployment rises. Paradoxically, though, some people will save and scrape, even at the lower end of the income scale, to see a doctor privately because it is felt that the SNS is providing only a second-rate service (Kadt, 1974). Second, a proportion of the poor and unemployed will receive virtually no medical attention, as the *consultario* service in many areas is practically unobtainable and the hospital out-patient and emergency services are too far from the patient's home. Third, a minority of the population will receive private treatment of a good standard.

Personal assessment

Particularly in a developing country, politics cannot be separated from health. It is unfortunate therefore that opposition to the fundamental and necessary changes in the organisation and structure of medical services always reveals the majority of the medical profession to be ignorant of the real needs of the country. This is partly because of their inappropriate medical education which makes them appear as a self-interested group intent on maintaining the standards of Western technological medicine. Such behaviour inevitably leads to accusations that doctors are imprisoned by their class origins (Waitzkin & Modell, 1974).

Even if the problem of poverty had been solved, there would be little prospect of an effective health service which would meet the needs of the people unless there was also a strengthening of the primary care sector. A specialist-orientated education in a hospital-dominated health service, in which primary care is carried out by reluctant specialists who have neither the desire nor the training to appreciate its dimensions, is a prescription for failure.

Finally, whatever improvements in medical education and organisation are made in the SNS, their effect on the health of the great mass of people would be limited. Until the fundamental problems of malnutrition (estimated by the Ministry of Health to affect between 5 and 10 per cent of children under six years and by independent paediatricians to affect nearer 20 to 25 per cent), poor housing, overcrowding, inadequate sanitation, poverty and unemployment have been faced by the government and its supporters, these factors will remain the major obstacles to even minimal health objectives.

CUBA

Cuba is an independent, socialist republic, set up in 1957 by Fidel Castro after the overthrow of the Batista regime. It is situated in the tropical zone of the Caribbean. The length of the island from east to west is 780 miles and its maximum width from north to south is 119 miles. Cuba has a multi-racial society with a population of

8 500 000, 73 per cent of whom are of white Spanish origin, and 27 per cent of black Afro-Cuban. It is a young country, as shown by the 1970 census figures, 37 per cent being under 15 years of age and only 6 per cent being 65 years or more. Again according to the same census, 60.5 per cent of the population live in urban areas, and the proportion of men to women is 51 to 49.

Structure of the health service

The country is divided into six provinces, but for the purpose of health administration there are seven, Oriente Province being divided into two. Each health province has a population of about 1 to 1.5 million, and is divided into regions covering populations of 200 000 to 300 000, which in turn are divided into health areas – the basic unit of administration and health care – with populations of between 25 000 and 30 000.

To provide a comprehensive service within reach of the community, the organisation has been firmly based on a rational use of resources, with clearly defined levels of care: primary at the area level, secondary (specialist) at the regional, and tertiary (super-specialist) at provincial level. In other words, the more specialised the care, the further it is from the patient's point of entry into the service (Figure 1). The polyclinic in urban areas and the rural hospital in the countryside are the most important elements in the whole system. All other health facilities and institutions are intended to support their activities, and great emphasis is laid on the importance of primary or first-contact care.

Pre-revolutionary situation

Even the most biased opponents of the Castro government could not disagree with the following assessment of health care at the end of the Batista period. Medicine functioned along the traditional pattern of the USA, showing many of its worst features and characteristics. This, of course, was and is the situation today in most South American countries.

(a) There was no health service. Perhaps 25–30 per cent of the population were able to obtain medical attention through private insurance, doctors being paid on an item-of-service basis. For the rest of the population, there was little hope of receiving medical care.

(b) Primary care or general practice was provided by general practitioners and specialists. The emphasis was almost entirely on curative rather than preventive medicine, because of the method of insurance payment.

(c) The hospital service was poorly organised, with no overall planning. There was confusion of function and maldistribution, inevitably leading to a duplication of some specialties and wide gaps in others.

(d) Maldistribution of doctors and nurses left a large proportion of

Figure 1   Structure of the Health Service

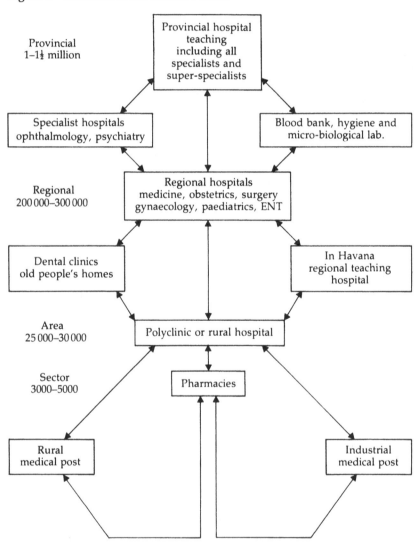

the population without even the possibility of medical attention. For example, in 1959, 63 per cent of doctors worked in Havana with only 22 per cent of the population (for comparable figures in other developing countries see Table 4).

(*e*) Medical education was totally divorced from the needs of the community: a situation, of course, in which Cuba was not alone.

Immediate post-revolution situation

(*a*) The state tried to provide a comprehensive (curative and preventive) service for the whole population, which was free at the time of use. There were and are prescription charges, with exemptions for children, pregnant women and old people.

(*b*) The health service should get away from the specialist-orientated, totally curative style of care, and concentrate more on the preventive aspect. However good the level of curative medicine, it was appreciated that alone it could not ensure the maintenance of a high standard of health.

(*c*) It was decided that total 'blanket care' could not be given immediately, and therefore well-defined priority groups and problems were focused upon, for example, nutrition – particularly of children, poor housing and sanitation, education and the specific medical priorities of ante-natal care and the supervision of confinements, perinatal and neonatal mortality and morbidity problems.

(*d*) Hospital resources were redistributed to rationalise their use and provide more equitable care. For example, in 1957, 54.7 per cent of hospital beds were in Havana with 22 per cent of the population, 15.5 per cent of beds were in Orente with 35 per cent of the population; in 1969, 40 per cent of beds were in Havana and 23 per cent of beds in Orente, with roughly similar proportions of the population. In 1971, there were 40 321 beds, 12 247 of which were set up in the ten years from 1960 to 1970. According to official figures from the Ministry of Health, new hospitals were built in areas of greatest need: 47 per cent of new hospital beds were in Orente province and only 8 per cent in Havana.

(*e*) Definite emphasis has been placed on the community or primary care services, in the hope that a more appropriate delivery system will be built up. In 1971, 236 polyclinics had been built or adapted from old buildings during the preceding ten years, and over 50 per cent of these had been provided in rural areas as rural hospitals.

(f) Re-allocation of medical and nursing personnel was a necessary step if resources were to be brought to the whole population. In 1959, there were 6300 physicians in Cuba, but by 1962 3000 had left the country, mostly for North America. This mass emigration caused enormous problems, and there followed an intensive campaign of recruitment over the next ten years.

Until 1962, there was one medical school – founded in 1728 in Havana – and this was quite inadequate to meet the acute shortage of doctors brought about by the 1962 exodus. Thus, in 1962, a new medical school was set up in Orente province, followed in 1965 by a third in Las Villas province. During the period 1962–72, 5079 doctors graduated from these three medical schools. In 1974, there were about 8000 doctors working in the health service. The decision to increase the output of doctors was made centrally by the government, who determine the intake of students into the various departments of the universities. During this period 30 per cent of all university entrants were for medicine, and of these about 50 per cent were women.

The ratio of doctor/population still varies enormously, in spite of the improvements which have taken place: 12.5 doctors per 10 000 population in Havana and 1.8 per 10 000 in some areas of Camaguey, the average for the whole country being 9.4 per 10 000. With the present intake of 1300–1500 students per year it is hoped by the end of the present decade to have a ratio of 13.9 per 10 000.

In 1958, only 6 nursing schools existed, with a total annual production of only 50 nurses. There are now 22 nursing schools with an average of 300 nurses qualifying annually. In addition there are 118 auxiliary nursing courses training 1000 to 1500 auxiliaries. The nurses' training lasts three years, beginning at the tenth school grade, while the auxiliary course is for one year only, the students having finished the sixth school grade.

Other auxiliary workers, such as physiotherapists and occupational therapists, are in very short supply.

(g) Participation by the people in the health service does in fact take place, and is not merely a vague promise or threat from the administrative bureaucrats. This is carried out principally at area level in the polyclinic or rural hospital, through such organisations as the Committee for the Defence of the Revolution, the Federation of Cuban Women, trade unions, and the Federation of Small Farmers. They are given responsibility for carrying out health education programmes, and follow up of such procedures as cervical smears, inoculations for children and for organising mother/child centres in which basic teaching is given in nutrition, hygiene and general welfare.

Primary medical care

The key to the provision of primary care is the polyclinic and the rural hospital. The actual structure and organisation of the polyclinic is similar to that found in Eastern Europe but does not follow the pattern of the USSR, where separate paediatric, adult, industrial and women's services exist. The doctor of first contact (as in Eastern Europe and the USSR) restricts his work to a particular age group or sex of patient. The exception to this rule is in rural areas, where the doctor in charge of the hospital acts as a general practitioner.

Polyclinic Julian Griman is situated on the outskirts of Havana. It serves a population of 31 000, which is divided into seven sectors with up to 5000 in each. Its permanent staff comprises six adult internists, ten paediatricians, three gynaecologists and visiting specialists from the local district hospital. It has an X-ray department (including contrast media) and a laboratory, but no facilities for physiotherapy. The chief nurse is assisted by ten auxiliary nurses and one social worker. The clinic staff carry out no home visits: if these are necessary, they are made by staff from the neighbouring district hospital, who are also responsible for emergency care at weekends and at night! This polyclinic is typical of those throughout the service.

In rural areas, primary care is provided by rural hospitals – in essence, polyclinics with beds. San Blas hospital in Las Villas province was built in 1960 and opened in 1961 – the first time the 6500 people of the area had had access to health care. The hospital is staffed by one doctor, one dentist, one nurse, three auxiliary nurses and one laboratory technician, who also acts as a radiographer. It contains 24 beds – 14 internal medicine, 6 paediatric and 4 obstetric. All surgical emergencies are transferred by ambulance to the nearest regional hospital. Doctors working in the rural health service are carrying out their compulsory three years' national service. They do not appear to resent this, feeling that it is quite reasonable that country districts should be so staffed. Again no home visits are carried out, all patients being transferred to the hospital for consultation and admission if necessary. The main emphasis is on paediatric and ante-natal care, the supervision of confinements and inoculation programmes. As in urban poly-clinics, the population has been further divided into two sectors which are staffed by a Red Cross worker (not a public health nurse as in urban areas) who is responsible for health education, simple medical care and some inoculations. The two sectors have been subdivided further into ten mini-sectors which are the responsibility of the Federation of Cuban Women.

Experiment in medical education

In July/August 1974, a new polyclinic was opened at Alamar, Havana. It has various experimental features, and it is intended that it should run without modification initially for six years. Its chief aim has been to change the emphasis in medical education from the hospital to the primary care service. Even in a revolutionary situation such as Cuba, old customs and traditions die slowly, particularly in medicine, and there has been the usual tendency to concentrate too much on hospital medicine.

The first reform in the curriculum took place in 1968, when the medical school in Havana decided to change from teaching by departments (internal medicine, surgery, paediatrics, obstetrics) to teaching by subjects (circulatory, digestive, reproductive and nervous systems). Next, it has been decided that, if community care is the cornerstone of the health service, then it is logical that there should be a further change of emphasis in education. At the Alamar polyclinic the exposure of students to primary care, as opposed to hospital medicine, has been increased considerably. For the first and second year, students spend four hours per day with teaching related to the needs of the locality and carried out by the permanent primary care staff of the polyclinic. In the third, fourth and fifth years, Alamar is planning for eight hours twice weekly. Such a complete change in conventional medical education has occurred nowhere else in the world (except China): its results will be watched with interest and hope by all those concerned with the training of doctors.

In addition, various weaknesses in the present organisation of primary care have been recognised, and it is hoped also that Alamar may help to rectify these. Because of the inevitable fragmentation of care at this level, the lack of continuity has affected the attitude of patients to the polyclinic service. It is intended to increase the doctor/patient ratio to one paediatrician per 1000 children, one internist per

2000 adults and one gynaecologist per 4000 women, so that, following the direct request from patients (through the Federation of Cuban Women) to the health authorities, home visits may be carried out by the polyclinic staff. It is hoped also to provide emergency care at night and at weekends at the polyclinic, rather than in the emergency room of the local hospital: in this way the quality of primary care should be improved.

So confident are the authorities that this is the correct policy, that they have built, since 1974, new teaching polyclinics in each of the provinces, and five additional ones in Havana. The increased doctor/patient ratios of the Alamar polyclinic are maintained, as half the working day of the permanent staff is now devoted to teaching. All non-teaching polyclinics are now called community polyclinics. (Rodriguez de la Vega & Sollett, 1976).

Personal assessment
There can be no doubt that without the overthrow of the Batista regime and the formation of a socialist government, no National Health Service would have been organised.

That the health of a nation depends more on the state of nutrition, housing, sanitation and employment than on the standard and organisation of its health service was appreciated by Fidel Castro's government, and priorities were decided quickly and accurately, particularly emphasising the feeding of all those under five years of age (Nuffield Trust, 1973). In fifteen years, the health indices of Cuba – infant and maternal mortality – have changed from those of a developing country almost to those of an advanced, industrialised society. The same cannot be said of Chile (Table 10).

It was realised that a fully comprehensive, free service would take many years to develop, so logically certain groups were given precedence – mothers and young children – and, in fact, they still remain the most important priority. Finally, it was appreciated that the building of large, prestige hospitals was not required and would not help the health of the mass of the people. The emphasis was placed on primary care.

One feature of health planning is both a surprise and, probably, a mistake: there is no intention of training and using medical auxiliaries, as is happening in many parts of both the developing and developed world. This is a surprise because in a revolutionary situation such as in

Cuba, the continuing professional and hierarchical dominance of doctors is contrary to the general ethos of society, and a mistake because it would seem certain that no developing country in the world can afford to train doctors to the exclusion of other paramedical personnel. Medical auxiliaries are an alternative to the highly trained doctor whose education, even in Cuba, is long and inevitably theoretical. 'Expensively trained physicians should be sensibly used in any country. To delegate suitable responsibilities to specially trained auxiliaries is not a detrimental dilution of standards of medical care. An adequate number of well-trained auxiliaries properly used must be better value than too few doctors desperately attempting the impossible.' (Elliott, 1971)

TABLE 10   *Health indices – Chile and Cuba*

	Birth rate	Death rate	Maternal mortality	Infant mortality
Chile				
1960	35.0	12.8	3.2	124.3
1965	31.5	10.5	2.8	107.1
1969	28.1	8.9	1.8	78.7
1972	27.5	8.8	1.6	71.1
Cuba				
1960	No reliable statistics			
1965	34.6	6.6	1.1	40.3
1969	26.6	6.7	0.9	47.7
1972	28.3	5.6	0.6	28.7

Source: Personal communication, Ministerio de Salud Publica, Santiago, Chile and Ministerio de Salud Publica, Havana, Cuba

Conclusion

Poor health in the Third World is directly related to poverty, malnutrition and underdevelopment: this is indisputable. But there are considerable differences of opinion about the cause of this poverty and the policies and actions which are thought necessary to improve this seemingly intractable problem. Many people state that the exploitation and oppression of the mass of the people by the economic, social and political impact of international capitalism is the main factor.

Others would counter this argument by maintaining that once the free-enterprise system is fully operational in developing countries, then poverty will be successfully, if slowly, defeated: the historical evidence for this is the success of the Western capitalist countries over the last two hundred years. Evidence against this thesis suggests that Western countries have consistently allied themselves to the local ruling class, thus helping to preserve oppressive social relations, particularly in the countryside (feudal, landlord, and tribal) which have held back the development process, even on a capitalist basis. Lack of resources and technical expertise, combined with an inability to manufacture products which can be sold on a world market is thought to play a part but, immediately, such a suggestion is opposed by the view that until economic development moves away from the manufacture of products for consumption in the Western world, there is no chance of economic self-sufficiency. Attitudes, both religious and social, may play a role that is ill-understood and often ignored by politicians and economists, leading to a passive process of underdevelopment – in other words poverty can, in some circumstances, be the result of primitiveness. Such a notion is totally unacceptable to many people who feel it is merely an excuse for governments and politicians to do nothing. Finally, there must be a redistribution of wealth by taking away the control of the economy from the small ruling class (including landowners) who also dictate the direction which society must take, and determine the pattern of Western-style consumption and aspirations. The aetiology of poverty in developing countries is extremely complex and only the most doctrinaire are able to see a simple lasting solution. Clearly poverty and health care cannot be separated and the causal relationship between them is fundamentally political. As a consequence, a number of disturbing questions remain unanswered. Can such changes in society as are necessary be brought about without the trauma of revolution? Is it still possible through evolution? Are the great mass of people prepared to wait patiently for changes that are necessary and inevitable? Only future historians can give the answer.

At the present time, health planning still emphasises the hospital-based, technically orientated specialist service with the corresponding Western-style medical education. The inevitable consequences are a health care system which does not meet the needs of the majority of people, with an over-concentration of doctors and nurses in the capital cities and larger towns and the migration of doctors and nurses to the developed world. Can a rational system of health care be provided in a developing country without innovations in education, training and organisation which run counter to the financial and social rewards of the present structure of society? Is it likely, or even possible, that such changes will be recommended by the medical profession? What conclusions can be drawn from the evidence available? It would seem that the societies which have followed the more egalitarian paths in their basic political, social and economic philosophies have also reaped the greatest benefits of improved health care for their people.

12

CONCLUSIONS

Few disagree, in theory at least, with the proposition that everyone should be provided with medical care and that there should be no barrier – either financial or geographical – for a patient in need of help. The success in achieving such an ideal depends on political leadership and action, professional cooperation by all health service workers and constant pressure from the general public. Such an egalitarian view will attempt to make a fair distribution of available resources so that priorities may be judged on medical need alone and fortuitous privilege will be abolished. When such a proposition is accepted, it produces a conflict between society and the individual and also between individual doctors and patients. How is it possible, even theoretically, to provide the best medical care for the individual and, at the same time, for society as a whole? Clearly there is no easy answer to this clash of values. But doctors can no longer ignore this dilemma without producing tensions within society. Eventually it will bring discredit upon themselves and a feeling of distrust amongst many patients if the problem is not honestly and openly faced. But, equally, patients must accept that, if there is an attempt at equality of access to medical care, then they, in their turn, must show responsibility in the use of this new-found access.

Demands, needs and resources

The reality of the insoluble equation of infinite demands measured against real needs and available resources exposes the most difficult problem facing medicine today and possibly for the next 25 years.

'There is virtually no limit to the amount of medical care an individual is capable of absorbing' (Powell, 1966) and because every society is seemingly prepared to devote a large and increasing share of their resources to the search for better health, it is essential to scrutinise more closely the way in which this money is spent.

One of the paradoxes of health care is that every advance produces further needs which are immediately translated into patient's demands. Quite obviously such a state of affairs may be both financially impossible and medically undesirable to implement. The spiralling costs of ever-expanding investigations and treatments, renders limited resources even more inadequate and this must inevitably lead to some form of rationing.

First, some effort must be made to assess and evaluate needs and demands. Every country must make decisions about what is possible and what is reasonable in the fields of both primary and secondary care, in the hope of curbing unrealistic and unnecessary demands (Sweden, p.165; USA, p. 271). It is here that the general practitioner is uniquely placed because he knows the patient's expectations and yet should understand the limitations of many investigations and treatments: he can, therefore, act as mediator. I do not believe that there should be any financial 'barriers', 'controls' or 'disincentives' on the availability of primary care. I do believe, however, that more time should be spent in trying to educate patients on the sensible use of a health service and away from the completely unreal and unrealistic expectations of 'instant cure' and a treatment for every 'dis-ease' and unhappiness.

Many primary care physicians are guilty of over-prescribing, over-investigation and over-treatment and the general public have been instilled with an almost 'blind faith' in the power and success of modern medicine. But it would be misleading to think that this is only a twentieth-century phenomena for

> a belief in medicine is a cultural myth we all share. Physicians have been honoured, respected and rewarded in almost all societies throughout history. Human society has always displayed a willingness to devote a large share of its resources to the service of beliefs that are based solely on an unshakeable faith. In modern society, medical services would seem to fall into this category. (Saward, 1977)

What *is* different, though, as we come to the last quarter of the twentieth century, is the sheer enormity of the expenditure of most developed societies, who are hypnotised by sophisticated medical and surgical technology involving high costs in money and manpower so that

> the vastly expensive hospital dominates. Gradually the demands of all types of intensive care, soak up staff and money to push other aspects of hospital work into the background. . . . Those who see that the most complicated techniques needed to save some lives will detract from the services required for the more numerous sick and disabled, should not be accused of assessing life in terms of money. They are only stating the facts. Moreover, the individual doctor may be so personally involved in the drama of his work that he is oblivious to the inordinate amount of nursing or laboratory time that makes his project possible. The more mundane aspects of personal medical care must be accorded equal status with the excitements of technical advance. Otherwise, it is the patient who gets left behind in the scientific rush. (JRCP, 1974)

As a consequence, health costs are rising steeply and the law of diminishing returns is regrettably a reality in many levels of medical care. As Dr Mahler, Director of WHO has said – 'The major and most expensive part of medical knowledge as applied today appears to be more for the satisfaction of the health professions than for the benefit of the consumers of health care. Priority must be given to the proven and effective form of medical care, to the common conditions which directly affect people and, finally, every effort should be made to bring that care within the reach of all.'

Relationship between spending and health

Since 1947 economists and politicians have been pointing out that there is no guarantee of improving a nation's health merely by increasing the allocation of money. In fact there is no statistical or proven correlation between health spending and the health of a nation as judged by the usual indices of maternal, neonatal, infant and general mortality rates. The Federal Republic of Germany, with a much higher standard of living, spends a greater percentage of its GNP on health than the UK (pp. 32, 86), and yet the UK comes much higher in the international health league tables (p. 58). Unless money is channelled in the right direction such anomalies will continue.

The major cost of any health service – both in money and manpower – is the hospital: this, of course, is inevitable. But if it is true that

between 80 and 90 per cent of all patient contacts can be seen, diagnosed and treated in the primary care situation, then it is surely a
mistake that the percentage spent on primary care is steadily decreasing in all developed countries. Over the last decade the actual decline
in the number of general practitioners seems to have been halted in
Western Europe, Scandinavia, Australia, New Zealand and North
America. But hospitals continue to swallow up an increasing proportion of young doctors and, as yet, primary care has not benefited
from the increasing output of medical schools. Clearly both these
continuing trends are a serious threat to the rational use of resources.
In 1976/7, Finland was the only country in the developed world which
was planning to increase the proportion of money and manpower
directed into primary care (p. 131).

What factors are responsible for the misuse of both financial and
manpower resources? The main culpability lies with the medical profession, which is basically responsible for advising and influencing the
actions of governments and opinions of patients. Until there is a radical
change in the training of doctors, particularly in undergraduate education, and in the attitudes of doctors involved in teaching, the present
dominance of hospital-orientated thinking will prevail. Sweden,
where 60 per cent of all patient contacts take place in hospitals, is a
salutary reminder of what can happen in these circumstances. It is
certainly not easy to alter the attitude of medical schools and universities, particularly when such change in the *status quo* will endanger
their élitism. This reluctance affects even the socialist countries of
Eastern Europe and the USSR, where there are rumblings of discontent amongst those who are working as primary care physicians.

Medical education

What is a good medical education? This is too vast a subject to
be considered here, and it must be stated immediately that there is no
'best buy' medical education, just as there is no 'best buy' health
service. Each country has its own particular requirements, influenced
and moulded by its past history and present social and economic
structure. But one error has been made which is common to all countries: no medical school appears to understand or considers itself
responsible for meeting the needs of the health service it is supply-
ing with doctors. Throughout the developed world the medical profession with its absolute insistence on educational freedom, has ignored

its responsibilities to society by producing too many doctors who are educated and trained to work in hospital.

Therefore, at the present time, specialist medicine maintains its stranglehold on education with a number of predictable consequences. The training received by most doctors is largely unsuited to the needs of first-contact care, where patients present with a mass of uncategorised symptoms and complaints. Students are increasingly taught by a multiplicity of super-specialists whose interests and horizons seldom extend beyond the sphere of their own specialty. There is a concentration on disease rather than on people and their problems. The epidemiology and spectrum of illness is inevitably distorted so that the day-to-day problems of primary care are a surprise to the newly qualified doctor. Impotence and frustration quickly follow – even a feeling of insecurity – and he immediately returns to the safety of the hospital and an environment he can understand.

It is easy to criticise the competence and standards of those working in primary care, particularly from the academic atmosphere of a teaching hospital where most doctors have no experience of general practice and are usually unaware of its particular problems. Is it, therefore, surprising that teachers and students alike believe that general practice is a second-class career carried out by second-class doctors. The increasing trend towards specialisation has enhanced the image and importance of hospital medicine *vis-à-vis* general practice. This has led to what can only be called a crisis of identity affecting both doctor and patient. Why are patients so ambivalent in their attitudes to general practice? In a number of countries I have found that, when patients have realised that I am a general practitioner, they have said, 'Oh, how we need more of your sort here'. And yet, on further questioning, it was obvious that should they have backache, they would want to consult an orthopaedic surgeon, eczema required a dermatologist, angina a cardiologist, a headache a neurologist and emotional disorders unquestionably a psychiatrist. If this is the attitude of patients, then it should be no surprise that general practitioners are steadily disappearing. During the last twenty-five years, through the medium of the press, television and wireless, the general public, and even doctors, have been persuaded that almost any illness, certainly those of clinical interest, can only be investigated and treated with the newest and most sophisticated equipment, which in turn requires specialist and hospital treatment. This lack of confidence in the general practitioner is most noticeable in Sweden, the USA and the large urban areas of most industrialised countries. Surprisingly, in Eastern Europe and the USSR, where there is at least a theoretical emphasis on primary care, the status of the primary care physician is also low compared with his specialist colleagues.

The majority of primary care physicians accept that there is a need for change in undergraduate education, and a need to promote vocational training and continuing education if primary care is to expand and flourish. Academic respectability is provided by departments of general practice in many countries – Canada, Denmark, Finland, the Republic of Ireland, the Netherlands, Norway, the UK and the USA. Vocational training is being organised with specially selected 'trainer general practitioners' or 'training practices' and continuing education is made relatively easy by well-organised clinical meetings, lectures and extended courses. But a number of disturbing trends are beginning to appear.

First, almost certainly as a reaction against the traditional disease-orientated medical education, many of the leaders in the newly formed university departments of general practice – particularly in Western Europe – have become almost exclusive followers of the sociological/behavioural/psycho-sexual view of medicine. Such a limited perspective is, of course, as distorted as the more traditional one from which they are trying to rescue general practice, and it is hoped that moderation and common sense will soon prevail.

Second, a conflict is developing between university departments of general practice and teaching practices on the one hand, and 'ordinary' general practitioners on the other, who feel that academic general practice is divorced from the pressures and realities of everyday life. This is inevitable with a heavy teaching commitment, but in addition their position has not been helped by the fact that a number of departments have become tainted with one of the modern status symbols of academic medicine – increasing attendances at meetings and conferences, both nationally and internationally. Such activities, until recently, have rarely been questioned, but there is little evidence to suggest that they are of much value. 'All sections of a medical school are involved in the conference game and amongst the newest and most enthusiastic members seem to be those from general practice and the behavioural sciences.' (*Hospital Update*, 1976)

Third, there is a danger that some general practitioners may become so imbued with the undoubted merits, interest and satisfaction of education for its own sake that they forget their *raison d'être* and ultimately form a self-perpetuating group of like-minded enthusiasts. Educators should always remember the basic requirements of primary care – availability, accessibility and continuity – otherwise the criticisms so often levelled against hospital medicine of merely satisfying the intellectual curiosity of doctors and forgetting the needs of patients, may soon apply equally to general practice. However well educated a doctor may be, however well he may understand the nuances of the doctor/patient relationship, however well attuned he is to the psycho-dynamics of illness, such qualifications are irrelevant to the patient if the doctor is unavailable or inaccessible. Teachers must teach by example. It is salutary to remember that there is no evidence from any part of the world that patients associate this increase in education and knowledge with a better service: in fact the reverse appears to be the case with increasing dissatisfaction about the inability to find a doctor, about deputising services, and the general level of care.

The need for organisation and planning

No health service functions efficiently or serves the needs of people effectively unless it has a well-organised system of primary care. Value for money is best effected in this way and those countries with a basically sound system of general practice – Denmark, Finland, the Republic of Ireland, the Netherlands, New Zealand and the UK – provide a safe, uncomplicated and relatively easy point of access for the patient. Contrary to what many of its critics say, the UK does as well as any country in the field of primary care particularly in view of its relatively low level of spending on health (Table 1).

TABLE 1   *Health expenditure as percentage of GNP, 1971*

Australia	8.3	Sweden	8.3
Finland	7.7	UK	4.9
Italy	7.4	USA	.7.6

Source: *World Health Statistics Report*, vol. 27, No. 11, 1974. WHO Geneva

On the other hand, unless primary care has specific and identifiable objectives, its influence will diminish and other health personnel will take over its work. It must demonstrate that there are certain roles that it can fulfil more effectively and appropriately than the specialist and hospital service. It must show that its objectives are achievable and then must be seen to be carrying out this work. Patients who cannot find a primary care physician will quickly turn for help to the emergency room or private specialist – depending on their social and economic status.

The point of entry into any health service must be correct: the more specialised the care the further it should be from direct access by the patient (see Chapter 2). First-contact care which is organised through hospitals or specialists lacks continuity and the patient is subjected to an inappropriate and often costly form of medical care. Furthermore, it is an inefficient and wasteful use of specialist training and manpower. In addition, primary care must be backed up by well-organised secondary and tertiary hospital services if it is to function well. Ideally the relationship between the general practitioner and specialist should be one of cooperation, not antagonism and competition. It is difficult to envisage an improvement in this direction in those countries which continue to use specialists as primary care physicians.

There are two main difficulties in relation to planning for primary care:

First, there is a basic lack of information and data: why are consultation rates so high in some countries, for instance Japan? What are the differences in patterns of work? Are morbidity statistics accurate and, if so, do they give a valid guide to patient's requirements? What is the content of work and is it much the same in every country? How different are the expectations of patients in differing societies? How many nurses and ancillary staff are needed? What is the ideal number of doctors and why is the figure so different between neighbouring countries : the Federal Republic of Germany (17.8 per 10 000 population in 1971), Italy (18.4), the Netherlands (13.2) and England and Wales (12.7)? Why is 2500 considered to be the ideal number of patients per general practitioner in the UK – why not 1500 or 3500? In every country such figures have been decided arbitrarily and have now become part of the 'folk-lore' of medical planning. Even in the USSR, where planning has always been a central feature of the health service, it is difficult to decide how many doctors are really required. Data concerning some of these questions have been collected by the WHO International Collaborative Study of Medical Care Utilization (Kohn & Kerr, 1976). This was concerned with twelve study areas involving seven countries in North and South America and Europe during a twelve-month period 1968–9. It is an excellent beginning but is unable to provide any firm conclusions on the relationship between needs and resources: it is to be hoped that the WHO will commission and stimulate further international investigations.

Second, as long as doctors working in primary care are largely independent and responsible only to individual patients, planning will remain a dream. Doctors wrongly equate planning with loss of clinical freedom and the imposition of a third party between themselves and their patients. In fact, it should create opportunities for a more rational organisation of their work which, in turn, should improve patient care.

Who should do the planning? If it is left to the medical profession, then the hospital service and the new, complicated, often dramatic investigation or treatment will be given priority, even though its efficacy is unproved. High technology is supported by the universities, medical schools and the medical establishments throughout the world. If it is left to the planners, then the danger of slow, inflexible bureaucratic decisions is very real. Plans which are administratively tidy usually please planners but rarely satisfy either the patients or the doctors. Arbitrary decisions by governments without reference to the people actually working 'at ground level' quickly demoralise any health service. If it is left to the patient the result is likely to be confused. Most patients are totally ignorant about what is feasible or desirable in matters of health policy. Equally, patients have their own vested interests and they are likely to support anything which may help to solve the particular problem facing their own family or one of their friends even if it is a minority issue. Patients, planners and members of the health professions must all be involved. To quote Dr Candau, a past Secretary-General of the WHO, 'We must have the courage and the skill to go to the consumer and put questions to him as to his needs and problems, and we must find out what are the conditions or factors that determine possible solutions.' It is the responsibility of doctors, and particularly general practitioners, to educate patients and planners about what is and is not possible with the resources available – clearly everyone cannot have everything and decisions must be made not to do certain things. It is the responsibility of the patients to tell the physicians (and other health professionals) and planners how satisfied they are with the service and where deficiencies lie.

In 1973, Sir Keith Joseph (then Minister of State for Health and Social Security in the UK) challenged the general public, and more particularly the medical profession when he said

> No-one can see better than doctors the needs of the patients and the shortcomings of the National Health Service, but they are not doing enough about it. I am not aware that there has been any steady, powerful informed medical pressure to remedy the really worst shortcomings. Nor am I aware that doctors have always responded to known needs by putting their own house in order. Medical leadership, sustained, synoptic, prepared to agree priorities in tackling the improvements of service to the public, has not been conspicuous. It often seems as if the National Health Service and the medical profession as a whole, are indifferent to the miseries they should be seeking to relieve. There has been, and is, too little money available, but there is no excuse for the sustained medical and lay indifference. (Joseph, 1973)

Sharp words indeed, but they apply to every country under consideration in this book.

The use of resources

Planning leads directly to the question of how available resources should be used. The 'inverse care law' (Hart, 1971) gives an objective and valuable insight into some of the reasons for the poor allocation of resources even in a state-organised national health service. The major problem facing all developed countries (with the possible exception of Eastern Europe and the USSR) in relation to primary care, is the difficulty in providing an adequate service in the centres of large cities. It is here that the maximum effort should be directed to overcome the almost insuperable problems of poverty, poor housing, underprivileged groups of workers and their families, increasing mobility of patients with the destruction of family life and its disastrous effect on the doctor/patient relationship, inadequate premises which are impossible to rebuild or replace because of the high cost of land and building, and finally the general lack of incentives for doctors, nurses and social workers to live and work under those conditions. How can this threat to urban medical care be solved? No country has the answer and only those governments which first tackle the evils of urban deprivation with energy, can hope for any success. Following this initiative it will be necessary to inject money to improve facilities and to provide incentives to try to persuade doctors to work in such areas. But, in my opinion, such incentives are unlikely to succeed and the outlook is gloomy, particularly in those countries where the general practitioner is totally independent and responsible to no-one but himself. By the end of the twentieth century, there is a real possibility that the standard of primary care in large urban areas will have deteriorated to such an extent that the emergency room of the local hospital will be the only provider of care.

In addition, it would seem that primary care is about to make the same mistake – at least in principle – as the specialist service has done in the past. Here, new expensive investigations and treatments have been introduced and have then become accepted as a necessary part of medical care without their efficacy and value having been decided. During the last few years screening has been established as a desirable objective, in the belief that early diagnosis will lead to more effective treatment with a reduction in morbidity and mortality. There is, therefore, a danger that it may become one of the accepted procedures of modern general practice without adequate evaluation in terms of clinical success and cost-effectiveness. Screening for a number of diseases – hypertension, diabetes mellitus, anaemia, urinary tract infections, obesity, depression, cancer of the breast and cervix – and for different groups of patients – babies and young children, the middle-aged (or the 'worried-well' as the Americans so aptly describe them) and elderly – should not be introduced on a wide scale until the usefulness of each procedure is firmly established, otherwise it could lead to the most extravagant waste of manpower and money. Unfortunately, the USSR which, through its 'dispenserisation scheme' (p. 171) has collected more information on screening than any other country, is unable or unwilling to provide the necessary evidence about its value. Rigorous and critical analysis of all screening programmes must be carried out to prevent their premature introduction, and to decide whether they are a necessity or a highly expensive luxury.

Requirements for sound primary care

An ideal system of primary care does not exist. Each country must decide its own organisation, taking into account such variables as population densities, the degree of urbanisation and the sophistication of transport facilities. But certain features are mandatory if there is to be any credence in its continuing existence.

First, without accessibility and availability, patients are only able to use the emergency room of the local hospital or the services of private medicine. This situation is clearly seen in Sweden, in the urban areas of Finland and Norway, in Japan and the USA, where routine consultations take place this way.

Second, continuity of care, a much valued ideal, is surely the essence of sound general practice: at least that is the view in those countries with a long tradition in this field – Denmark, the Republic of Ireland, the Netherlands, New Zealand and the UK. The value of continuity to the doctor and patient is the building of a relationship which facilitates ease of communication and gradually establishes empathy between them. The advantage to the doctor of knowing the history, the family and social background of the patient is obvious. To know that he will, as far as possible, always see the same doctor (provided there is choice and the ability to change if desired), gives the patient a security and reassurance which grows with each consultation. Many doctors will disagree with this view and maintain that episodic interviews make no difference to the success of patient management. I would suggest that anyone who makes such a claim has never been closely involved in continuity of care: indeed I believe that those systems which discourage or make continuity almost impossible are imposing serious disadvantages both on the patient and the doctor as well as increasing costs by the inevitable reduplication of investigations. Of course there are other obstacles, mainly arising from the increasing mobility of patients and doctors, and from the formation of group or health centre practice, where patients are encouraged to see any doctor in the group: this is unfortunately the situation in many parts of the UK. I have found in talking to patients, in places as far afield as Tokyo and Alta in Arctic Norway, Prague and Charleston, South Carolina, Ornsköldsvik in Sweden and Irkutsk in Eastern Siberia, that one of the things they want from any health service is a 'personal' doctor who will care for the whole family.

The following points, although by no means an absolute requirement, are ingredients of primary care which allow it to function more effectively. Adequate facilities for examination, investigation and treatment should be available. It is not always easy to strike the correct balance between under-investment in radiological and physiotherapy facilities, as in the Republic of Ireland and the UK, which leads to long waiting-times for patients and often unnecessary referrals to specialists, or over-investment, as in the Federal Republic of Germany, Japan and the USA, which leads to unnecessary over-investigation as being the only means whereby the practitioner can recoup his capital expenditure within a reasonable time. Perhaps Canada, Denmark, Finland and Sweden, Eastern Europe and the USSR have found a satisfactory balance.

Gradually it is being accepted that teamwork between nurses, health visitors, midwives, social workers, receptionists and doctors is necessary for a comprehensive primary care service. Each member of the team has differing professional skills which are often necessary for the total care of patients in the community. Each worker must define his or her role and then carry out his appropriate tasks. There are obstacles to the team approach. First, doctors may believe that, in fact, it leads to a lowering of standards because inevitably it changes the doctor/patient relationship (France, 79) and furthermore it is claimed that the majority of patients do not relish such a change as it diminishes the likelihood of personal care and raises a feeling of disquiet concerning confidentiality. The expectations of patients obviously vary from country to country but it has been shown in the UK that if patients are forewarned and educated about the changes that are likely to take place then, in general, they are pleased with the service they receive (DHSS, 1971). Group practices and health centres must always aim at personalised care which, in the past, has always characterised general practice at its best. The opponents of the this type of practice will relish the experience of a specialist in the UK who, on enquiring the name of a patient's doctor, was told 'Oh, we don't have a doctor, we only belong to a health centre' (McCormack, 1977). Second, if doctors are paid by item-of-service, as in Australia, Belgium, France, the Federal Republic of Germany, Japan and the USA, there is a definite financial disincentive for any form of cooperation.

The use of auxiliaries is a vexed question, but there is now sufficient evidence from Canada, Sweden, the UK, the USA and the USSR to show that they can be used without any drop in standards: 'In the developing world the insistence of the medical profession that only physicians can evaluate and treat the sick has had a paralysing effect on the design and implementation of health services and is one of the

most serious obstacles to the effective use of limited health resources.'
(Bryant, 1969) This attitude is also true of developed countries and it is
difficult to see any rapid changes in this direction: perhaps economic
difficulties will eventually force the issue.

The arguments for and against home visiting by doctors are well
known. There is no statistical evidence that the virtual abolition of
home visits in Finland and Sweden has done any harm, especially
when it is acknowledged that these two countries have the very best
health statistics in the world. The evidence is subjective and defies
statistical analysis; it is concerned more with caring than curing, more
with the patient than the disease. To refuse a home visit in certain
categories of illness or in some circumstances to the very young or the
elderly, affects the quality of care. I have accompanied primary care
physicians on home visits in very differing parts of the world – a small
fishing village on the Izu peninsula in Japan; a collective farm in
Armenia; the residential areas of Sofia and Budapest; the Arctic fjords
of Northern Norway; and a country town in New York State – and
without exception such visits were greatly appreciated by the patient
even if in strictly medical terms they might have been considered
unnecessary by many physicians; particularly in countries in which
home visits are a rarity, one of the things most requested by patients is
the assurance that a doctor will visit their sick child or elderly relative
should it be necessary. Without doubt the willingness of general practitioners to do home visits is prized very highly by patients – and will
often obscure the more obvious defects in a doctor's training or pattern
of work. Visiting has now been reduced in most countries to the
absolute minimum and general practitioners would be foolish to
reduce this any further and run the risk of alienating their patients
even more.

Another cause of the growing, universal dissatisfaction with
primary care services is the generally poor quality of 'out of hours'
services. The use that is made of them is related to a number of factors.
First, if the availability, accessibility and general standard of primary
care during normal working hours is poor or inadequate, then work
collects for the emergency service; in other words, the number of
out-of-hours and night calls is often a direct reflection on the general
standard of day-to-day care. The introduction of the shorter working
day in countries such as Finland and Sweden has produced an apparent shortage of doctors so that it is impossible to organise a satisfactory

08.0–16.00 hours service: at the present time there is often a waiting time of anything between one and four weeks to see a doctor – inevitably in these circumstances there is a 'spill over' of routine work onto the emergency service. Similar situations exist in the USA, particularly in the large urban areas where no-one is responsible for anyone, or in the 'lock-up' type practices and, increasingly, in partnership and group practices in a number of cities in the UK, and in Denmark, where the emergency service is now accepted as an alternative and continuing system of primary care. As a result, the patient must rely on either the hospital emergency room, or emergency services of differing degrees of efficiency and acceptability. A wide variation in the organisation of 'out-of-hours' care exists. In the USSR (and in Copenhagen) there is a completely separate, highly efficient and well-organised emergency service in all large cities; in Denmark, the Netherlands, Norway and the UK, deputising services are springing up though, unfortunately, not staffed by doctors experienced in general practice; in Australia, Canada, Sweden and the USA, many patients have only the emergency room at the local hospital. Each of these systems bring their own problems, and probably the best compromise, both for patient and doctor, is a rota system between a limited number of doctors which provides extended cover by the personnel who are responsible for the ordinary day-to-day care. By this method some continuity of care is provided and experienced general practitioners are doing the work with quite obvious advantages. In fact this system is widely used in Canada, France, the Federal Republic of Germany, the Republic of Ireland, the Netherlands, rural areas of Norway, New Zealand, in 'small town' practices in the USA and in some parts, particularly rural areas, of the UK.

Each country must decide what it wants. If it is decided that doctors should work fixed seven- to eight-hour shifts, as in Eastern Europe, Finland, Sweden and the USSR, then the Soviet system would seem to be the best, provided there are sufficient personnel. If, on the other hand, society would like general practitioners to be responsible and provide cover which involves long hours of 'on call' duty, then there must be some incentive for the doctor and a recognition by society that his service is really valued.

Generalist or specialist?

The importance of the family for the health and happiness of present and future generations can scarcely be exaggerated. Healthy families make healthy people. The child's relationship with the family foreshadows his relationship in society. Yet in many parts of the world today the medical establishments, obsessed as they are with a concern for marginal disease, are doing far from enough to provide health care for the family. (Mahler, 1975)

Health has its roots in the family which is now subjected to many pressures: both parents may go out to work; there is a lack of support from grandparents and other relatives which was so often a feature of the extended family; a feeling of isolation and insecurity associated with the self-imposed pressures of a materialistic secular society is all pervasive.

What type of doctor is best suited for primary care and for looking after the family – a generalist or specialist?

> Most people live in small family units. Almost everybody is born into and grows up in a family which largely conditions them in the physical, psychological and social spheres of their later life. The family has a great impact on the health of its members and a general practitioner is in a position to note the constant interaction between individual illness and the family. He also knows from experience that illness is not spread at random over his practice population but seems to be concentrated not only in certain individuals, but even more in certain families who seem to pass on ill-health. (Huygen, 1976)

In my view one of the crying needs in medicine is for there to be one person, often a physician, to whom a family can turn. Such a physician is able to provide some continuity and stability in their troubled lives; he should be able to investigate, diagnose and treat the majority of illness that is brought to him, and he should be in a position to carry out simple preventive measures and give straightforward health education. Such a physician can exist only if he has been trained adequately and appropriately, if he works in a reasonably organised health care system, if he is paid in a way which will allow him to act beyond the restricted confines of curative medicine, and if he has the support, not competition, of his specialist colleagues. I believe that a generalist is more likely to succeed in this role for reasons which have already been discussed (Chapter 2, p. 18). Furthermore, I think that the generalist should act as a family doctor: a concept which is out of fashion at the present time, though it might help to resolve the dilemma felt by many doctors – the need to care for the individual as well as the need to care for the whole community. If the idea of a family doctor could be re-introduced, it might form a basis of compromise between two apparently irreconcilable positions: the individual and the community.

The general practitioner and the hospital

The relationship between the general practitioner (or primary care physician) and the hospital service is extremely varied and is seldom the result of organised planning: rather it has developed in a haphazard manner for historical and geographical reasons. The acceptance or rejection of general practitioners working in hospitals depends largely on custom and traditions which in turn are reflected in the expectations of both patients and physicians.

Those countries which involve their general practitioners in the care of 'hospital patients' can be divided into two main groups. First, in Australia, Canada, Japan and the USA practically all primary care physicians (including general practitoners) have hospital privileges alongside their specialist colleagues and many general practitioners are still involved in active surgery up to an intermediate level; cholecystectomy, gastrectomy, hysterectomy. Obstetric care in hospital, particularly in the USA, is an accepted part of everyday life for rural and some urban general practitioners. In Canada and the USA, every doctor must submit an application for 'hospital admitting rights' which is scrutinised by the appropriate department, while in Australia and Japan there is no such attempt at medical audit.

In the second group the extent of clinical involvement is much less and is restricted to medical and sometimes normal obstetric care; it is rare for even minor surgery to be undertaken. The hospitals are much smaller – averaging between 40 and 50 beds – and are staffed exclusively by general practitioners; specialist involvement being only in an advisory and visiting capacity. Because of the geographical situation of these hospitals, there is no question of applying for 'admitting privileges', as the only physicians who can staff them are the local general practitioners (or primary care physicians in the USSR). In Finland, France and Norway such hospitals are predominantly in rural areas and are increasingly concerned with the care of the elderly, although in very remote parts of Finland emergency and routine minor surgery (hernias, varicose veins, haemorrhoids) is carried out. In the UK, 'cottage' or general practitioner hospitals are the result of historical accident and largely grew up at the end of the nineteenth and beginning of the twentieth century, through the initiative and foresight of local communities. There are 400 scattered throughout England and Wales. They continue to flourish and are staffed by general practitioners with specialists acting in an advisory capacity as well as holding out-patient clinics and carrying out operating sessions. In addition, general practitioners play a very limited role, in the staffing of district general hospitals by acting as 'clinical assistants' to specialist colleagues in a number of different departments – medicine, rheumatology, dermatology, geriatrics, paediatrics, anaesthetics and obstetrics. Their clinical responsibility is limited and they are under the supervision of the appropriate specialist. Theoretically the intention of such posts is to re-integrate the general practitioner into the hospital service and also to act as an 'educational aide' in any particular branch of medicine which is of particular interest to him. In fact it is now felt by many doctors that such attachments are merely a means of filling a number of hospital posts which would otherwise, almost certainly, remain empty. In the Republic of Ireland, local district hospitals are now mainly concerned with chronic, long-stay geriatric care. 'Clinical assistantships' are also a part of the hospital service and, as in the UK, general practitioners believe that they are employed merely to prop up an ailing hospital service. The rural hospital in the USSR is the key to the whole rural health service and combines the function of a polyclinic (out-patient facilities) with in-patient care. It is staffed by primary care physicians (*uchastock* therapist, paediatrician and gynaecologist with sometimes a dentist and surgeon/radiologist) and has a noticeably high bed-per-population ratio compared with all other developed countries. Because of this, many patients are unnecessarily admitted for comparatively minor reasons as it is the easiest way (at least for the doctor) to care for them.

What is there to learn from these differing methods of organisation and work? First, it is impossible to be dogmatic since the relationship between specialist and primary care physicians differs so markedly in each country. This relationship often mirrors the traditions of medicine and the expectations of society and is related to the conservative nature of the profession, the rivalry between specialist and general practitioner, the method of payment of doctors, and the indoctrination of society over the last 25 years that many illnesses now need ever-increasing levels of expertise in diagnosis and treatment which can only be provided by a specialist. It is obvious that such misconceptions and obstacles are a serious impediment to a rational solution of this problem. But progress is being made in some countries. In the UK, cooperation and understanding between the Royal College of Physicians and the Royal College of General Practitioners are growing. In October 1976, a general practitioner was invited by the Royal College of Physicians of London to reply to an address which had been given by the President of the Royal College of Physicians at the previous Spring Meeting of the Royal College of General Practitioners. In this thoughtful paper the reasons for the doubts and antipathy between specialist and general practitioner are given; the complementary nature of their roles in patient care are described; and finally an ideal new relationship between hospital physician and family doctor is put forward and the essential conditions for the realisation of this relationship are outlined (Horder, 1977).

Second, if there is to be any planning for the future, two questions must be asked and answered within the context of each country's health care system. What is the function of the hospital in the overall strategy of patient care? For instance, is it reasonable that the overemphasis on hospital care in the USA and the USSR (for entirely different reasons) results in many patients being needlessly admitted to hospital? Is it economic or medical sense that patients with uncomplicated illness should be admitted to hospitals where all the latest techniques for diagnosis and treatment are available? Having decided such questions, it is then necessary to ask – is there any place for the primary care physician in the hospital? In those countries which have excluded him entirely from hospital work, has there been any advantage for the patient? If it is decided to give general practitioners full clinical responsibility for the patients in hospital, then they must be able to provide care superior or at least equal to that of their specialist colleagues and must resist work which is beyond their competence. Working in hospital should be an extension of the routine work in the consulting room or patient's home and should never become an obstacle to their basic function of providing first-contact care. Clearly, in many countries, the conflicting demands of practice and partnership, to say nothing of the distance and the time involved, may put hospital work, however desirable or deserved, beyond the reach of many conscientious general practitioners (*Practitioner*, 1973).

Registration of patients

Formal registration of patients by law or by agreement with health insurance agencies only occurs in Eastern Europe, the USSR, the Republic of Ireland (the full eligibility group representing 37 per cent of the population), the UK, Denmark (Class A patients representing 90 per cent) and the Netherlands (Zkw representing 70 per cent). In Denmark, patients must register with one doctor for at least one year, while in Ireland, the Netherlands and the UK, there is no time limit, so the arrangement can be terminated by patients or doctors at any time. In Eastern Europe and the USSR, under exceptional circumstances, it is also possible for patients to change their *uchastock* doctor, but it is not encouraged and formal application must be made to the chief doctor of the local polyclinic.

There is considerable opposition to registration by the medical profession, perhaps typified most eloquently by the 'liberal tradition of medicine' in France, where it is seen as an infringement of the rights of both patient and doctor, a curtailment of clinical freedom and an inevitable step towards total government control with a consequent lowering of standards and massive bureaucratic involvement.

How justified are these fears? Certainly registration in Denmark, the Republic of Ireland, the Netherlands and the UK has not produced a loss of clinical freedom nor has it produced any outcry from patients, even in Denmark where they must remain with the same doctor for a year. The claustrophobic and demoralising effect of bureaucracy and government control which is felt by some doctors in the UK is in no way related to registration and is an entirely separate issue.

What are the benefits of registration? It can prevent the chaotic and wasteful use of medical resources when patients 'shop around' from one doctor to another and it also encourages continuity of care. From the patient's point of view he has a doctor with whom he can immediately identify and, in addition, he has the safeguard that the doctor is not only morally but also legally responsible for him. Patient's records can be kept more easily and in the UK they are automatically transferred from one doctor to the next whenever the patient moves from one area to another or changes his doctor. This is a tremendous asset, particularly for the doctor, who then has a complete record of the patient's past investigations and treatment. Without registration, it is difficult to carry out any effective research into the requirements, needs and problems of primary care. From personal experience I know of no cogent reason against registration and, on balance, I believe that it should be seriously considered by governments and insurance agencies as a simple means of rationalising and improving primary care.

Methods of payment of doctors

There is quite obviously no perfect way of paying doctors either in hospital or in general practice. If society is materialistic and greedy, without ideals and ethical values, then medicine will reflect these values whatever method of payment is used. But differing methods do affect primary care by encouraging or discouraging certain aspects of organisation and patterns of work.

The most widely adopted method is by item-of-service payment. Undoubtedly this is most popular with doctors for it ensures a high income even though most fees are negotiated by insurance agencies, governments and the profession. The more services a doctor performs, the more he earns. From a politician's and a patient's point of view, this should be a cause for concern as it is, in effect, an open-ended contract in favour of the doctor. He alone decides how many investigations should be carried out and how often treatment should be given, which inevitably leads to an uncontrolled rise in health costs. In Australia, Belgium, Canada, France, the Federal Republic of Germany, Italy, Japan and the USA the item-of-service payment is heavily weighted in favour of technical and therapeutic medicine, and insurance agencies must share some of the blame for this situation. Thoughts of teamwork with nurses, health visitors, midwives and social workers, and even cooperation between doctors, is alien to the philosophy of medical care in these countries, and some responsibility for this must lie with this method of remuneration. Lastly, maldistribution of manpower can never be solved as long as it is possible for doctors to earn a satisfactory living in overdoctored areas by involving their patients in overinvestigation and unnecessary treatment. On the other hand, patients are not subjected to the same waiting time for radiological investigation as in the Republic of Ireland, Norway and the UK. One of the biggest complaints from Japanese patients living in the UK, and using the National Health Service, is the long waiting time for contrast media radiography and for non-urgent routine hospital admission (Maeda, 1972).

Capitation fees are used as the method of payment in Denmark

(Copenhagen only), the Netherlands (70 per cent), Italy (50 per cent) and the UK. One of the problems of this system is the encouragement it gives the doctor to look after too many patients; this can be rectified either through the government or insurance agency by limiting the number of patients for which the doctor is paid. As well as looking after too many patients, the criticism is also levelled that doctors do as little as possible for their patients by referring an unnecessarily large number to specialists or the hospital service on the slightest pretext. Certainly this was and possibly may still be the situation in the UK. Likewise there was little financial encouragement in the UK to provide a good service until 1966, when a 70 per cent reimbursement scheme for receptionists', secretaries' and nurses' salaries was introduced (p. 37): until that time, the less the doctor or group of doctors spent on practice expenses, the larger was their actual income. Capitation payment penalises a doctor who has a large number of elderly patients on his list. They are likely to require much more care and attention than the younger age groups and this anomaly has been rectified in the UK by increasing the capitation fee for the 65–75 and 75-and-over age groups. Maldistribution of general practitioners is much less likely to happen with capitation payment than with an item-of-service payment while the capitation method associated with registration of patients creates the right atmosphere for encouraging continuity of care.

Payment by salary is the method favoured by all countries of Eastern Europe, the USSR, Finland and Sweden. In Norway, a part of the district doctor's income is also paid in this way. To the majority of the medical profession this symbolises the dead hand of state intervention and control with the added danger of political conformity. This particular fear is no greater in Sweden than in Japan – what, of course, matters is the general political freedom enjoyed by society at large, and this is in no way associated with payment by salary.

A salary, like the capitation fee, may encourage laziness just as the item-of-service may stimulate greediness. The rate of work in Eastern Europe, the USSR, Finland and Sweden is slow compared with other countries that I visited. This is compensated for in Eastern Europe and the USSR by the highest doctor/patient ratio in the world (except Israel) and they are thus able to cope not only with a slow work rate but also with a 6–7-hour shift system. In Finland and Sweden, however, the health authorities do not have this extra manpower and by introducing office hours in the early 1970s, they have created a relative and spurious shortage of doctors. Consequently, long waiting times to see primary care physicians are now commonplace so that for a long time to come the private sector will flourish, and the emergency departments of hospitals will be overwhelmed because the salaried service has proved unresponsive to the needs of the situation. If a colleague is ill, on holiday or on study leave, there is no increase in work rate by the remaining doctors, and, in discussion, I found that few doctors saw any reason to respond in such a manner as there is no incentive to do so; in short, the salaried service is proving counter-productive. Finally, the salary may be unacceptably low and this is a real fear. What can be done in such circumstances? In a free society, resignation, followed by emigration or entry into private practice, is the only solution, and this bogey is held up as the final warning for anyone who supports this method of payment. But, on the credit side, with a salary it is possible to recognise experience, special training and responsibility, whereas with the other methods this is rather difficult.

There is no perfect arrangement, but a system which incorporates some means of control on the doctor either by a health insurance agency or the government (capitation or salary) and also provides some incentive for hard work, item-of-service payment is probably the best combination for the providers and recipients of health care. In my view the closest to this ideal is the payment of the district medical officer in Norway.

Monitoring, evaluation and audit

The idea of medical audit is most attractive, certainly to the patient who hopes that he will receive a better service and standard of care, and to governments and insurance organisations who hope they will get better value for money. The problem is whether this idea can be translated into a workable reality.

Peer review has been practised in Canada and the USA for a number of years, and in the USA this activity has been federally organised by Professional Standard Review Organisation who are responsible for monitoring diagnosis, treatment, cost-effectiveness and workload in hospitals although not, as yet, in primary care. Limitation of admitting privileges, depending on experience and training, are also imposed on all doctors, particularly in relation to surgical procedures. Their colleagues decide what they can and cannot do: compare this with

Australia and Japan where there is almost no control on what a doctor may attempt. But is there any evidence that the quality of care is different in these countries?

Can a similar system be used in primary care? The evaluation of such activities as prescribing habits, requests for investigation, the quality of clinical records, and hospital referral letters would almost certainly improve the standard of care. The effectiveness of diagnosis and treatment, the cost to the patient, insurance company or the state, the level of patient satisfaction as well as the value of sympathetic patient management, warrant close scrutiny. But who should do the evaluation and how should it be organised? Would it be cost-effective or would it produce its own self-perpetuating and increasing bureaucracy? In the current situation, because so few conditions seen in general practice lend themselves to a definite diagnosis, it is highly unlikely that any accurate assessment of outcome can be measured. According to one practice in the UK, two-fifths of all attendances are undiagnosed and recover spontaneously (Thomas, 1975). Many doctors would say that this is a conservative figure and that an even higher proportion of illness remains undiagnosed. How, therefore, can audit be applied to this situation? Nobody can answer these questions with any certainty. New techniques for measuring clinical performance must be studied so that this aspect of primary care, which is only in its infancy, can be developed – initially on a national basis and then internationally.

Quality of care

Health care does not lend itself easily to objective measurement because in the light of present-day knowledge such measurements are usually only an indication of disease. Mortality rates are of no help in evaluating the quality of care as death is not the only consequence of disease, and it is possible to have a situation where the mortality rate may be low and yet there is still a high incidence of disease. In addition, international mortality rates are of limited value owing to differences in classification and nomenclature. Similarly, morbidity rates are imprecise and are too crude a guide. Clearly, quality of care is difficult to define and yet we all know when we have received it.

The quality and effectiveness of hospital care are marginally easier to measure than those of primary care. Clinical medicine has a clearly defined pathology, requiring routine examination and specific investigation in order to produce a diagnosis, followed by appropriate treatment to effect a cure or at least alleviate symptoms. In a sense there is a beginning and an end. The investigation and treatment can often be defined in scientific terms and measured qualitatively.

In primary care the situation is different. There is no baseline of accepted subject-matter nor is there any agreement about its nature. To some it is the summation of the basic knowledge of a number of clinical specialists, while to others it is almost exclusively concerned with the effects of social, psychological and emotional forces on interpersonal relationships and ultimately on disease. How, therefore, is it possible to measure the care provided by primary care physicians when there are no agreed guidelines to help? Most information is, at present, limited to consultation rates, workload, morbidity patterns, methods and scope of work, time allowed per consultation, the use of ancillary staff and the relevance of home visits. Interesting and important as this information may be, there is little evidence to suggest an absolute correlation between such factors and the quality of care. It is easy, although inaccurate, to equate efficiency with quality, although they are interdependent. Equally, the effectiveness and acceptability of the organisation of medical services by patients gives some indication of quality. Similarly the professional knowledge and technical expertise of the medical profession greatly affect quality and it is the responsibility of the profession to guarantee its own competence.

And yet, vital as all these factors are, aspects of care remain untouched. Why is it that in spite of all the improved planning and an increasing awareness of the problems of primary care, patients remain critical and dissatisfied? For too long governments and their advisers have failed to recognise, or ignored, these warning signs. In all the countries I visited there was only one consistent answer to my question 'What is your main criticism of general practice?' The answer: 'Some doctors don't care, don't listen, don't understand and aren't interested.' In that universal answer lies the essence of what we are trying to define. Why does the sense of vocation, which is so strong in many young doctors, so quickly disappear? Does the selection of students, or an inappropriate medical education, or the stimulation of unrealistic and unrealisable expectations play a part? Or is it merely a reflection of many societies which place so little value on, and even scorn, a sense of vocation? Motivation and dedication are qualities which should not be denigrated and, in fact, require urgent study.

At the present time the success of any health service is judged almost exclusively by its care of mothers and children and by the generally rising life expectancy, both for men and women. The monopoly of concern, both by individual countries, and international organisations such as the WHO, with such statistics, although appropriate for developing countries, has tended to obscure some of the more important problems facing the developed world which, in turn, are directly related to the quality of care. If, in fact, maternal and infant mortality rates were the main indicators of success, then there might be a strong argument for the abolition of primary care, or at least its assimilation into the hospital service, for no country in the world can boast better maternal, neonatal and infant mortality rates than Sweden. But, in reality, many Swedish people are becoming increasingly dissatisfied with their health service and its serious limitations brought about by the steady decline of general practice over the last twenty years.

Such health statistics are of course of limited value for two main reasons. First, they depend as much upon the general socio/economic status of a country as on the adequacy of its health service. Second, they do not measure the worldwide 'present-day disenchantment with physicians, which, at a time when they can do more than ever in history to halt and repair the ravages of serious illness, probably reflects the perception by people that they are not being cared for' (Eisenberg, 1977). Primary care has a leading role to play in responding to this need, and in the future must direct its attention towards the care of the chronic sick, the elderly and, most important of all, the management and terminal care of the dying, so that through such a renaissance the quality of care will be improved.

APPENDIX*

Dr Ayvin Aarflot, Director, Division of Local Health Services, Det. Kangelige Sosialdepatement, Postboks 80 111, Oslo 1, Norway.

Dr Juhani Aer, Assistant Chief, Department of Primary Care, National Board of Health, Siltasaarenkatu 18, 00 530 Helsinki, Finland.

Dr Peter Anjou, Hill Hospital, Lower Hill, New Zealand.

Dr Aoki, Prefecture Health Department, Osaka, Japan.

Associate Professor S. Asakura, Department of Public Health, University Medical School, Osaka, Japan.

Dr Ian Bailey, Consultant Physician, Southmead Hospital, Bristol, UK.

Miss E. M. Ball, Regional Officer, USSR/Eastern Europe Department, The British Council, 65 Davies Street, London W1Y 2AA.

Professor Hugo Behm, formerly Director, Department of Public Health, University of Santiago, Chile: imprisoned in 1974 and now believed to be living in Costa Rica.

Dr Niels Bentzen, J. B. Winsløwsvej 15, DK-5000 Odense, Denmark.

Mrs Irena Bochenska, Swigtokrzyska, 25, Krakow, Poland.

Professor Dr and Mrs R. B. Boelaert, Katholieke Universiteit te Leuven, Minderbroedersstraat 17, 3000 Leuven, Belgium.

Dr Lilian Bourilkova, Slavianska 5a, Sofia, Bulgaria.

Professor Neville Butler, Department of Child Health, University of Bristol, Bristol, UK.

Professor Chachava, General Hospital No. 2, Tbilisi, Republic of Georgia, USSR.

Dr Tomoo Cho, 8–11 Shoraiso, Nishinomiya, Japan.

Dr Alexandra Ciuca, Str. Aviator Papa Marin Nr. 3, Bucharest, Romania.

Dr H. A. Clegg, past Editor of the *British Medical Journal*, late International Relations Department, Royal Society of Medicine, 2 Queen Ann Street, London W1.

Dr Nicolai Constantinescu, Str. Bujoveni 23, Bucharest, Romania: he has now moved to the West and has eventually settled in the Netherlands.

Professor Hiram Curry, Department of Family Practice, Medical University of South Carolina, 80 Barre Street, Charleston, South Carolina 29140, USA.

* See Acknowledgements, p. xv.

Mr Davey, Scientific Counsellor, British Embassy, Havana, Cuba.

Dr Stevan Dilanian, Ministry of Health, Yerevan, Republic of Armenia, USSR.

Dr H. Dodo, Prefecture Health Department, Osaka, Japan.

Dr Florea Duna, Director, Ministere de la Sante et de la Prevoyance Sociale, 2 Lt. Lemnea, Bucharest, Romania.

Dr Eristavi, Protocol Department, External Relations, Ministry of Health, Moscow, USSR.

Dr and Mrs Armand J. D'Errico, 31 First Avenue, Gloversville, New York, USA.

Professor Eugene Farley, Jacob W. Hillier, Family Medicine Centre, 885 South Avenue, Rochester, NY 14620, USA.

Mr William Ferratti, Vice-President for Medical Affairs, Hunterdon Medical Centre, Flemington, New Jersey 08 822, USA.

Dr J. Fog, Sundhedsstyrelsen, 1 St Kongensgade, DK 1264, Copenhagen, Denmark.

Dr P. Fox, Department of Health Education and Welfare, Bethesda, Maryland, USA.

Dr Flemming Frølund, Laevkevej 14, 4000, Roskilde, Denmark.

Dr S. Gallie, 11 Küküllo, U8 1026 Budapest, Hungary.

Dr Sidney Garfield, Kaiser-Permanente Medical Care Programme, Oakland, California 94 612, USA.

Professor K. Gargov, Department of the Organisation of Health Services, Institute of Postgraduate Training, Sofia, Bulgaria.

Mr T. Garrett, Scientific Attaché, British Embassy, Moscow, USSR.

Dr and Mrs C. Gunnarson, Nygaton 12, 891 000 Ornsköldsvik, Sweden.

Dr Romnald Gutt, ul Lubertowieza 3a Bielsko Biala, Poland.

Dr Gustav Haglund, Health and Medical Care Centre, S-240 10, Dalby, Sweden.

Dr and Mrs Hamanaka, Minami-Izu Village, Shizuoka, Japan.

Dr Michael Hegarty, The Abbey, Rosscarberry, County Cork, Republic of Ireland.

Dr and Mrs Hillered, Kung Alles väg 2, 5161 41 Bromma, Sweden.

Dr Hirai, Higashisumiyoshitu, Japan.

Dr J. P. Horder, 98 Regents Park Road, London NW1, UK.

Professor Dr Sigurd Humerfelt, Instituutt for Almenmedisin, Ulriksdol 8C, 5000 Bergen, Norway.

Dr John Hunt, 82 Sloane Street, London SW1, UK.

Dr George Jbaltuadze, Head of Department of Preventive Medicine, Ministry of Health, Tbilisi, Republic of Georgia, USSR.

Mrs Anna Jones, Lep Travel, Bristol.

Dr Bogoslav Juricic, International Relations Department, Ministry of Health, Santiago, Chile.

Dr Emanuel de Kadt, The Institute of Development Studies, University of Sussex, Brighton BN1 9RE, UK.

Dr K. Kanada, Department of Public Health, University Medical School, Osaka, Japan.

Dr William Kane, Duke University Medical Centre, Durham, North Carolina 27 710, USA.

Dr K. Kimura, Department of Public Health, University Medical School, Osaka, Japan.

Dr B. M. Kleczkowski, Chief Medical Officer, Resource Group, Division of Strengthening of Health Services, WHO, 1211 Geneva 27, Switzerland.

Dr Jos Kohl, Ministère de la Societé Publique, 48 rue Auguste Lumière, Luxemburg.

Dr A. Kuzmanic, Luis Pasteur 6249 Carilla, 16 191 Santiago, Chile.

Dr Jan-Ivor Kvamme, Alta, Finmark, Norway.

Dr and Mrs J. Lincoln, 3828 – 49th Avenue North East, Seattle, Washington, 98 105, USA

Dr Valentina Nikolalvina Litvinova, Director of District Health Service (Rayon) Irkutsk, Eastern Siberia, USSR.

Associate Professor N. Maeda, National Institute of Public Health, Tokyo, Japan.

Dr Mahmudov, General and Paediatric Hospital No. 2, Tashkent, Republic of Uzbekistan, USSR.

Dr Mario Martinez, International Relations Department, Ministry of Health, Havana, Cuba.

Dr Orbi Mkhitarian, Ministry of Health, Yerevan, Republic of Armenia, USSR.

Dr and Mrs J. Moore, Route 2, Box 519, Chapel Hill, North Carolina 27 514, USA.

Dr Conor Morgan, Drimoleague, County Cork, Republic of Ireland.

Professor Muhamedov, Paediatric Research Institute, Tashkent, Republic of Uzbekistan, USSR.

Dr H. Nesterova, Chairman, Public Health Department, Odessa, Republic of the Ukraine, USSR.

Dr Finn Nilsson, Klokkarvik, Norway.

Professor Nosov, Paediatric Research Institute, Moscow, USSR.

Dr Nusche, Der Bundesminister für Jugend, Familie und Gesundheit, Kennedyalle 105–7, 53 Bonn-Bad Godesberg 1, Federal Republic of Germany.

Dr John O'Connor, Department of Health, Custom House, Dublin 1, Republic of Ireland.

Dr Michael O'Donnell, Editor, World Medicine, 26/7 Oxenden Street, London SW1Y 4EL.

Dr E. Pelrene, Ministere van Volkesgezonheid en Van Het Gezin Rijksadminstratref Centrum Vesaluns-Gebo, Oratorienberg 20, Brussels, Belgium.

Professor T. J. Phillips, Department of Family Medicine, University of Washington, Seattle, Washington 98 195, USA.

Dr Boris Ivanovitch Poblinkov, Deputy Director of Regional Health Services (Oblast) Irkutsk, Eastern Siberia, USSR.

Dr Sandor Rado, 11 Küküllo, U8 1026 Budapest, Hungary.

Dr A. M. Reynolds, 9 Avenue Jean-Joures, 91 120 Palaisean, France.

Dr Bruce Jones Sams, The Permanent Medical Group, 1924 Broadway, Oakland, California, 94 617, USA.

Dr R. Schackelford, Mount Olive, North Carolina, USA.

Dr and Mrs Schaffarzick, 2837 Rivera Drive, Burlingame, California 94 010, USA.

Miss Birgitta Schmidt, National Board of Health and Welfare, Stockholm, Sweden.

Dr and Mrs S. Schuman, 1019 Scotland Drive, Mount Pleasant, South Carolina 29 464, USA.

Dr Malcolm Segall, Ministry of Health, Maputo, Moçambique.

Professor Tei Seki, Dean, University Medical School, Osaka, Japan.

Dr F. Simon, La Division des Rélations Internationales, Ministère de la Santé, 14 Avenue Duguesne 75 700, Paris, France.

Dr John Smellie, Assistant to the Executive Director, The Permanente Medical Group, 1924 Broadway, Oakland, California 94 617, USA.

Dr Roberto Sollett, 15 Street No. 9, Apartment 13, Vedado, Havana, Cuba.

Dr Dag Søvik, Health Centre, Askøy 5300, Kleppestø, Norway.

Dr T. Suzuki, Centre for Adult Diseases, Osaka, Japan.

Miss Karin Svenninger, Health and Medical Care Centre, S-240, 10 Dalby, Sweden.

Dr Marianne Szatamari, Visegradi U47/C, 32 Budapest, Hungary.

Dr Jo Telje, Institute of Social Medicine, University of Tromsø, Norway.

Dr Glyn Thomas, Regional Officer for the Organisation of Medical Care, WHO, 8 Scherfigsvej, DK-2100 Copenhagen, Denmark.

Dr and Mrs K. H. Torp, Sentralsykehuset, Tromsø, Norway.

Dr J. Torres, Depto 201, Holanda 05, Santiago, Chile.

Professor H. J. van Aalderen, Huisartsen Instituut, Vrije Universiteit, Amsterdam, the Netherlands.

Professor Dr J. C. Van Es, Rijksuniversiteit Utrecht, Marihoek 5–6, Utrecht 2501, the Netherlands.

Dr Kina Vardanian, Collective Farm, Garni, Republic of Armenia, USSR.

Dr Vasiljerna, Polyclinic No. 22, Kiev, Republic of the Ukraine, USSR.

Professor Carlo Vetere, Vice-Direttore, Generale dei Servizi di Medicina Sociale, Minstero della Sanità, Rome, Italy.

Professor Hannu Vuori, Department of Community Health, University of Kuopio, Kuopio 70 101, Finland.

Mr and Mrs Lloyd Westcott, Hunterdon Hill, Holsteins Inc., Rosemont, New Jersey, USA.

Dr Giorgobiani Zuzal, County Hospital, Mtskheta, Republic of Georgia, USSR.

REFERENCES

Chapter 1
Illich, I. D. (1975). *Medical Nemesis*. London: Calder & Bowyers.

Chapter 2
BMA (1970). *Primary Medical Care*. Planning unit report No. 4. British Medical Association.
Elliott, K. (1971). Using medical auxiliaries: some ideas and examples. *Health Manpower and the Medical Auxiliary*. London: Intermediate Technology Development Group.
Fry, J. (1969). *Medicine in Three Societies*. Lancaster: Medical Technical Publishing Co. Ltd.
Fry, J. (ed.) (1977). *Trends in General Practice 1977*, p. 188, London: *British Medical Journal*.
Gish, O. (1971). *Towards an Appropriate Health Care Technology*. London: Intermediate Technology Development Group.
Haglund, G. (1974). Who helps the doctor? The work of the nurse in Sweden. *Update*, April.
Heller, R. (1976) 'Priest-Doctors' as a rural health source in the age of enlightenment. *Medical History*, **20**, 361–83.
Jonas, S. (1973). Some thoughts on primary care: problems of implementation. *International Journal of Health Services*, **2**, 178.
JRCGP (1973). Present state and future needs of general practice. Report from general practice No. 16. *Journal of the Royal College of General Practitioners*.
Knox, J. (1970). Introduction to new general practice. *British Medical Journal*, **2**, viii.
McWhinney, I. R. (1964). Postgraduate preparation for family medicine in the USA and other aspects of general practice. Report to the Nuffield Foundation.
Marsh, G. N. (1969). Visiting nurse – analysis of one year's work. *British Medical Journal*, **4**, 42–4.
Marsh, G. N. *et al*. (1972). Survey of home visiting by general practitioners in North-east England. *British Medical Journal*, **1**, 487–92.
Marsland, D. W., Wood, M. & Mayo, F. (1976). Content of family practice. *Journal of Family Practice*, **3**, 1–14.
Spitzer, W. O. *et al*. (1974). The Burlington randomized trial of the nurse practitioner. *New England Journal of Medicine*, **290**, 251–6.

Weston-Smith, J. & Mottram, E. M. (1967). Extended use of nursing services in general practice. *British Medical Journal*, **4**, 672.
Weston-Smith, J. & O'Donovan, J. B. (1970). *British Medical Journal*, **4**, 673.
WHO (1970). *The Role of the Primary Physician in Health Services*. Geneva: World Health Organisation.

Note: Some of the information in this chapter was collected from the following publications:
Role of the Primary Physician in Health Services. World Health Organisation, Copenhagen, 1971.
Trends in the Development of Primary Care. World Health Organisation, Copenhagen, 1973.
Further Organisation of Medical Practice in Europe. Council of Europe. Strasbourg, 1973.

Chapter 3
Barber, J. H., Robinson, E. T., Morey, S. & Hass, E. (1974). Health centre X-ray unit. *British Medical Journal*, 25 May, pp. 423–7.
Bradford, T. C. (1975). *Journal of Royal College of General Practitioners*, **25**, 445–50.
Burns, C. (1971). Ballymoney Health Centre. *Journal of Royal College of General Practitioners*, **21**, 86.
Cartwright, A. (1967). *Patients and their Doctors*. London: Routledge & Kegan Paul.
Cartwright, A. & Scott, R. (1961). The work of a nurse employed in general practice. *British Medical Journal*, **1**, 807–13.
Collings, J. (1950). Report on general practice in the United Kingdom. *Lancet*, 25 March, p. 555.
Connolly, M. M. (1966). The health visitor and nurse in general practice. *Practitioner*, **197**, 159–62.
Crombie, D. L. (1957). The contribution of the nurse in general practice. *British Journal of Preventive and Social Medicine*, **1**, 41–4.
Dawson of Penn (1920). Intermediate report on the future provision of medical and allied services. *Ministry of Health, Card 193*. London: HMSO.
DHSS (1969). *Functions of the District and General Hospital*. Department of Health and Social Security. London: HMSO.
DHSS (1970). *National Health Service Notes*. Department of Health and Social Security. London: HMSO.
DHSS (1973). *Health Trends*, vol. 5, No. 4. Department of Health and Social Security. London: HMSO.
DHSS (1974a). *Health Trends*, vol. 6, No. 1. Department of Health and Social Security. London: HMSO.
DHSS (1974b). *General Medical Services, 1973*. Report of joint working party. Department of Health and Social Security. London: HMSO.
DHSS (1974c). *National Health Service. Development of Health Services. Community Hospitals*. Department of Health and Social Security. London: HMSO.
DHSS (1975). *State of the Public Health for the Year 1975*. Department of Health and Social Security. London: HMSO.
DHSS (1976). *Annual Report 1975*. Department of Health and Social Security. London: HMSO.
Evans, J. W. (1969). Social workers and general practice. *British Medical Journal*, **1**, 44–6.

Forsyth, G. (1973). United Kingdom. In *Health Service Prospects*, pp. 1–35. London: *Lancet* and Nuffield Provincial Hospital Trust.

Freedman, G. R., Charlewood, J. E., Dodds, P. A. & York, K. (1975). Physiotherapy in general practice. *Journal of Royal College of General Practitioners*, 25, 587–91.

Fry, J. (1969). *Medicine in Three Societies*. Lancaster: Medical Technical Publishing Co. Ltd.

Godber, G. (1975). The health service: past, present and future. *Health Clark Lectures, 1973*. London: Athlone Press.

Hawthorn, P. J. (1971). *The Nurse Working with the General Practitioner – an Evaluation of Research and a Review of the Literature*. Department of Health and Social Security. London: HMSO.

Horder, J. (1969). Education after the Royal Commission. *Journal of Royal College of General Practitioners*, 18, 9–21.

Howie, V. (1974). The evaluation of an X-ray unit in a health centre. *Scottish Health Service Studies No. 30*. Scottish Home & Health Department.

Israel, S. & Draper, P. (1971). *British Medical Journal*, 1, 452–6.

JRCGP (1965). Special vocational training for general practice. Reports from General Practice No. 1. *Journal of Royal College of General Practitioners*.

Kernick, D. P. & Davies, P. (1977). *British Medical Journal*, 6 Nov., pp. 348–51.

Kyle, D. (1971). Contribution of a general practitioner hospital. *British Medical Journal*, 4, 348–51.

Lennon, E. A. (1971). How general practitioners use X-ray departments. *Health Trends*. Department of Health and Social Security. London: HMSO.

Lord, W. J. H. (1965). The general practitioner, the social worker and the health visitor. *Journal of Royal College of General Practitioners* 10, 247–56.

McDonald, M. D., Morgan, D. C. & Tucker, A. M. (1974). Patients' attitudes to the provision of medical care from a health centre. *Journal of Royal College of General Practitioners*, 24, 29.

McKeown, T. (1965). *Medicine in Modern Society*. London: Allen & Unwin.

Mair, W. J., Berkeley, J. S., Gillanders, L. A. & Allen, W. M. C. (1974). Use of radiological facilities by general practitioners. *British Medical Journal*, 3, 732–4.

Marsh, G. N. (1969). Visiting nurse: analysis of one year's work. *British Medical Journal*, 4, 42–4.

Norman, P., Clifton, H., Williams, E. & Nichols, P. J. R. (1975). Access by general practitioners to the physiotherapy department of a district general hospital. *British Medical Journal*, 4, 220–1.

Patterson, J. S. (1975). *Health Bulletin*, 33, 52.

Roberts, E. R. M. (1969). Personal communication.

Stephen, W. J. (1969). What do students want? *Journal of Royal College of General Practitioners*, 18, 132.

Stranraer Health Centre (1968). *Journal of Royal College of General Practitioners*, 16, 484.

Taylor, S. (1954). *Good General Practice*. London: Oxford University Press.

Wade, O. L. & Elmes, P. C. (1969). *Update*, June.

Wallace, B. B., Millward, D., Parsons, A. S. & Davis, R. H. (1973). Unrestricted access by general practitioners to a department of diagnostic radiology. *Journal of Royal College of General Practitioners*, 23, 337.

Waters, W. H. R. *et al.* (1975). *Journal of Royal College of General Practitioners*, 25, 576–84.

Weston-Smith, J. & Mottram, E. M. (1967). Extended use of nursing services in general practice. *British Medical Journal*, 4, 672.

Weston-Smith, J. & O'Donovan, J. B. (1970). *British Medical Journal*, **4**, 653–6.
Wilkinson, B.R. (1968). *British Medical Journal*, **1**, 436–8.
Woods, J. O. *et al.* (1974). *Journal of Royal College of General Practitioners*, **24**, 23–7.

Chapter 4
Bentzen, N. (1976). Personal communication.
Bentzen, N. *et al.* (1976). *Journal of Royal College of General Practitioners*, **26**, 37–45.
Boelaert, R. B. (1976). Personal communication.
Caylon, J. S. (1975). *Trends in the Evaluation of Medical Care and Hospital Services in France*. International Series, vol. 2. Beckenham: Ravenswood Publications Ltd.
Consultative Council (1973). *General Medical Services*, p. 22. Report of Joint Working Party. London: HMSO.
Consultative Council (1975). *General Practitioner in Ireland*. Report of Joint Working Party. Dublin: Stationery Office.
Cornillot, P. & Bonamour, P. (1973). France. In *Health Service Prospects*, pp. 55–79. London: *Lancet* and Nuffield Provincial Hospital Trust
de Bruïne, T. J. L. A. (1973). *British Medical Journal*, 17 Nov., p. 399.
de Melker, R. A. (1974). The relationship between the family doctor and the hospital. *Journal of Royal College of General Practitioners*, **24**, 703–9.
Eichhorn, S. (1973). German Federal Republic. In *Health Service Prospects*, pp. 81–92. London: *Lancet* and Nuffield Provincial Hospital Trust.
Eimerl, T. S. (1967). A general practitioner looks at Denmark. *Journal of Royal College of General Practitioners*, **14**, 203.
Fog, J. (1976). Personal communication.
Frølund, F. (1976). Personal communication.
Groot, L. M. J. (1972). Postindustrial Europe and its health care: views of an insider. *International Journal of Health Services*, **2**, 479–90.
Grunberg, C. (1976). Personal communication.
Hall, D. W. (1975). *Journal of Royal College of General Practitioners*, **26**, 19–34.
Häussler, S. (1973). Germany. *British Medical Journal*, 17 Nov., pp. 396–411.
Hornuil & Poulsen, E. F. (1971). *Ugeskrift for Laeger*, **133**, 1601.
Janssens, H. (1974). Family practice symposium. Adjustment and acceptance of change. *Update*, Dec., pp. 1692–8,
Jones, R. V. H. (1974). A week with a French country doctor. *Journal of Royal College of General Practitioners*, **24**, 689–93.
Juel, S. (1972). Primary health services: Denmark. *Danish Medical Bulletin*, **19**, 182.
Koch, J. H. (1974). Health service in Denmark. Lecture at Kings Fund Centre, London.
Maynard, A. (1975). *Health Care in the EEC*, pp. 157, 159. London: Croom Helm.
Muri, S. (1976). Personal communication.
Nusche (1976). Personal communication.
O'Connor, J. (1975). Personal communication.
Reynolds, A. M. (1976). Personal communication.
Simon, F. (1975). Personal communication.
van Aalderen, H. J. (1976). Personal communication.
van Aalderen, H. J. (1977). Personal communication.

Van Es, J. C. (1976). Personal communication.
van Zonneveld, R. J. (1975). The Netherlands. *Geriatric Care in Advanced Societies*. Lancaster: Medical Technical Publishing Co. Ltd.
Waldman, H. (1973). West Germany. *British Medical Journal*, Nov., p. 479.
WHO (1975). *Fifth Report of the World Health situation 1969–74*. Geneva: World Health Organisation.
Wolff, G. (1970). Arztstatistik im zehn-Jahre vergleich. *Deutsches Ärzteblatt*, Dec.
Wright, A. T. (1975). Primary medical care in France. *Journal of Royal College of General Practitioners*, **25**, 664–9.
Zanchetti, A. (1973). Italy. *British Medical Journal*, 17 Nov., p. 409.

Chapter 5
Aer, J. (1976). Personal communication.
Berg, K. (1975). *Journal of Royal College of General Practitioners*, **25**, 305–7.
Borchgrevink, C. F. (1970). Current problems of general practice in Norway. *Den Norske Laegeforening*, **90**, 1149–50.
Brunsgaard, D. (1974). Primaërlege Norge. *Den Norske Laegeforening*, **94**, 923–7.
Forsdahl, A. & Telje, J. (1976). Personal communication.
Freedman, D. L. (1975). *Journal of Royal College of General Practitioners*, **25**, 302–4.
Gunnarson, C. (1976). Personal communication.
Haglund, G. (1974). Primary care in Sweden. *Update*, Oct., pp. 1104–5.
Hall, D. W. (1976). The off duty arrangements of general practitioners in four European countries. *Journal of Royal College of General Practitioners*, **26**, 19–34.
Hümerfelt, S. (1976). Personal communication.
Kasari, K. (1975). Community health care and its costs in 1974. *The Finnish Communities*, **19**, 1128. Helsinki.
Kekki, P. (1975). Changing status of doctors in Finland. *British Medical Journal*, **4**, 273–5.
Kekki, P. (1976). Some goals – different philosophy. *British Medical Journal*, **1**, 204–5.
Kvamme, J. I. (1976). Personal communication.
Lindmark, C. (1976). Personal communication.
Stockholm City Council (1976). Personal communication.
Telje, J. (1976). Personal communication.

Chapter 6
Barisova, V. (1971). Personal communication.
Bobakhoddzaev, I. (1971). *Sovetskve zdravookhranenie*, **6**, 22–7.
Bradshaw, A. B., Ryan, T. M. & Thomas, I. B. (1975). Primary medical care in the Ukraine 1975. *Journal of Royal College of General Practitioners*, **25**, 753–60.
Poblinkov, Z. & Litvinova, V. (1972). Personal communication.
Popov, G. A. (1969). *Sovetskoe zdravookhranenie*, **4**, 18–20.
Popov, G. A. (1971). *Principle of health planning in the USSR*. Public health paper No. 43, World Health Organisation, Geneva.
Revutskaya, R. G. (1975). *Geriatric Care in Advanced Societies*, p. 131. Lancaster: Medical Technical Publishing Co. Ltd.
Romenskii, A. A. (1970). *Sovetskoe zdravookhranenie*, **12**, 25–7.
Ryan, T. M. (1972). Primary medical care in the Soviet Union. *International Journal of Health Services*, vol. 2, No. 2.
Vasilperna, B. (1971). Personal communication.

Vasilperna, B. *et al.* (1971). Personal communication.
Venedikkov, D. (1973). *Health Service Prospects*. International survey. London: *Lancet* and Nuffield Provincial Hospital Trust.
WHO (1960). *Health Service in the USSR*. Public health paper No. 3. Geneva: World Health Organisation.

Note: Some of the material for this chapter has been taken from my articles published in *Update* (1973), 1 March, pp. 749–53; 15 March, pp. 817–24.

Chapter 7
Bratanov B. & Vulchev, A. (1966). Extract symposium of postgraduate medical education. *Sofia Medicina*, pp. 183–97. Fizkultura publishing house. pp. 183–97.
Ezban, A. (1975). *World Health*. Geneva: World Health Organisation.
Gargov, K. (1970). Personal communication.
Inst. Soc. Med. (1972). *The Patient and the Health Community; Doctor/General Practitioner*. A study of the relationship between the citizen and the primary health care facilities. Prague: Institute of Social Medicine and the Organisation of Health Services.
Kaser, M. (1976). *Health Care in the Soviet Union and Eastern Europe*. London: Croom Helm.
Lingeman, J. G. (1973). *Youth Health Care in Czechoslovakia*. Report of the World Health Organisation's fellowship van Nahuysplein 12, Zwolle, Netherlands.
MOH, Prague (1966). *On Health Care of the People*. Act No. 20 of March 17, 1966. Prague: Ministry of Health.
Ošanec, F. (1973). Personal communication.
Stich, Z. (1962). *Czechoslovak Health Services*. Prague: Ministry of Health.
Szatmari, M. (1976). Personal communication.
Weinerman, E. R. (1969). *Social Medicine in Eastern Europe*. Cambridge Massachusetts: Harvard University Press.

Chapter 8
AMA (1976). *Profile of Medical Practice 1975/76*. Centre for Health Services Research and Development, Chicago. American Medical Association.
Andreopoulos, S. (1974). *Primary Care: Where Medicine Fails*, p. 36. New York: Wiley.
Curry, H. B. (1977). Personal communication.
Curry, H. B. *et al.* (1974) *Twenty Years of Community Medicine*. New Jersey: Columbia Publishing Company Inc.
DHEW (1972). *Proceedings and Debates of 92nd Congress, First Session*. Congressional Record H 10974–5 vol. 117. 11 November 1971. Department of Health, Education & Welfare.
Fox, P. (1977). Options for National Health Insurance: an overview. *Policy Analysis*, Winter.
Fry, J. (1969). *Medicine in Three Societies*, pp. 54, 133. Lancaster: Medical Technical Publishing Co. Ltd.
Garfield, S. (1970). The delivery of Medicare care. *Scientific American*, **222**, 15–23.
Garfield, S. (1977). Personal communication.
Garfield, S., Collen, M. F., Feldman, R. (1976). Evaluation of an ambulatory medical care delivery system. *New England Journal of Medicine*, **294**, 426–31.
Goldsmith, S. (1977). Personal communication.
Kaiser, R. G. (1976). *Russia: the People and the Power*. New York: Atheneum.

Lawrence, D. (1977). Personal communication.

Luria (1977). Personal communication.

Marsh, G. N., Wallace, R. B. & Whewell, J. (1976). Anglo-American contrasts in general practice. *British Medical Journal*, **1**, 1325.

Marsland, D. W., Wood, M. & Mayo, F. (1976). *Journal of Family Practice*, **3**, 1.

Maxwell, R. (1975). *Health Care: the Growing Dilemma*, p. 30. New York: McKinsey & Co.

O'Donnell, M. (1975). The American alternative. *World Medicine*, 12 Feb., pp. 22–31.

Parker, A. W. (1974). *Primary Care: Where Medicine Fails*, ed. S. Andreopoulos, p. 36. New York: Wiley.

Piore, N. (1975). *Community Hospital and the Challenge of Primary Medical Care*, pp. 15, 21. Centre for Community Health Systems, Columbia University, New York.

Rabin, D. & Spector, K. (1976). *Roles and Functions of Physicians' Assistants*. Final Report. Contrast No. 1 – MB – 44172. Bureau of Health Manpower. Department of Health, Education & Welfare.

Schwartz, H. (1972). *The Case for American Medicine*: New York: McKay.

Shinefield, H. R. & Smillie, J. G. (1973) Prepaid groups practice and the delivery of health care. *Advances in Paediatrics*, **20**, 206.

Smith, H. (1976). *The Russians*. New York: Quadrangle/The New York Times Book Co.

Smith, R. (1972). Family medicine in the USA. *International Journal of Health Services*, **2**, 208.

Van der Post, L. (1965). *Journey into Russia*. Harmondsworth: Penguin Books.

Chapter 9

Anyon, C. P. (1976). Personal communication.

Australian Govt. (1970). *National Health Act*. Australian Government Publication.

Australian Medical Association (1973). Unpublished survey.

CFPC. *Research Awareness Publication*.

Collyer, J. A. (1975). *Canadian Medical Association Journal*, **12**, 1357–60.

Farrar, F. (1977). Personal communication.

McWhinney, I. R. (1972). *International Journal of Health Services*, **2**, 229–37.

Medimail Pty. Ltd (1976). Statistical data.

N.Z. Govt. (1974). *A Health Service for New Zealand*. New Zealand Government White Paper.

RACGP (1976). The Australian General Practice Morbidity and Prescribing Survey, 1969–1974. Royal Australian College of General Practitioners. *Medical Journal of Australia Special Supplement*.

Rice, D. (1977). Personal communication.

Ryan. J. G. P. (1972). *International Journal of Health Services*, **2**, 273–84.

Spitzer, W. O. *et al*. (1973). *Canadian Medical Association Journal*, **108**, 991–5, 988–1003, 1005–16.

Spitzer, W. O. *et al*. (1974). *New England Journal of Medicine*, **290**, 251–6.

Wolfe, S. & Badgely, R. F. (1972). *The Family Doctor*. Milbank Memorial Fund. Q. 50., No. 2.

Chapter 10

Seki, T. (1972). Personal communication.

Stephen, W. J. (1972). A study of the health service in Japan with particular reference to primary medical care. Report to the Nuffield Foundation.

Takemi, T. (1970*a*). *The Medical Practitioner in Japan*. Japanese Medical Association.
Takemi, T. (1970*b*). Group practice in Japan. New horizons in health care. *Proceedings of the First International Congress on Group Medicine*. Winnipeg.

Note: Some of the material in this chapter has been taken from my articles published in *Update* (1974) 1, 15 April, 1, 15 May.

Chapter 11
Banerji, D. (1973). Health behaviour of rural populations. *Economic and Political Weekly*, **8**, 2261–8.
Committee on the International Migration of Talent (1970). *International Migration of High-level Manpower*, pp. 695–6. New York: Praeger.
DHEW (1975). *International Migration of Physicians and Nurses*. Department of Health Education and Welfare, USA.
Djukonovic, V. & Mach, E. P. (1975). *Alternative Approaches to Meeting Basic Health Needs in Developing Countries*. Geneva: World Health Organisation.
Elliott, K. (1971). Using medical auxiliaries: some ideas and examples. In *Health Manpower and the Medical Auxiliary*, ed. O. Gish. London: Intermediate Technology Development Group.
Gish, O. (1971). Towards an appropriate health care technology. *Health Manpower and the Medical Auxiliary*. London: Intermediate Technology Development Group.
Hamilton, P. J. S. & Anderson, A. (1965). *An Analysis of Basic Data on Admissions in 1963 and 1964 to Mulago Hospital. Kampala*. Report for the Ministry of Health, Uganda.
Heller, T. (1976). Medical goals at home and away. *Contact 33* Christian Medical Commission, World Council of Churches, Geneva.
Kadt, E. de (1974). *Discussion Paper No. 17*. Institute of Development Studies, University of Sussex.
King, M. H. (1966). *Medical Care in Developing Countries*. London: Oxford University Press.
King, M. H. (1972). Medicine, red and blue. *Lancet*, **1**, 679.
Lancet, Editorial (1973). How many doctors? *Lancet*, **1**, 367.
Ministerio de Salud Publica (1974). XIX Conferencia Sanitaria Panamerica. Santiago, Chile.
Morley, D. C. (1973). *Paediatric Priorities in the Developing World*. London: Butterworths.
Mukerjee, S. N. (1975). *The Murre Hospital, Nagpur, India*. Geneva: World Health Organisation.
Newell, K. W. (1975). *Health by the People*. Geneva: World Health Organisation.
Nuffield Trust (1973) *Health Service Prospects*. London: *Lancet* and Nuffield Provincial Hospital Trust.
OHE (1972). *Medical Care in Developing Countries*. Office of Health Economics, London.
Rodriguez de la Vega, A. & Sollett, R. (1976). Personal communication.
Roemer, M. I. (1972). India, Rural Health Training Centre, Najafgesh. The services from a primary centre (1964). Cited in *Evaluation of Community Health Centres*, 25. Geneva, World Health Organisation.
Schulpen, T. W. J. (1975) *Integration of Church and Government Medical Services in Tanzania. Effects at District Level*. African Medical Research Foundation, Nairobi.

Senewiratne, B. (1975). *British Medical Journal*, 1, 618–20.

Stephen, W. J. (1974). Personal communication with Chilean doctors wishing to remain anonymous.

Stevenson, D. (1975). Health manpower in Nepal and Malawi. Seventh All Nepal Conference at Bis Hospital, Katmandu.

UN (1971). *World Economic Survey 1969–70*. Geneva: United Nations.

Waitzkin, H. & Modell, H. (1974). *New England Journal of Medicine*, 25 July.

World Bank (1976). *Village Water Supply*, p. 96. World Bank Paper. Washington DC.

Note: Some of the material on Chile and Cuba has been taken from my articles published in *Update* (1975) September; (1976) June.

Chapter 12

Bryant, J. (1969). *Health and the Developing World*, p. 163. New York: Cornell University Press.

DHSS (1971). *Nurse Working with the General Practitioner*. Department of Health and Social Security. London: HMSO.

Eisenberg, L. (1977). The search for care. *Daedalus*, Winter, p. 238.

Hart, J. T. (1971). *Lancet*, 1, 405–8.

Horder, J. P. (1977). Physicians and family doctors: a new relationship. *Journal of Royal College of Physicians*, 11, 311–22.

Hospital Update, (1976). Editorial. December.

Huygen, F. J. A. (1976). Editorial. *International General Practice*, No. 3.

Joseph, K. (1973). Marsden Lecture at the Royal Free Hospital.

JRCP (1974). Editorial. *Journal of Royal College of Physicians*, 8, 100.

Kohn, R. & Kerr, L. W. (1976). *Health Care: An International Study*. London: Oxford University Press.

McCormack, M. P. (1977). Personal communication.

Maeda, N. (1972). Personal communication.

Mahler, H. (1975). *World Health*, August/September p. 3. Geneva: World Health Organisation.

Powell, J. E. (1966). *Medicine and Politics*, p. 4. London: Pitman Medical.

Practitioner (1973). Editorial. *Practitioner*, 210, 735.

Saward, E. M. (1977). Institutional organisation, incentives and change. *Daedalus*, Winter, p. 193.

Thomas, K. B. (1975). *Lancet*, 1, 1086.

BIBLIOGRAPHY

Medical care in developing countries

Bryant, J. H. (1969). *Health in the Developing World*, New York: Cornell University Press.

King, M. H. (1966). *Medical Care in Developing Countries*. Nairobi: Oxford University Press.

Morley, D. (1973). *Paediatric Priorities in the Developing World*. London: Butterworths.

General

Djukonovic, V. & Mach, E. P. (1975). *Alternative Approaches to Meeting Basic Health Needs*. A joint Unicef/WHO study. Geneva: World Health Organisation.

References 396

Includes accounts of Bangladesh, China, Cuba, Tanzania, Venezuela, Yugoslavia, India, Niger and Nigeria.

Kind, M. H. (1971). The auxiliary – his role and training. *Journal of Tropical Medicine and Hygiene*, **73**, 336–46.

Rosinstein, E. F. & Spence, F. J. (1969). *The Assistant Medical Officer*. Chapel Hill: University of North Carolina Press.

World Health Organisation (1975). *Health by the People*. Geneva. Includes accounts of China, Cuba, Guatemala, India, Central Java, Iran, Niger, Tanzania and Venezuela.

Africa

Barlow, R. (1976). Application of a health planning model in Morocco. *International Journal of Health Services*, **6**, 103–21.

Bennett, F. J., Hall, S. A., Lutwama, J. S. & Rado, E. R. (1965). Medical manpower in East Africa: prospects and problems. *East African Medical Journal*, **42**, 149–61.

Chang, W. P. (1970). Health manpower development in an African country. The case of Ethiopa. *Journal of Medical Education*, **45**, 26–39.

Rodney, W. (1972). *How Europe underdeveloped Africa*. Tanzanian Publishing House.

Schulpen T. W. J. (1975). *Integration of Church and Government Medical Services in Tanzania. Effects at District Level*. African Medical Research Foundation. Nairobi, Kenya.

Asia

Biddulph, J. (1969). Medical assistants. *Papua: New Guinea Medical Journal*, **12**, 22–5.

Bryant, J. H. & Arnstein, G. (1965). *Report to Thailand on Health Service, Health Personnel and Medical Education*. New York: Rockefeller Foundation.

Christian Medical Commission (1971). The Koje Do Project, South Korea. *Contact 5*. Geneva.

Christian Medical Commission (1976). Community health care in rural Java. *Contact 31*. Geneva.

Christian Medical Commission (1976). Rural health care in Bangladesh. *Contact 34*. Geneva.

Dutt, P. R. (1962). Rural health services in India. *Primary Health Centres*. Central Health Education Bureau. Ministry of Health, New Delhi.

Horn, J. S. (1969). *Away with all Pests*. London: Hamlyn.

Horn, J. S. (1972). Building a rural health service in the People's Republic of China. *International Journal of Health Services*, **2**, 377–83.

Lee, W. C. (1970). Medical education and medical practice in Korea. *Journal of Medical Education*, **45**, 283–92.

Segall, M. (1973). In *Disaster in Bangladesh: Health Crises in a Developing Nation* ed. L. C. Chen. London: Oxford University Press.

Segall, (1975). *International Journal of Health Services*, **5**, 521–5.

Sidel, V. W. (1972). Some observations on the health services in the People's Republic of China. *International Journal of Health Services*, **2**, 385–95.

Smith, A. J. (1974). Medicine in China. *British Medical Journal*, **2**, 367–71, 492–4.

Smith, A. J. & Adey, E. M. (1974). Medicine in China. *British Medical Journal*, **2**, 603–5.

Takulia, H. S. (1967). *The Health Care Doctor in India*. Baltimore: Johns Hopkins.

Taylor, C. E. (1976). The doctor's role in rural health care (India). *International Journal of Health Services*, **6**, 219–30.

Taylor, C. E. et al. (1976). *Doctors for the Villages*. New York: Asia.

South America

Behm, H., Gutiérrez, H. & Regnena, M. (1972). Demographic trends, health and medical care in Latin America. *International Journal of Health Services*, **2**, 1.

Christian Medical Commission (1974). The Chimaltenango development project, Guatemala. *Contact 19*. Geneva.

Hall, T. L. (1969). *Health Manpower in Peru. A Case Study in Planning*. Baltimore: Johns Hopkins.

Navarro, V. (1974). The underdevelopment of health or the health of underdevelopment: an analysis of the distribution of health resources in Latin America. *International Journal of Health Services*, **4**, 5–27.

INDEX